T0309169

American Psychiatric Association Task Force on Electroconvulsive Therapy

Task Force Members

Christopher C. Abbott, M.D., M.S.C.R.
Ethan O. Bryson, M.D.
M. Justin Coffey, M.D.
Laura J. Fochtmann, M.D., M.B.I.
Mustafa M. Husain, M.D.
Charles H. Kellner, M.D.
Andrew Krystal, M.D.
Sarah H. Lisanby, M.D.
Shawn M. McClintock, Ph.D., M.S.C.S.
William M. McDonald, M.D.
Georgios Petrides, M.D.
Joan Prudic, M.D.
Richard D. Weiner, M.D., Ph.D.

The Practice of Electroconvulsive Therapy

Recommendations for Treatment, Training, and Privileging

Third Edition

A Task Force Report of the
American Psychiatric Association

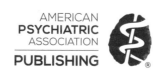

If you wish to buy 50 or more copies of the same title, please go to www.appi.org/specialdiscounts for more information.

Copyright © 2025 American Psychiatric Association Publishing
ALL RIGHTS RESERVED
Third Edition
Manufactured in the United States of America on acid-free paper
28 27 26 25 24   5 4 3 2 1
American Psychiatric Association Publishing
800 Maine Avenue SW, Suite 900
Washington, DC 20024–2812
www.appi.org

Library of Congress Cataloging-in-Publication Data
Names: American Psychiatric Association. Task Force on Electroconvulsive Therapy, author.
Title: The practice of electroconvulsive therapy : recommendations for treatment, training, and privileging / American Psychiatric Association Task Force on Electroconvulsive Therapy.
Description: Third edition. | Washington : American Psychiatric Association, 2024. | Includes bibliographical references and index.
Identifiers: LCCN 2024014438 (print) | LCCN 2024014439 (ebook) | ISBN 9780890426678 (paperback) | ISBN 9780890427125 (ebook)
Subjects: MESH: Electroconvulsive Therapy—standards
Classification: LCC RC485 (print) | LCC RC485 (ebook) | NLM WM 412 | DDC 616.89/122—dc23/eng/20240430
LC record available at https://lccn.loc.gov/2024014438
LC ebook record available at https://lccn.loc.gov/2024014439

British Library Cataloguing in Publication Data
A CIP record is available from the British Library.

Contents

Contributors

Christopher C. Abbott, M.D., M.S.C.R. Dr. Abbott, a psychiatrist, is the Division Chief of Neuromodulation and ECT Medical Director at the University of New Mexico. He is the Edward and Sophie Schmider Professor of Psychiatry in Neuromodulation. He has published on ECT imaging and is involved with the Global ECT MRI Collaboration (GEMRIC). He has been the principal investigator on several National Institute of Mental Health (NIMH) ECT imaging projects, with a research focus on electric field modeling and neuroimaging correlates of clinical outcomes. He is an Associate Editor for *Frontiers in Human Neuroscience—Brain Imaging and Stimulation*.

Ethan O. Bryson, M.D. Dr. Bryson, an anesthesiologist, is Professor in the Department of Anesthesiology, Perioperative and Pain Medicine and the Department of Psychiatry at the Icahn School of Medicine at Mount Sinai. He has published on anesthesia for ECT as well as issues related to addiction in health care professionals. He has been a coinvestigator on a grant funded by the NIMH. He has received royalties from Springer Science and Business Media, Cambridge University Press, and New Horizon Press.

M. Justin Coffey, M.D. Dr. Coffey, a neuropsychiatrist, is Professor of Psychiatry at Geisinger Commonwealth School of Medicine and Chief Medical Officer of Workit Health.

Laura J. Fochtmann, M.D., M.B.I. Dr. Fochtmann, a psychiatrist, is SUNY Distinguished Service Professor in the Departments of Psychiatry, Pharmacological Sciences, and Biomedical Informatics at Stony Brook University and Deputy Chief Medical Information Officer for Stony Brook Medicine. She has published on the neurobiology of ECT and on clinical practice guidelines in psychiatry. She has been a coinvestigator on a grant funded by the NIMH. and is an Editorial Board Member of the *Journal of ECT*. She also consults for the American Psychiatric Association on the development of practice guidelines.

Mustafa M. Husain, M.D.   Dr. Husain, a psychiatrist, is tenured Professor of Psychiatry, Neurology, and Biomedical Engineering; Director of the Neurostimulation Research Lab; and Fellow at Peter O'Donnell Brain Institute at the University of Texas Southwestern Medical Center at Dallas. Dr. Husain has authored several book chapters and published numerous peer-reviewed articles in national and international scientific journals. He also is on the editorial board for the *Journal of ECT* and serves as a reviewer for major professional journals and grant-funding agencies. Dr. Husain is involved in training, education, and research in general psychiatry; aging and geriatric issues; and novel treatments for major depressive disorder, including magnetic stimulation therapy, vagus nerve stimulation, and deep brain stimulation. His research funding has included several federally funded grants as well as multiple foundation funded research studies. He has also received research funding from Cyberonics, Neuronetics, BrainsWay, and Advanced Neuromodulation Systems as well as equipment from MagVenture.

Charles H. Kellner, M.D.   Dr. Kellner, a psychiatrist and neurologist, is Professor Emeritus in the Department of Psychiatry and Behavioral Sciences at the Medical University of South Carolina. He has published extensively on ECT, was the Editor-in-Chief of the *Journal of ECT* from 1994 to 2004, and now serves on its editorial board. He has been principal investigator on grants funded by the NIMH. He receives royalties from Cambridge University Press for the textbook *Handbook of ECT* (2019), fees for writing/editing ECT topics in UpToDate, and fees for teaching in an ECT course at Northwell Health.

Andrew D. Krystal, M.D., M.S.   Dr. Krystal is the Ray and Dagmar Dolby Distinguished Professor of Psychiatry and Neurology at the University of California, San Francisco, where he is also Vice-Chair for Research in Psychiatry, Director of the Dolby Family Center for Mood Disorders, Director of the Sleep Disorders Program, Director of the Interventional Psychiatry Program, and Director of the Programs in Transcranial Magnetic Stimulation and Transcranial Focused Ultrasound. He is also Professor Emeritus in the Department of Psychiatry and Behavioral Sciences at the Duke University School of Medicine. Over the course of his career, his research has focused on the development of biomarkers for mood disorders and sleep disorders and the use of these biomarkers in developing novel, personalized brain stimulation and pharmacological treatments for these conditions. In the past 15 years, he has been principal investigator on research grants funded by NIH, the Ray and Dagmar Dolby Family Fund, Sunovion, Novartis, Neosync, ANS St. Jude, Astellas, Abbot, Pfizer, Takeda, Cephalon, Sepracor, Somaxon, Organon, Evotec, Respironics, Merck, Sanofi, Aventis, Neuronetics, Neurocrine, Brainsway, Teva, Janssen, Jazz, Stanley Foundation, Axsome, Reveal Biosensors, Attune, and Eisai. He has received royalties for serving on advisory boards from Adare, Axsome Therapeutics, Big Health, Eisai, Evecxia, Ferring Pharmaceuticals, Galderma, Harmony Biosciences, Idorsia, Janssen Pharmaceuticals, Jazz Pharmaceuticals, Millenium Pharmaceuticals, Merck, Neurocrine Biosciences, Neurawell, Pernix, Otsuka Pharmaceuticals, Sage, Takeda, Angelini, Cephalon, Sunovion, Sepracor, Novarrtis, Organon, Respironics, Pfizer, Sanofi, and Aventis. He owns options from Big Health and Neurawell. He is inventor on patents on ECT held by Duke University, for which he receives no royalties.

Sarah Hollingsworth Lisanby, M.D.   Dr. Lisanby, a psychiatrist, is Professor Emeritus in the Department of Psychiatry and Behavioral Sciences at the Duke University School of Medicine and a Distinguished Life Fellow of the American Psychiatric Association. She is the Director of the Noninvasive Neuromodulation Unit and the Division of Translational Research at the NIMH. She has published widely on ECT and related topics and chaired the American Psychiatric Association's Task Force to Revise the Practice on Electroconvulsive Therapy. In the past 15 years, she has been principal investigator on research grants, with a focus on ECT and other neuromodulation devices, from Advanced Neuromodulation Systems; Brain Behavior Research Foundation; Brainsway; Cyberonics; Defense of Defense; Lieber Center; NeoSync Inc.; Neuronetics; New York State Office of Science, Technology and Academic Research; NexStim; NIH; Stanley Medical Research Institute; and Tourette Syndrome Association. She is inventor on patents and patent applications on electrical and magnetic brain stimulation therapy systems held by the NIH and Columbia University, for which she receives no royalties. She has received royalties from Oxford University Press for editing a textbook on transcranial stimulation. She serves on the FDA Neurological Devices Advisory Panel; the Scientific Advisory Board for the Aalto University School of Science, Netherlands; the Scientific Council of the Brain Behavior Research Foundation; the Scientific Advisory Board of the German Center for Brain Stimulation, a research consortium funded by the German Ministry for Education and Research; the Scientific Advisory Committee of the Burroughs Wellcome Fund (BWF) Career Awards for Medical Scientists (CAMS); and the editorial board of the *Journal of ECT*. The opinions expressed in this article are the author's own and do not reflect the views of the NIH, the Department of Health and Human Services, or the United States government.

Shawn M. McClintock, Ph.D., M.S.C.S.   Dr. McClintock, a clinical neuropsychologist, holds the Lydia Bryant Test Distinguished Professorship in Psychiatric Research and is Professor with tenure in the Department of Psychiatry at the University of Texas Southwestern Medical Center. He also is the Scientific Director of the Perot Neuroscience Translational Research Center in the Peter O'Donnell Jr. Brain Institute at UT Southwestern Medical Center as well asthe Director of Research Training in the Clinical Psychology Doctoral Program in the UT Southwestern Medical Center Graduate School of Biomedical Sciences. Dr. McClintock is a globally recognized expert in the neurocognitive effects of major depressive disorder and antidepressant neuromodulation therapeutics. He has published more than 100 peer-reviewed articles and 12 book chapters and is Co-Editor of the book *Neuropsychology of Depression*, which centers on his program of research focused on the intersection of clinical neuropsychology, depression, and antidepressant therapeutic development. Dr. McClintock is an Editorial Board Member of the *Journal of ECT* and is an Associate Editor for the journal *Neuropsychology Review*. He has received grant funding from the National Institutes of Health and the Brain and Behavior Foundation. He is also a consultant to Pearson Assessments and receives royalties from Guilford Press.

William M. McDonald, M.D.   Dr. McDonald, a psychiatrist, is the Chair of Psychiatry and Behavioral Sciences at Emory University School of Medicine. He is also the J. B. Fuqua Chair for Late-Life Depression and Reunette W. Harris Chair for Psychiatry. Dr. McDonald is a past member of the American Psychiatric Association Council on Research representing ECT and Neuromodulation Therapies. Dr. McDonald is compensated as the chair of the data safety and monitoring board for a National Institute of Aging–sponsored multicenter study. He is on the Board of Skyland Trail and 3Keys. He has been a paid consultant for Signant Health and Sage Therapeutics. He has received past funding from the Stanley Foundation, Soterix, Neuronetics, NeoSync, and Cervel Neurotherapeutics. He is a deputy editor of the *American Journal of*

Psychiatry and is on the editorial boards of the *American Journal of Geriatric Psychiatry* and *Personalized Medicine in Psychiatry.*

Georgios Petrides, M.D.   Dr. Petrides, a psychiatrist, is the Chair of Behavioral Health and Psychiatry at Trinitas Regional Medical Center of RWJBarnabas Health in New Jersey. He is a past Director of the Division of ECT at the Zucker Hillside Hospital of Northwell Health in New York, one of the busiest in North America, performing more than 6,500 treatments annually. He has published extensively in various aspects of the clinical practice of ECT, as well on depression and schizophrenia. Dr. Petrides is currently the co-chair of the Task Force for ECT of the World Federation of Societies for Biological Psychiatry and serves on the Editorial Board of the *Journal of ECT.* He has served as an officer, as well as member and chair of the Board of Directors, of the International Society for ECT and Neurostimulation (ISEN). He has also directed a week-long certificate course for ECT practitioners at the Zucker Hillside Hospital and is a faculty member of the ECT certificate course offered by ISEN. He has been the principal or co-principal investigator of multiple grant awards from the National Institute of Mental Health, National Institute of Aging, Stanley Foundation, the U.S. Department of Veterans Affairs, and the National Alliance for Research on Schizophrenia and Depression (NARSAD). He has also participated in clinical studies funded by Corcept Therapeutics, Gennaissance, Pfizer, Bristol Meyers Squibb, Novartis, and Abbott.

Joan Prudic, M.D.   Dr. Prudic, a psychiatrist, is Clinical Professor of Psychiatry, Columbia University Irving Medical Center. She has published on various aspects of the treatment of patients with ECT, including the effectiveness of the treatment, the mitigation of adverse effects of ECT, continuation therapies post ECT, and the use of brain imaging to investigate the mechanisms of the treatment. She is Associate Editor of the *Journal of ECT* and serves on the Board of the International Society for ECT and Neurostimulation. She has been a principal investigator and coinvestigator on grants funded by the NIMH, the National Association for Research on Schizophrenia and Depression, the Dana Foundation, Cyberonics, Advanced Neuromodulation Systems, and the Alzheimer's Association.

Richard D. Weiner, M.D., Ph.D.   Dr. Weiner, a psychiatrist, is Professor Emeritus in the Department of Psychiatry and Behavioral Sciences of the Duke University School of Medicine. He has published widely on ECT topics and chaired the American Psychiatric Association's Task Forces responsible for the prior two editions of this volume (1990 and 2001). He has received past research funding from the NIMH and the U.S. Department of Veterans Affairs and is co-inventor on a Duke University patent licensed to Mecta Corporation, a manufacturer of ECT devices, but has not received royalties.

The Task Force Report authors have worked to ensure that all information in this book is accurate at the time of publication and consistent with general psychiatric and medical standards. The findings, opinions, and conclusions of this report do not necessarily represent the views of the officers, trustees, all members of the committee, or all members of the American Psychiatric Association (APA). Task Force Reports are considered a substantive contribution of ongoing analysis and evaluation of problems, programs, issues, and practices in a given area of concern.

Task Force Reports 1) do not set a standard of care and are not inclusive of all proper treatments or methods of care; 2) are not continually updated and may not reflect the most recent evidence because new evidence may emerge between the time information is developed and when the guidelines are published or read; 3) address only the question(s) or issue(s) specifically identified; 4) do not mandate any particular course of medical care; 5) are not intended to substitute for the independent professional judgment of the treating clinician; and 6) do not account for individual variation among patients. As such, it is not possible to draw conclusions about the effects of omitting a particular recommendation, either in general or for a specific patient. Furthermore, adherence to information in this Task Force Report will not ensure a successful outcome for every individual, nor should this document be interpreted as including all proper methods of evaluation and care or excluding other acceptable methods of evaluation and care aimed at the same results. The ultimate recommendation regarding a particular assessment, clinical procedure, or treatment plan must be made by the clinician directly involved in the patient's care in light of the psychiatric evaluation, other clinical data, and the diagnostic and treatment options available. Such recommendations should be made in collaboration with the patient, whenever possible, and incorporate the patient's personal and sociocultural preferences and values in order to enhance the therapeutic alliance, adherence to treatment, and treatment outcomes. For all of these reasons, the APA cautions against the use of Task Force Reports in litigation. Use of this Task Force Report is voluntary. APA provides Task Force Reports on an "as is" basis and makes no warranty, expressed or implied, regarding them. APA assumes no responsibility for any injury or damage to persons or property arising out of or related to any use of this Task Force Report or for any errors or omissions.

CHAPTER 1

Introduction

The American Psychiatric Association (APA) first presented recommendations on the practice of electroconvulsive therapy (ECT) in 1978 with the publication of the landmark report *Electroconvulsive Therapy* (American Psychiatric Association 1978). Following a consensus conference on ECT sponsored by the National Institutes of Health (NIH) and the National Institute of Mental Health (NIMH) in 1985, the APA determined that updated practice recommendations for ECT would be beneficial, as would development of recommendations on education, training, and clinical privileging of ECT staff (Consensus Conference 1985). Accordingly, in the late 1980s, a new APA Task Force on ECT was charged with developing these recommendations with partial financial support from the NIMH.

In 1990, the APA published the first edition of *The Practice of Electroconvulsive Therapy: Recommendations for Treatment, Training, and Privileging*, a comprehensive set of recommendations for the practice of ECT (American Psychiatric Association 1990). This work influenced clinical practice in meaningful ways, including the encouragement of guideline development by other groups within the United States (Fink et al. 1996) and elsewhere (Gangadhar 1992; Royal Australian and New Zealand College of Psychiatrists 1992; Royal College of Psychiatrists 1995). In the ensuing decade, the field of ECT continued to advance, with hundreds of relevant publications and a substantial amount of new scientific and clinical information appearing each year.

Because of this growing knowledge base, the Task Force on ECT was asked to update the 1990 report. The revision process for the second edition of *The Practice of Electroconvulsive Therapy: Recommendations for Treatment, Training, and Privileging* was extensive. Published in 2001, the second edition served as an important resource for education and training in ECT and as a reference guide for safe and effective ECT practice.

Over the past two decades, the body of literature on the safety and efficacy of ECT has been increasing, including results of major multicenter randomized controlled trials sponsored by the NIMH. These advances suggested the need for revision of the 2001 edition, and the APA appointed a new Task Force on ECT for this purpose.

As was done for each of the previous editions, we have made the scope of these recommendations as comprehensive as possible, including coverage of the important issues of education, training, and privileging (Chapters 6 and 7). We also cover the significant advances that have occurred in the past two decades, citing the most recent literature (Espinoza and Kellner 2022), including new information on ECT anesthesia (Chapter 12) and on the detection and management of adverse effects (Chapter 19), including cognitive side effects (Chapter 20). We now have increasing evidence for the use of stimulus dose titration and the safety and efficacy of ultrabrief width pulse stimulation (Chapter 14). Significant research has also been done on the efficacy of continuation and maintenance treatment after ECT (Chapter 23), which we refer to as maintenance treatment in the remainder of the document. We have also included a discussion of the 2018 U.S. Food and Drug Administration reclassification of ECT devices and the implications of the reclassification on clinical ECT practice (Chapters 2 and 10).

For the first time, we have included a chapter on other neuromodulation techniques, including transcranial magnetic stimulation, vagus nerve stimulation (VNS), deep brain stimulation (DBS), transcranial direct current stimulation, and other investigational techniques (Chapter 24). In Chapter 24 we focus on the role of ECT in the continuum of neuromodulation treatment options. We also cover situations in which ECT may be carried out during treatment with other neuromodulation modalities, specifically VNS and DBS.

In each section, applicable background information, with pertinent updated literature citations, are followed by recommendations. This format matches closely with that of the 2001 report and allows integration of the recommendations with their justification.

In writing recommendations for a complex procedure such as ECT, it is impossible to cover all situations or deal with all possible exceptions. Accordingly, there will be times when overriding factors lead a reasonable and prudent practitioner to alter practice from that recommended here. It is also apparent that courses of action may exist that are reasonable alternatives to those presented in these recommendations.

Where applicable, attempts have been made to describe several such alternatives. Furthermore, new, clinically relevant information is continually appearing and should be readily incorporated into clinical practice whenever it is shown to either maximize efficacy or minimize adverse effects. Statutory and regulatory requirements related to ECT, such as informed consent procedures (Chapter 10), also vary considerably among jurisdictions and over time. Consequently, these recommendations may not always be compatible with all requirements of present or future statutes. Practitioners should seek out information on relevant regulations before beginning practice of ECT and should be aware of substantive statutory changes as they unfold.

As before, the bibliography and appendix provide additional resource material of use to practitioners. Consistent with the literature review noted above, the bibliography in this revised report has been updated, with representation of those articles published within the past two decades. In addition to citations focused on specific topics, a number of general texts on ECT for practitioners are available (Ferrier and Waite 2019; Ghaziuddin and Walter 2013; Kellner 2019; Mankad et al. 2010; Rasmussen 2019; Weiss 2018). Other books or monographs are oriented to the layperson (Dukakis and Tye 2007; Fink 2009; Hersh 2010; Kivler 2018).

The overall intent of this report is to offer a comprehensive yet practical overview of the safe and effective use of ECT, with recommendations that should be applicable across a wide spectrum of clinical settings. We encourage practitioners and trainees in psychiatry as well as those in related disciplines to read this document and integrate its recommendations into their clinical practice.

CHAPTER 2

Indications for the Use of Electroconvulsive Therapy

2.1. General Issues

A substantial body of clinical literature has established the efficacy of electroconvulsive therapy (ECT) in specific psychiatric and medical disorders (Ali et al. 2019; Luchini et al. 2015; Pagnin et al. 2004). The decision to recommend ECT derives from a risk-benefit analysis for the specific patient as discussed in the informed consent process (see Chapter 10). This analysis considers the patient's preferences, diagnosis, type and severity of symptoms, treatment history, and the likely speed of action, efficacy, and safety of ECT and other treatment options.

In 2018, the U.S. Food and Drug Administration (FDA) Center for Devices and Radiological Health reclassified ECT devices, and manufacturers' labeling of ECT devices now notes that ECT is indicated in "catatonia or severe major depressive episode (MDE) associated with major depressive disorder (MDD) or bipolar disorder (BPD) in patients ages 13 years and older who are treatment resistant or who require a rapid response due to the severity of their psychiatric or medical condition" (U.S. Food and Drug Administration 2018b). Although the FDA final order did not provide a definition of "treatment resistant" or "requiring a rapid response to treatment," it notes that "comments by healthcare professionals generally indicated that the terms are well understood" and "can be based on clinical judgment." In addition, the FDA classification applies to the marketing of ECT devices by manufacturers and does not limit use of ECT devices by psychiatrists providing care for other indications within a doctor-patient relationship (Kellner et al. 2019).

2.2. Timing of the Use of ECT

As an important somatic treatment in psychiatry with well-defined indications, ECT should not be reserved for use only as a "last resort" (Beale and Kellner 2000). Such practice may deprive patients of an effective treatment, may delay response and prolong suffering, and may possibly contribute to treatment resistance (Ghio et al. 2014; Hung et al. 2017; Riedel et al. 2011). Tools, such as pre-ECT neuroimaging or genomics, may eventually improve our ability to predict ECT response but have not yet achieved the accuracy necessary for clinical care (Redlich et al. 2016; Soda et al. 2020; van Waarde et al. 2015).

The speed and efficacy of ECT are factors that influence its use. Severe major depression with psychotic features and catatonia are conditions for which there is a clear support for early reliance on ECT (American Psychiatric Association 2010; Sienaert et al. 2014; U.S. Food and Drug Administration 2018b). It is common for patients to manifest appreciable improvement after a few treatments (England et al. 2011; Husain et al. 2004). In addition, the time to achieve maximal response to ECT is often more rapid than with psychotropic medications (Kho et al. 2003; C. H. Lin et al. 2018; Quitkin et al. 1996). Furthermore, the likelihood of obtaining significant clinical improvement is often more certain with ECT than with other treatment alternatives (Pagnin et al. 2004). Therefore, ECT should be considered when a rapid or a higher probability of response is needed, such as when patients have severe medical conditions or are at risk of harming themselves or others.

ECT is most often used in patients who have not responded to other treatments. Although evidence is mixed, medication resistance may predict a poorer clinical outcome with ECT (de Vreede et al. 2005; Dombrovski et al. 2005; Haq et al. 2015; Prudic et al. 1996). Nonetheless, in individuals with a diagnosis of major depression, a lack of response to one or more antidepressant medication trials does not preclude a favorable response to ECT (Pinna et al. 2018; Prudic et al. 1996). Indeed, compared with other treatment alternatives, the probability of response to ECT is favorable among patients with medication-resistant depression. During the course of pharmacotherapy, reasons to consider using ECT include lack of clinical response, intolerance of side effects, deterioration in psychiatric condition, inanition, or development of suicidal ideas or behaviors (American Psychiatric Association 2010; Fink 2014). Regardless of diagnosis, patients who have not responded to psychotherapy alone should not be considered to have treatment-resistant illness in the context of a referral for ECT.

Additional considerations for the use of ECT relate to the patient's medical status, treatment history, and treatment preference. Depending on the patient's medical status, ECT may be characterized by a more favorable risk-benefit profile than other therapeutic options (Sackeim 1998; Weiner et al. 2000). This circumstance most commonly arises among persons who are physically debilitated, among geriatric patients, and during pregnancy (see Chapter 9). Positive response to ECT in the past, particularly in the context of medication resistance or intolerance, also should lead to early consideration of ECT. At times, patients will prefer ECT over other treatment options, but commonly the opposite will be the case. Patient preferences should be discussed and considered before making treatment recommendations.

2.3. Principal Diagnostic Indications

MDE and catatonia are the principal diagnostic indications for ECT. Use of ECT in the treatment of other psychiatric conditions, including schizophrenia, mania, and other psychiatric diagnoses, is discussed in section 2.4.

2.3.1. Major Depression

2.3.1.1. Efficacy

The efficacy of ECT in depressive disorders is documented by a substantial body of research, including the open trials of the 1940s (Kalinowsky and Hoch 1946; Sargant and Slater 1954), the comparative ECT-pharmacotherapy trials of the 1960s (Greenblatt et al. 1964; Thiery and Medical Research Council 1965), comparisons of ECT and sham ECT (Brandon et al. 1984; Freeman et al. 1978; Gregory et al. 1985; Johnstone et al. 1980; Lambourn and Gill 1978; West 1981), studies contrasting variations in ECT technique (Kellner et al. 2010; Loo et al. 2014; Sackeim et al. 1987a, 1993, 2000, 2008; Sienaert et al. 2009), and studies examining maintenance strategies after an acute course of ECT (Kellner et al. 2016a; Petrides et al. 2011; Sackeim et al. 2001a). The efficacy of ECT in depression has also been demonstrated in studies comparing ECT with newer forms of neuromodulation, particularly transcranial magnetic stimulation (TMS; Chen et al. 2017; Rasmussen 2011; Ren et al. 2014).

Shortly after ECT became available, it was found to be especially effective in patients with depressive and manic states. In the 1940s and 1950s, ECT was a mainstay of treatment for such patients, with response rates between 80% and 90% commonly reported (Kalinowsky and Hoch 1946; Sargant and Slater 1954). The results of these early, largely open-label, studies have been summarized by experts in the field (Abrams 2002; American Psychiatric Association 1978; Elias et al. 2021; Fink 1979; Kiloh et al. 1988; Mukherjee et al. 1994).

With the introduction of the tricyclic antidepressants (TCAs) and monoamine oxidase inhibitors (MAOIs), random assignment trials were conducted in patients with depression in which ECT was used as the "gold standard" for measuring efficacy of these medications. Three such studies involved random assignment and blinded ratings, and each found a significant therapeutic advantage for ECT over TCAs and placebo (Gangadhar et al. 1982; Greenblatt et al. 1964; Thiery and Medical Research Council 1965). Other studies also reported ECT to be equal to or more effective than TCAs (Bruce et al. 1960; Davidson et al. 1978; Fahy et al. 1963; Hutchinson and Smedberg 1963; Kristiansen 1961; McDonald et al. 1966; Norris and Clancy 1961; Robin and Harris 1962; Stanley and Fleming 1962; Wilson et al. 1963) or MAOIs (Davidson et al. 1978; Hutchinson and Smedberg 1963; Kiloh et al. 1960; King 1959; Stanley and Fleming 1962). In a meta-analysis of this work (Janicak et al. 1985), the average response rate to ECT was 20% higher than that of TCAs and 45% higher than that of MAOIs. A subsequent systematic review and meta-analysis was conducted by the FDA and concluded that ECT was equal to or better than some antidepressant medications (U.S. Food and Drug Administration 2015).

Other studies have contrasted the clinical outcome of depressed patients who received inadequate or no pharmacotherapy with that of patients who received ECT. These studies usually focused on depressed patients who were receiving their first somatic treatment during the acute episode. Although few of these early comparative trials used aggressive pharmacotherapy by current criteria in terms of dosage or duration (Quitkin 1985; Rifkin 1988; Sackeim et al. 1990), most studies indicated that ECT resulted in decreased illness chronicity, morbidity, and rates of mortality (Avery and Winokur 1976; Babigian and Guttmacher 1984; Black et al. 1989b; Philibert et al. 1995; Wesner and Winokur 1989). In much of this work, the advantages of ECT were particularly pronounced in geriatric patients. For example, in a retrospective comparison of geriatric depressed patients treated with ECT or pharmacotherapy, significant depressive symptoms and a higher rate of mortality were observed in the pharmacotherapy group at long-term follow-up (Philibert et al. 1995). In a small randomized controlled trial (RCT) of patients who did not respond to monotherapy with a TCA, the efficacy of ECT was comparable to that of a combination of a TCA and lithium carbonate (Dinan and Barry 1989).

One study has compared the efficacy of ECT with that of the selective serotonin reuptake inhibitor (SSRI) paroxetine in patients with medication-resistant depression and found ECT to be markedly superior to paroxetine in short-term benefit (Folkerts et al. 1997). More recently, a pooled analysis of two open-label studies found ECT to be superior to fluoxetine in symptom improvement and quality of life (C. H. Lin et al. 2018). No studies have compared the efficacy of ECT with that of other antidepressant medications such as bupropion, mirtazapine, nefazodone, or venlafaxine. However, no study has ever found an antidepressant medication regimen to be more effective than ECT. Among patients who received ECT as a first-line treatment or who received inadequate pharmacotherapy during the index episode because of medication intolerance, response rates were reported in the range of 80%–90% (Prudic et al. 1990, 1996; Rasmussen et al. 2007c). Among patients who did not respond to one or more adequate antidepressant trials, the response rate was substantial, in the range of 50%–60% (Prudic et al. 1996; Sackeim et al. 2000) or greater.

The time to achieve full symptomatic improvement with antidepressant medications is typically estimated as 4–6 weeks (Quitkin et al. 1984, 1996). This delay until response may be longer in older patients (Salzman et al. 1995). In contrast, the average course of ECT for major depression consists of eight or nine treatments (Kellner et al. 2010; Prudic et al. 2004; Sackeim et al. 2000, 2008). Thus, when ECT is administered at a schedule of three treatments per week, full symptomatic improvement may be more rapid than with pharmacological treatment.

During the late 1970s and 1980s, a set of double-blind randomized assignment trials was conducted in England that contrasted "real" ECT with "sham" ECT—the repeated administration of anesthesia alone without electrical stimulation. With one exception (Lambourn and Gill 1978), real ECT was found to be consistently more efficacious than sham treatment (Brandon et al. 1984; Freeman et al. 1978; Gregory et al. 1985; Johnstone et al. 1980; West 1981). The single exception (Lambourn and Gill 1978) used a form of real ECT involving low stimulus intensity and right unilateral electrode placement that is now known to be ineffective (Sackeim et al. 1987a, 1993). In preparation for discussion of the classification of ECT devices, the FDA conducted a meta-analysis of the extant RCT literature comparing ECT with sham ECT, which included these studies as well as studies conducted earlier and later than this series. This meta-analysis concluded that ECT was more effective than sham ECT or placebo (U.S. Food and Drug Administration 2015). Furthermore, these real-versus-sham ECT studies suggested that antidepressant effects of ECT require administration of an effective electrical stimulus capable of eliciting a generalized seizure.

Subsequent studies have examined variations in ECT technique and compared outcomes in patients with major depression. Although each of these approaches involved electrical stimulation with production of a generalized seizure, it is now clear that clinical outcome with ECT in the treatment of major depression depends on interactions of multiple factors, including electrode placement, stimulus dosing, and pulse duration, when bipolar pulse waveforms are used (Loo et al. 2014; Mayur et al. 2013; McCall et al. 2000; Sackeim et al. 1987a, 1993, 2000, 2008). Thus, technical factors in ECT administration can strongly influence efficacy (see Chapter 14).

Although there now are comparisons of ECT with other forms of brain stimulation, only vagus nerve stimulation and TMS are FDA approved for treatment of major depression (see Chapter 24). Several meta-analyses confirmed the therapeutic benefit of ECT compared with TMS (Berlim et al. 2013; Minichino et al. 2012; Ren et al. 2014). Although TMS had fewer cognitive side effects, particularly for memory and verbal fluency (Chen et al. 2017; Mutz et al. 2019; Ren et al. 2014), both TMS and ECT were well tolerated, with similar rates of treatment discontinuation frequency. Furthermore, ECT was superior to high-frequency TMS in terms of response (64.4% vs. 48.7%, risk ratio [RR]=1.41, $P=0.03$) and remission (52.9% vs. 33.6%, RR=1.38, $P=0.006$; Ren et al. 2014). In an accompanying subgroup analysis, high-frequency TMS was as effective as ECT in persons with nonpsychotic depression, whereas ECT was superior to high-frequency TMS in those with psychotic depression (Berlim et al. 2013).

2.3.1.2. Prediction of Response

ECT is an effective somatic treatment in patients with an MDE regardless of whether it occurs in the context of MDD or bipolar disorder (Aronson et al. 1988; Black et al. 1986, 1993; Dierckx et al. 2012; U.S. Food and Drug Administration 2018b; Zorumski et al. 1986). However, it is not yet possible to predict ECT outcomes or personalize treatment recommendations for ECT using clinical, biological, and/or procedural variables (Soda et al. 2020). Biological predictors are being actively explored, with functional connectivity and genomics most actively studied, but most published studies have small sample sizes and limited predictive power (Sota et al. 2020).

Race, sex, and socioeconomic status do not have predictive value; however, older age has been associated with better ECT outcome in most (Black et al. 1993; Coryell and Zimmerman 1984; Dominiak et al. 2021b; Folstein et al. 1973; Gold and Chiarello 1944; Greenblatt et al. 1962; Mendels 1965a, 1965b; Nystrom 1964; O'Connor et al. 2001; Roberts 1959a, 1959b; Spashett et al. 2014; Strömgren 1973; Tew et al. 1999) but not all (van Diermen et al. 2020) relevant studies.

In the 1950s and 1960s, a series of studies in patients with depression suggested that outcome was related to the pattern of symptoms that patients exhibited (Abrams 2002; Black et al. 1987a; Carney et al. 1965; Hamilton and White 1960; Hobson 1953; Mendels 1967; Nobler and Sackeim 1996; Rose 1963). This work emphasized the importance of vegetative symptoms and melancholic features in determining the response to ECT. Although some evidence indicates that psychomotor agitation (van Diermen et al. 2020) or psychomotor retardation (Buchan et al. 1992; Heijnen et al. 2019; Hickie et al. 1990, 1996; Sobin et al. 1996; van Diermen et al. 2020) may predict a favorable response to ECT in patients with depression, melancholic symptoms or an endogenous subtype of depression do not appear to predict ECT response (Abrams et al. 1973; Black et al. 1993; Coryell and Zimmerman 1984; Fink et al. 2007; Prudic et al. 1989; Sackeim and Rush 1995; Veltman et al. 2019; Zimmerman et al. 1985, 1986).

In the majority of studies that have examined the rate of response to ECT, patients diagnosed with psychotic depression had a higher response rate than did nonpsychotic patients (Avery and Lubrano 1979; Buchan et al. 1992; Clinical Research Centre 1984; Heijnen et al. 2019; Hobson 1953; Lykouras et al. 1986; Mandel et al. 1977; Pande et al. 1990; Petrides et al. 2001; Sobin et al. 1996; Spashett et al. 2014; van Diermen et al. 2020), and rates of suicide decreased after ECT treatment in individuals with psychotic depression (Rönnqvist et al. 2021). This finding is of particular importance because patients with psychotic depression commonly have severe symptoms and are at increased risk for suicide (American Psychiatric Association 2010; Gournellis et al. 2018; Roose et al. 1983). In addition, psychotic depression has a relatively low rate of response to monotherapy with an antidepressant or antipsychotic medication (Farahani and Correll 2012; Kroessler 1985; Parker et al. 1992; Rothschild 2013), and many patients with psychotic depression have not had an adequate medication trial before being referred for ECT (Mulsant et al. 1997; Nelson et al. 1986; Rasmussen et al. 2006).

The duration of a depressive episode is often interconnected to an incomplete response to prior treatment, but the duration of the depressive episode also appears to affect the likelihood of response to ECT. As is true of pharmacological treatment response, several studies have noted that patients with a long episode duration are less likely to respond to ECT (Haq et al. 2015; Kho et al. 2005; Kukopulos et al. 1977; Magni et al. 1988; Perugi et al. 2012; Pinna et al. 2018; Prudic et al. 1996; van Diermen et al. 2020) than do those with a short episode duration, although results are not homogeneous (Dombrovski et al. 2005; Pluijms et al. 2006). It remains unclear whether the longer period of time in an episode or ineffective treatment actively contributes to treatment resistance (Ghio et al. 2014; Hung et al. 2017; Riedel et al. 2011). Nonetheless, depressed individuals with a long episode duration are likely to have experienced more trials of medication and other treatments before being referred for ECT (de Vreede et al. 2005; Dombrovski et al. 2005; Haq et al. 2015; Prudic et al. 1996).

The definition of psychotropic medication resistance and its implications with respect to a referral for ECT have been the subject of considerable discussion (Prudic et al. 1996; Réus et al. 2019; Voineskos et al. 2020). At present, there are no universally adopted standards by which to define medication resistance. In practice, when assessing the adequacy of pharmacological treatment, psychiatrists rely on factors such as the type and dosage of medication used, blood levels (when available), duration of treatment, adherence to the medication regimen, adverse effects, degree of therapeutic response, and type and severity of clinical symptoms (Prudic et al. 1996). In general, patients with a diagnosis of major depression who have not responded to one or more antidepressant medication trials may have a poorer clinical outcome of ECT compared with patients treated with ECT who have not received an adequate medication trial during the index episode (Prudic et al. 1990, 1996; Shapira et al. 1996). The relationship between medication resistance and ECT outcome may be stronger with TCAs than with SSRIs (Prudic et al. 1996), but little information is available about the predictive significance of resistance to other pharmacological agents (e.g., mirtazapine, nefazodone, venlafaxine). Importantly, the presence of medication resistance does not preclude a favorable response to ECT (Avery and Lubrano 1979; Magni et al. 1988; Paul et al. 1981; Prudic et al. 1996). Indeed, among patients with medication-resistant depression, the probability of response to ECT is likely to be more favorable than with other treatment alternatives. However, a greater number of ECT treatments may be required to achieve symptomatic improvement among some patients with substantial histories of treatment resistance.

Individuals with major depression often have concomitant psychiatric disorders or other co-occurring medical conditions. Uncontrolled studies suggest that patients with secondary depression, which appears to be related to another psychiatric or medical disorder, respond less well to somatic treatments, including ECT, than do patients with primary depression (Black et al. 1993; Coryell et al. 1985; Krystal and Coffey 1997). Although dysthymia (persistent depressive disorder) is not typically treated with ECT, individuals with a history of dysthymia preceding a major depressive episode may be referred for ECT. The response to ECT may be lessened by the presence of persistent depression or dysthymia (Dombrovski et al. 2005), but many such patients will show a robust response. There is also evidence suggesting that the degree of residual symptoms after ECT is equivalent in some patients with major depression superimposed on a dysthymic baseline (i.e., double depression) compared with patients with major depression without a history of dysthymia (Prudic et al. 1993).

Some studies have observed that patients with comorbid personality disorder may be more likely to be referred for ECT because of complexity and refractoriness of their mood symptoms (Patel et al. 2019; Peltzman et al. 2020). Although patients with major depression and a concomitant personality disorder may have a reduced probability of ECT response, this correlation may depend on the type of personality disorder (Popiolek et al. 2019; Prudic et al. 2004; Rasmussen 2015). In a population-based registry study, persistence of suicidal ideation after ECT was associated with younger age and a concomitant personality disorder, although the clinical response to ECT and reduction of suicidal ideation were still substantial (Sienaert et al. 2022). A systematic review also suggested that rates of response to ECT may be lower if borderline personality disorder is present as compared with patients without this comorbidity (Nicolini and Sienaert 2023). Nevertheless, outcomes with ECT may still be positive, and use of ECT should not be precluded by the presence of a personality disorder (e.g., borderline personality disorder) or other psychiatric disorder (e.g., anorexia nervosa) when comorbid with major depression (Kaster et al. 2018; Lee et al. 2019; Shilton et al. 2020).

In individuals referred for ECT, cognitive impairment may result from a concomitant psychiatric diagnosis (e.g., dementia) or may be a manifestation of MDD itself (Ahern and Semkovska 2017; Butters et al. 2000; Izquierdo-Guerra et al. 2018; Lim et al. 2013; Lisanby et al. 2020; McClintock et al. 2010, 2014; Semkovska and McLoughlin 2010; Semkovska et al. 2011; Zakzanis et al. 1998). A subgroup of depressed patients will exhibit cognitive impairment that resolves with treatment of the MDE (Alexopoulos et al. 1993; Butters et al. 2000; Dybedal et al. 2015; Grützner et al. 2019; Verwijk et al. 2014). Occasionally, this cognitive impairment may be sufficiently severe as to mask the presence of mood symptoms. When such patients have been treated with ECT, recovery has often been dramatic (Allen 1982; Bulbena and Berrios 1986; Burke et al. 1985; Fink 1990; Grunhaus et al. 1983; McAllister and Price 1982; O'Shea et al. 1987; Pier et al. 2012; Wagner et al. 2011). Nevertheless, among patients with major depression without known neurological disease, the extent of pre-ECT cognitive impairment appears to predict the severity of amnesia following ECT (Sackeim et al. 2008; Sobin et al. 1995). Thus, patients with baseline cognitive impairment related to major depression may show improved global cognitive function in conjunction with the improvement in depressive symptoms; however, they may also be at risk for retrograde amnesia (Martin et al. 2015; Sobin et al. 1995). Furthermore, preexisting neurological impairments, including dementia, may increase the risks for ECT-induced delirium and for more severe and persistent amnestic effects (Figiel et al. 1990, 1991; Krystal and Coffey 1997; Mulsant et al. 1991). In Chapter 20, we provide further discussion of the interactions of preexisting cognitive or neurological impairments with depressive and cognitive outcomes of ECT treatment.

2.3.2. Catatonia

Catatonia may occur with or without other psychiatric comorbidity, but it is commonly associated with mood disorder, psychosis, or autism spectrum disorder (American Psychiatric Association 2022; Connell et al. 2023; Fink 2013; Mormando and Francis 2020; Rasmussen et al. 2016; Sienaert et al. 2014; Wachtel 2019). Although controlled studies are lacking, observational reports support the fact that catatonia is responsive to ECT with effectiveness in the range of 80%–100% (Dutt et al. 2011; England et al. 2011; Luchini et al. 2015; Raveendranathan et al. 2012). Case reports also suggest that ECT is effective in the treatment of catatonia in adolescents and children, as well as in adults (Dhossche and Withane 2019; U.S. Food and Drug Administration 2018b; Wachtel 2019).

ECT is most often indicated when catatonia is severe and potentially life-threatening (i.e., malignant or lethal catatonia), or when catatonia has not responded to pharmacological approaches, typically a course of benzodiazepines (Bush et al. 1996b; Dhossche et al. 2009; Rogers et al. 2023; Sienaert et al. 2014; U.S. Food and Drug Administration 2018b). The combination of ECT and benzodiazepines has also been reported to be effective for catatonia (Cronemeyer et al. 2022; Petrides et al. 1997; Unal et al. 2013, 2017).

Comorbidity of catatonia with a mood disorder may be a more favorable prognostic characteristic (Luchini et al. 2015; Rohland et al. 1993) than comorbidity with schizophrenia, particularly chronic catatonia in individuals with schizophrenia (Tharyan and Adams 2005; Ungvari et al. 2010). Younger age, autonomic dysregulation, and shorter episode duration have also been correlated with better prognosis for the use of ECT in the treatment of catatonia (Luchini et al. 2015; van Waarde et al. 2010). A longer duration of catatonia has been associated with the need for a longer course of ECT (Malur et al. 2001).

Catatonia may also be associated with medical conditions (Ali et al. 2008; Denysenko et al. 2018; Kamigaichi et al. 2009; Oldham 2018; Rogers et al. 2019), including autoimmune conditions (Bica et al. 2015; Boeke et al. 2018; Fricchione et al. 1990; Mischel et al. 2020), particularly anti-*N*-methyl-D-aspartate encephalitis (Dalmau et al. 2008; Espi Forcen et al. 2022; Giné-Servén et al. 2022; Levy et al. 2023; Marques Macedo and Gama Marques 2020; Sarkis et al. 2019; Serra-Mestres et al. 2020); epilepsy, including status epilepticus (Ogyu et al. 2021); drug intoxication and withdrawal (Oldham and Desan 2016; Yeoh et al. 2022); and abnormal metabolic states (Espi Forcen et al. 2022; Taylor and Fink 2003). A growing number of reports suggest that catatonia can also develop subsequent to infection with coronavirus disease 2019 (COVID-19) (Austgen et al. 2022; Deocleciano de Araujo et al. 2021; Kaur et al.

2021; Scheiner et al. 2021; Torrico et al. 2021). In addition, some patients may have multiple potential factors that could contribute to developing catatonia (Jaimes-Albornoz et al. 2022).

Although catatonia associated with neurological conditions seems less responsive to ECT than catatonia that occurs in association with other psychiatric conditions (Luchini et al. 2015; Swartz et al. 2003; Tripodi et al. 2021), catatonia as a feature of medical illness can be responsive to ECT. Most frequently, ECT is used when treatment of the associated illness fails to resolve catatonic symptoms (Bush et al. 1996b; Fink et al. 2016; Fricchione et al. 1990; Rummans and Bassingthwaighte 1991).

2.4. Other Diagnostic Indications

The evidence base for the use of ECT is most extensive and definitive for major depression, but ECT has been used successfully in treating other conditions as well (American Psychiatric Association 2001; Kellner et al. 2020; Rosenquist et al. 2018). The evidence for use of ECT in primary psychotic disorders and bipolar mania is substantial, although subject to some qualification. In other, rarer circumstances, ECT has been used on a more individualized basis to treat other psychiatric disorders or other medical conditions. Most such usage involves patients who have exhausted other treatment options, who present with extremely severe or life-threatening symptoms, and for whom there is some expectation of benefit from ECT. Accordingly, controlled studies would be difficult to conduct, and available evidence is primarily from case reports. Although these indications would be considered "off label" in the context of the FDA's final order for ECT devices (U.S. Food and Drug Administration 2018b), the FDA classification applies to the marketing of the machines by manufacturers and does not limit the use of the machines by psychiatrists providing care within a doctor-patient relationship (Kellner et al. 2019). As with any clinical intervention, the evidence for the efficacy of ECT in these conditions should be considered along with the potential benefits and risks for each individual patient as part of the consent process (see Chapter 10).

2.4.1. Schizophrenia and Schizophrenia Spectrum Disorders

Convulsive therapy was first used as a treatment for schizophrenia (as reviewed by Fink 1979). Early in its use, it became evident that the efficacy of ECT was greater in mood disorders than in schizophrenia. The introduction of effective antipsychotic medications markedly reduced the use of ECT in patients with schizophrenia. Despite this, schizophrenia has remained a common diagnostic indication for the use of ECT worldwide (Leiknes et al. 2012). In developed countries, ECT continues to be effective in patients with schizophrenia who do not respond to pharmacological treatment and who have particularly severe symptoms or course of illness (Pompili et al. 2013; Teodorczuk et al. 2019).

The earliest reports on the efficacy of ECT in patients with schizophrenia largely comprised uncontrolled case series (Danziger and Kindwall 1946; Guttmann et al. 1939; Kalinowsky 1943; Kalinowsky and Worthing 1943; Kennedy and Anchel 1948; Kino and Thorpe 1946; Miller et al. 1953; Ross and Malzberg 1939; Zeifert 1941), historical comparisons (Bond 1954; Currier et al. 1952; Ellison and Hamilton 1949; Gottlieb and Huston 1951), and comparisons of ECT with milieu therapy or psychotherapy (Goldfarb and Kiene 1945; MacKinnon 1948; Palmer et al. 1951; Rachlin et al. 1956; Wolff 1955). These early reports lacked operational criteria for diagnosis, and patient samples and outcome criteria were often poorly characterized.

Several trials have used a real-versus-sham-ECT design to examine efficacy in patients with schizophrenia. Studies prior to 1980 did not demonstrate a therapeutic advantage of real ECT relative to sham treatment (Brill et al. 1959a, 1959b, 1959c; Heath et al. 1964; Miller et al. 1953; Ulett et al. 1954, 1956). In contrast, later studies all found a substantial advantage for real ECT in short-term therapeutic outcome (Abraham and Kulhara 1987; Brandon et al. 1985; Goswami et al. 1989; Masoudzadeh and Khalilian 2007; Sarkar et al. 1994; Taylor and Fleminger 1980; Ukpong et al. 2002). The early studies focused more on patients with a chronic, unremitting course, whereas patients with acute exacerbations were more common in the more recent studies. More recent studies also administered antipsychotic medications in both the real ECT and the sham groups, which likely increased treatment efficacy, as discussed below.

The utility of monotherapy with ECT or antipsychotic medication was compared in a variety of retrospective (Ayres 1960; Borowitz 1959; De Wet 1957; Rohde and Sargant 1961) and prospective (Bagadia et al. 1970, 1983; Baker et al. 1958, 1960; Childers 1964; Exner and Murillo 1973, 1977; King 1960; Langsley et al. 1959; May and Tuma 1965; May et al. 1976, 1981; Murillo and Exner 1973; Ray 1962) studies of patients with schizophrenia. Overall, short-term clinical outcome in schizophrenia with antipsychotic medication was found to be equivalent or superior to that of ECT, which contributed to the decreased use of ECT as a first-line acute treatment for schizophrenia.

More recently, a randomized open-label study compared acute ECT followed by maintenance ECT with clozapine and found greater benefit of ECT in reducing symptoms and improving general functioning (Mishra et al. 2022). Other prospective studies have compared the efficacy of combination treatment using ECT and antipsychotic medication with that of monotherapy using antipsychotic medication (Ali et al. 2019; Grover et al. 2019; Petrides et al. 2015; Sanghani et al. 2018). In one prospective randomized trial, individuals with schizophrenia that had not responded to clozapine were either continued on clozapine or treated with 20 sessions of bilateral ECT over 8 weeks in combination with clozapine (N=39; Petrides et al. 2015). Of patients in the ECT plus clozapine group, half showed a reduction in psychotic symptoms of at least 40%, whereas none of the clozapine-only patients met this response criteria. During an open-label phase, those who had continued the clozapine were also administered ECT, with response occurring in 47% (Petrides et al. 2015).

Meta-analyses have also found an advantage for the combination of ECT with antipsychotics as compared with continued antipsychotic monotherapy (Lally et al. 2016; Wang et al. 2018; Zheng et al. 2016). This advantage seemed particularly pronounced when clozapine was the antipsychotic used (Ahmed et al. 2017). When restricting these analyses to RCTs, a Cochrane Collaboration systematic review concluded: "Moderate-quality evidence indicates that relative to standard care, ECT has a positive effect on medium-term clinical response for people with treatment-resistant schizophrenia" (Sinclair et al. 2019, p. 2).

Since publication of the earliest research, the clinical feature most strongly associated with the therapeutic outcome of ECT in patients with schizophrenia has been the duration of the episode of illness. Patients with acute onset of psychotic symptoms and shorter episode duration are more likely to benefit from ECT than are patients with persistent, unremitting symptoms (Chanpattana and Sackeim 2010; Cheney and Drewry 1938; Danziger and Kindwall 1946; Herzberg 1954; Landmark et al. 1987; Pawełczyk et al. 2014). Nevertheless, recent observational studies suggest that a significant fraction of individuals with schizophrenia will respond to ECT (Plahouras et al. 2021). In addition, ECT is associated with a reduction in the number of inpatient hospitalizations (Joo et al. 2022; Ying et al. 2021) and improvements in functioning and quality of life (Tor et al. 2021) in patients with schizophrenia. Thus, it has also been argued that such patients should not be denied a trial of ECT, especially in the presence of markedly severe symptoms (Grover et al. 2018).

Limited evidence is available on the effects of ECT on other diagnoses on the schizophrenia spectrum. Treatment studies have typically not distinguished individuals with schizoaffective and schizophreniform disorder from those with schizophrenia when assessing outcomes of ECT (e.g., Ali et al. 2019). In addition, diagnostic conceptualizations of these disorders have evolved over time (American Psychiatric Association 2022), further confounding the interpretation of results. Nevertheless, the available evidence suggests that ECT may be considered in the treatment of patients with schizoaffective or schizophreniform disorder (Ali et al. 2019; Black et al. 1987b, 1987c; Pope et al. 1980; Ries et al. 1981; Tsuang et al. 1979). Many practitioners believe that the presence of mood symptoms in patients with schizophrenia is predictive of positive clinical outcome; however, the evidence supporting this view is inconsistent (Dodwell and Goldberg 1989; Folstein et al. 1973; Wells 1973).

2.4.2. Mania

Mania is a syndrome with a wide range of clinical expressions, but in its most severe form, it can be life-threatening because of its attendant exhaustion, excitement, and potential for violence. Early case reports first suggested that ECT is rapidly effective in mania and also has mood-stabilizing effects (Impastato and Almansi 1943; Kino and Thorpe 1946; Smith et al. 1943). A number of observational studies either included naturalistic case series or compared outcomes with ECT with those with lithium carbonate or chlorpromazine. This literature supports the efficacy of ECT in acute mania and suggested that ECT had equivalent or superior antimanic properties relative to lithium and chlorpromazine (Mukherjee et al. 1994; Versiani et al. 2011).

Three prospective comparative studies of ECT in acute mania have been published. One study compared ECT primarily with lithium treatment (Small et al. 1988); another compared ECT with combined treatment with lithium and haloperidol (Mukherjee et al. 1988, 1994); and the third study compared real and sham ECT in patients receiving antipsychotic treatment (Sikdar et al. 1994). Although each of these prospective studies had small samples, the findings supported the conclusion that ECT was efficacious in acute mania; ECT was associated with remission or marked clinical improvement in approximately 80% of patients (Mukherjee et al. 1994). In addition, ECT resulted in better short-term outcomes than did pharmacotherapy with lithium or first-generation antipsychotic medications (Mukherjee et al. 1994). There have been no comparisons of ECT and newer antimanic medication regimens (Fornaro et al. 2020). Several trials have compared the use of different bilateral electrode placements and dosing strategies in the ECT treatment of mania and found comparable response rates in the range of 72%–92% (Barekatain et al. 2008; Hiremani et al. 2008; Mohan et al. 2009).

In current practice, ECT has been reserved for patients with acute mania whose symptoms do not respond to adequate pharmacological treatment (e.g., lithium, anticonvulsants, antipsychotic medications including clozapine) or who have severe episodes frequently characterized by uncontrolled agitation. As with major depression, medication resistance appears to predict a somewhat poorer response to ECT in acute mania (Mukherjee et al. 1994). Nonetheless, evidence from retrospective and prospective studies has indicated that a substantial number of patients whose mania has not responded to medications will benefit from ECT (Black et al. 1986; Mukherjee et al. 1988; Perugi et al. 2017). Using a combination of ECT and medication may have greater benefit than medication alone in these circumstances (Zhang et al. 2021). Consequently, clinical practice guidelines have listed the use of ECT as an appropriate treatment when other options have not been beneficial (American Psychiatric Association 2002; Fountoulakis et al. 2020; Goodwin et al. 2016; Malhi et al. 2021).

Episodes of BPD with mixed features can be particularly resistant to psychopharmacological treatments. The evidence for using ECT in this context includes retrospective series and reviews (Devanand et al. 2000; Gruber et al. 2000; Palma et al. 2016) as well as several larger prospective observational studies (Ciapparelli et al. 2001; Medda et al. 2010, 2014; Perugi et al. 2017). In these reports, responses to ECT of patients with mixed features were at least as favorable as the response of patients with bipolar depressive episodes (Perugi et al. 2020). In addition, for patients with mania who cycle rapidly and may be particularly unresponsive to medications, ECT represents a potentially effective treatment option (Minnai et al. 2011; Vanelle et al. 1994).

Other than medication resistance, few attempts have been made to examine the clinical features predictive of ECT response in acute mania (Mukherjee et al. 1994). One study suggested that symptoms of anger, irritability, and suspiciousness were associated with poorer ECT outcome (Schnur et al. 1992). In rare instances, individuals with severe mania may present in a confused state, which has been termed *manic delirium*. In such individuals, ECT is rapidly effective, with a high margin of safety (Detweiler et al. 2009; Fink 1999; Jacobowski et al. 2013; Karmacharya et al. 2008; Strömgren 1997), and may be indicated as a first-line treatment.

2.4.3. Mental Disorders Due to Medical Conditions

Severe mood syndromes, psychosis, and certain types of delirium that are due to a medical condition may be responsive to ECT. The use of ECT in such circumstances is rare and should be reserved for patients who require an urgent response, are intolerant of more standard medical treatments, or have symptoms that have not responded to treatment. Prior to ECT, attention should be given to determining the underlying etiology of the medical condition, and treatment should be targeted at the specific causes.

It is largely of historical interest that ECT has been reported to be of benefit in conditions such as alcoholic delirium (Dudley and Williams 1972; Kramp and Bolwig 1981); toxic delirium due to phencyclidine (PCP; Dinwiddie et al. 1988; Rosen et al. 1984); and in psychiatric syndromes caused by enteric fevers (Breakey and Kala 1977; Hafeiz 1987; O'Toole and Dyck 1977), head injury (Kant et al. 1995), and other causes (Strömgren 1997). This use of ECT to treat delirium is very rare in the United States but continues occasionally in Scandinavia (Nielsen et al. 2014), although the available evidence is limited (Lupke et al. 2023).

2.4.4. Medical Conditions

The physiological effects associated with ECT may result in therapeutic benefit in certain medical conditions, independent of antidepressant, antimanic, and antipsychotic actions. Because other effective treatments are usually available for these disorders, ECT should be reserved for use when a patient's symptoms have not responded to standard treatments.

There is now considerable experience in the use of ECT in patients with Parkinson's disease, particularly for depression as a feature of the illness (Borisovskaya et al. 2016; Kellner et al. 1994a; Riva-Posse et al. 2013). Independent of effects on psychiatric symptoms, ECT can result in general improvement in motor function (Faber and Trimble 1991; Grover et al. 2018; Kennedy et al. 2003; Takamiya et al. 2021). Patients with "on-off" phenomenon, in particular, may show considerable improvement (Andersen et al. 1987). However, the beneficial effects of ECT on the motor symptoms of Parkinson's disease are limited and are variable in duration, generally up to a month. Preliminary evidence indicates that maintenance ECT may be helpful in prolonging therapeutic effects (Popeo and Kellner 2009). With the advent of second-generation antipsychotics to treat side effects of dopaminergic therapies and deep brain stimulation as a better targeted and more durable form of neuromodulation for Parkinson's disease, ECT is only rarely used for features of Parkinson's disease other than depression.

ECT has marked anticonvulsant properties (Coffey et al. 1995b; Sackeim 1999), and its use as an anticonvulsant has been reported in patients with seizure disorders since the 1940s (Ahmed et al. 2018; Fink et al. 1999; Zeiler et al. 2016). ECT may be of value in patients with intractable epilepsy or status epilepticus, particularly severe super-refractory status epilepticus that is unresponsive to pharmacological or other treatments (García-López et al. 2020; Katzell et al. 2023; Pinchotti et al. 2018; San-Juan et al. 2019; Schneegans et al. 2019; Singla et al. 2022; Tan et al. 2020; Woodward et al. 2023). The benefit of ECT under these circumstances varies depending on the underlying pathophysiology and the degree of brain tissue damage already sustained during the period of status epilepticus.

Neuroleptic malignant syndrome (NMS), which some believe to be similar to malignant catatonia (Carroll et al. 2001; Fricchione et al. 2000; Koch et al. 2000), has been shown to improve after ECT in case reports and case series (Bhanushali and Tuite 2004; Davis et al. 1991; Morcos et al. 2019; Nisijima and Ishiguro 1999; Trollor and Sachdev 1999). ECT is usually considered when pharmacological approaches to NMS have been ineffective, symptom severity necessitates immediate intervention, or NMS features overlap with catatonia. ECT has also been used in patients with current or past history of NMS who need to avoid treatment with dopamine-blocking agents but whose underlying psychiatric illness is expected to be responsive to ECT.

Recommendations

2.1. General Issues

1. The decision to recommend ECT derives from a risk-benefit analysis for the specific patient as discussed in the informed consent process.
2. Referrals for ECT are based on a combination of factors, including the patient's preferences; diagnosis; type and severity of symptoms; treatment history; and the likely speed of action, efficacy, and safety of ECT and other treatment options.

2.2. Timing of the Use of ECT

1. In most individuals, ECT is used after there is inadequate response to treatment with psychotropic medications or if symptoms are so severe that acute intervention is needed.
2. Early use of ECT in a course of treatment is indicated when illness is so severe that there is a need for a rapid alleviation of critical symptoms, such as precipitous deterioration, inanition, catatonia, disabling manifestations of psychosis, and/or suicidal ideation or behaviors.
3. Other factors supporting earlier use of ECT include patient preference, intolerance or poor response to psychotropic medications, past history of positive response to ECT, and/or a risk-benefit analysis that favors ECT over other therapeutic options.

2.3. Principal Diagnostic Indications

1. ECT is an efficacious treatment, supported by a substantial evidence base, for MDEs that occur in individuals with MDD or BPD.
2. ECT is a highly efficacious treatment, supported by strong expert consensus and observational evidence, for acute catatonia.
3. The presence of a concomitant psychiatric condition should not deter the use of ECT in an individual with an MDE or catatonia.

2.4. Other Diagnostic Indications

1. ECT may be indicated for the treatment of schizophrenia in combination with antipsychotic medications when there is a past history of positive response to ECT, symptoms have not responded to anti-

psychotic medications including clozapine, and/or symptoms are very severe (e.g., violence toward self or others driven by hallucinations and delusions, significant associated disability).

2. Although the evidence base is more limited, ECT can be considered for the treatment of schizophrenia spectrum disorders (e.g., schizophreniform disorder, schizoaffective disorder) when there is a past history of positive response to ECT, symptoms have not responded to psychotropic medications, and/or symptoms are very severe.

3. ECT is an efficacious treatment for manic episodes in individuals with BPD but is generally recommended when episodes have not responded to pharmacotherapy or are unusually severe.

4. The neurobiological effects of ECT may produce therapeutic benefits in a small number of medical conditions, including Parkinson's disease (and its associated on-off phenomenon), NMS, and status epilepticus, particularly severe super-refractory status epilepticus when standard treatment approaches have been unsuccessful and with appropriate neurological consultation.

CHAPTER 3

Staffing

3.1. The ECT Treatment Team

3.1.1. Members

Electroconvulsive therapy (ECT) is a complex procedure that requires a well-trained, competent staff of professionals if it is to be administered in a safe and effective fashion. The ECT treatment team functions as a unit and typically consists of a psychiatrist (termed here the ECT psychiatrist), an anesthesiologist, one or more recovery nurses, and one or more ECT treatment nurses. When properly qualified, the ECT psychiatrist may also perform the duties of the ECT treatment nurse, although having a distinct ECT treatment nurse is strongly encouraged. Furthermore, at least two health care professionals should be in the treatment area during the administration of ECT. For each role on the treatment team, the pool of available staff members should be kept as small as possible to maximize continuity of care and to ensure that each individual has sufficient ongoing experience to maintain proficiency in their work.

All physicians administering ECT should be privileged in the performance of ECT-related duties by the organized medical staff of the facility under whose auspices ECT will be delivered (see Chapter 7). In addition, all anesthesiologists and other anesthesia providers involved in anesthesia administration for ECT should be privileged to deliver general anesthesia for the age groups of patients who are being treated. Nursing staff members involved in ECT should also receive adequate training and assessment of competency before assuming ECT-related duties. Psychiatric, anesthetic, and nursing trainees may assist in the performance of ECT-related duties only under the direct supervision of appropriately privileged attending physicians or credentialed staff and only at a level commensurate with the level of relevant training they have received.

3.1.2. Responsibilities

3.1.2.1. ECT Psychiatrist

Because their training and experience in ECT is the most comprehensive, the ECT psychiatrist should maintain overall responsibility for the administration of ECT. The ECT psychiatrist is also responsible for 1) assessing the patient prior to beginning ECT (see Chapters 8 and 11), 2) ensuring that the pre-ECT evaluation has been completed (see Chapters 8 and 9), 3) determining that ECT is still indicated prior to each ECT treatment (see Chapters 2, 11, and 17), 4) verifying that the patient has provided informed consent for ECT (see Chapter 10), 5) identifying changes in psychiatric symptoms or health status that would influence ECT-related decision-making (see Chapters 8, 17, 19, and 20), 6) instituting appropriate modifications to the ECT course or technique, as indicated (see Chapters 12, 13, 14, and 17–22), 7) ensuring that the delivery of ECT is compatible with established policies and procedures, and 8) making sure that evaluation and treatment results are properly documented (see Chapter 5).

Practice varies as to whether the ECT psychiatrist also oversees all other aspects of the patient's mental health care during and immediately after the ECT course or whether a separate mental health clinician fulfills this latter function. When such roles are separate, it is important for both individuals to agree on treatment decisions such as the rationale for ECT, the choice of an inpatient versus an outpatient setting, the electrode placement, the number of ECT treatments, and the choice of a maintenance treatment. However, except for some aspects of anesthetic management, the ECT psychiatrist should maintain overall responsibility for the conduct of ECT, including determination of how each treatment is administered.

3.1.2.2. Anesthesiology Providers

Even for a procedure as brief as ECT, the administration of anesthesia requires skill in airway management, use of ultrabrief anesthetic and relaxant agents, cardiopulmonary resuscitation, and management of acute adverse events. The anesthesia provider must be capable of managing acute medical emergencies that could occur during and immediately after ECT (see Chapter 12) and must also be familiar with relevant emergency medications and emergency life support. A certified registered nurse anesthetist (CRNA), physician assistant anesthetist (PAA), or anesthesiologist assistant (AA) may administer anesthesia for ECT if trained and competent to perform the tasks described above as well as appropriately privileged by the facility (see Chapter 7). Supervision of a CRNA, PAA, or AA is generally conducted by an anesthesiologist; however, in jurisdictions where this is not required, the ECT psychiatrist needs to be skilled in advanced cardiac life support (ACLS) and airway management to be able to provide any required physician supervision. Furthermore, a qualified anesthesiologist should be present when treating high-risk patients who need more complex anesthetic management.

The provision of anesthetic care is inextricably linked to the safety and efficacy of ECT. Although the anesthesia provider has primary responsibility for emergency management of cardiopulmonary function and maintaining life support, it is critical that the ECT psychiatrist and anesthesia provider agree on the patient's medical management. This includes discussing the type and dosage of medications for the ECT procedure and interventions for adverse events. The patient's recovery from anesthesia is also overseen by the anesthesia provider.

3.1.2.3. ECT Treatment Nurse

The specific duties of the ECT nurse may vary at different ECT programs (Burns and Stuart 1991; Froimson et al. 1995; Gunderson-Falcone 1995; Hannigan 2019; Jewell et al. 2017; Kavanagh and McLoughlin 2009; Munday et al. 2003), but these responsibilities should be consistent with the nurse's training and clinical competence as well as reflecting up-to-date knowledge of psychiatric–mental health nursing (American Nurses Association 2014; Jewell et al. 2017; LoBiondo-Wood and Haber 2018).

Typically, the ECT nurse is a registered nurse whose responsibilities include overseeing the availability of ECT-related equipment and supplies, readying the treatment area for ECT, assessing and documenting the patient's status before each treatment, helping patients to and from the treatment area, applying stimulus and monitoring electrodes, monitoring vital signs, and assisting the ECT psychiatrist and anesthesia provider in duties such as coordinating treatment logistics. The role of the ECT nurse may additionally include conducting standardized clinical ratings, providing patient and family education, promoting positive ECT attitudes and education, assisting with informed consent procedures, educating clinical staff about ECT treatment, implementing continuous quality improvement programs, providing clinical or financial case management, and managing outpatient ECT programs. At the advanced practice level, nurses may be involved with other activities to the extent of their institutionally established privileges or clinical competencies. Such activities may include ordering and interpreting laboratory and diagnostic studies and procedures; prescribing, monitoring, managing, and evaluating psychopharmacological and related medications; and conducting clinical research (American Nurses Association 2014; Jewell et al. 2017; LoBiondo-Wood and Haber 2018).

3.1.2.4. Recovery Nurse

The recovery nurse, a registered nurse, provides care for patients in the recovery area (now often termed the *postanesthesia care unit* or PACU). The recovery nurse may be a critical care registered nurse (CCRN) or a psychiatric–mental health nurse with training in ACLS and principles of recovery care. The recovery nurse monitors patients when they are still under the effects of anesthesia and provides constant care for 30 minutes to a few hours immediately following the ECT treatment until the patient is stable enough either to be transported to their hospital room or discharged as an outpatient. The recovery nurse is also the primary patient advocate following treatment.

Patient monitoring is an essential role of the recovery nurse. On a regular basis, they monitor the patient's vital signs, pulse oximetry, and mental status. The nurse ensures that the patient is breathing properly, suctions the patient, administers oxygen when needed, and reacts rapidly to any significant changes in patient status by calling for assistance and beginning cardiopulmonary resuscitation if necessary. The nurse also observes patients to assess their comfort level, asks about a patient's level of pain, administers pain medications that have been prescribed, and notifies the ECT psychiatrist or anesthesia provider if more pain medication appears to be needed. Recovery nurses assess the patient's orientation, provide supportive care for postictal disorientation, and assess the patient's ability to safely ambulate after treatment. They make complete notes on the charts and communicate information in verbal or written form to the ECT team concerning time for reorientation, any postictal agitation, effectiveness of pain relief, and any other considerations important to patient safety and comfort. Recovery area staffing should be sufficient to ensure adequate performance of these duties at all times. Accordingly, if multiple patients will be in the recovery area simultaneously, it is preferable to have more than one recovery nurse available, with the nurse-to-patient ratio compatible with the institutional policy for recovery care staffing.

3.2. Administrative Staffing

Facilities offering ECT should designate a psychiatrist privileged in administering ECT to develop, update, and oversee adherence to policies and procedures for ECT, including those related to staffing, equipment, and supplies (see Chapter 4). This psychiatrist should work with the director of nursing and anesthesia providers to ensure that the staffing needs of the ECT unit are met using individuals who have appropriate credentials and training. This individual or another clinician with responsibility for quality improvement should implement an ECT quality improvement program, with correction of any observed deficiencies. Examples of quality improvement activities include monitoring clinical outcomes, tracking occurrences of major adverse effects, and ensuring adherence to policies and procedures.

Recommendations

3.1. The ECT Treatment Team

3.1.1. Members

1. The ECT treatment team typically consists of an ECT psychiatrist, an anesthesia provider, one or more recovery nurses, and one or more ECT treatment nurses.
2. All physicians involved in the delivery of ECT should be privileged in the performance of clinical ECT-related duties.
3. Nursing staff members involved in ECT should receive adequate training and assessment of competency before assuming ECT-related duties.
4. The ECT recovery nurse should be a registered nurse who is a CCRN or a psychiatric–mental health nurse with training in ACLS and principles of recovery care.
5. Psychiatric, anesthetic, and nursing trainees may assist in performing ECT-related duties only under direct supervision and only at a level commensurate with the level of relevant training they have received.

6. Staffing levels should be sufficient to ensure adequate performance of ECT-related duties at all times.

3.1.2. Responsibilities

3.1.2.1. ECT Psychiatrist

1. The ECT psychiatrist should maintain overall responsibility for the proper administration of ECT.
2. The ECT psychiatrist's responsibilities include

    a. Assessing the patient before the first treatment
    b. Confirming that the pre-ECT evaluation has been completed
    c. Determining that ECT is indicated before each treatment
    d. Verifying that the patient has provided informed consent for ECT
    e. Identifying changes in psychiatric symptoms or health status that would influence ECT-related decision-making
    f. Instituting appropriate modifications to the ECT course or technique as indicated
    g. Ensuring that the delivery of ECT is compatible with established policies and procedures
    h. Ensuring that evaluation and treatment results are properly documented

3.1.2.2. Anesthesiology Providers

1. The anesthesiologist or other anesthesia provider is responsible for the maintenance of an airway and oxygenation as well as oversight of the patient's recovery from anesthesia.
2. Additional responsibilities of the anesthesiologist or other anesthesia provider include

    a. Administering and making decisions about anesthetic, relaxant, and adjunctive agents
    b. Management of emergent adverse reactions in collaboration with the ECT psychiatrist
    c. Managing foreseeable medical emergencies, including provision of emergency medications, emergency management of cardiopulmonary function, and emergency life support until other appropriate personnel are available

3.1.2.3. ECT Treatment Nurse

1. The ECT treatment nurse is responsible for providing evidence-based nursing care compatible with their training and competencies.
2. Specific duties of the ECT treatment nurse vary but typically include
   a. Overseeing the availability of ECT-related equipment and supplies
   b. Readying the treatment area for ECT
   c. Assessing and documenting the patient's status before each treatment
   d. Helping patients to and from the treatment area ·
   e. Applying stimulus and monitoring electrodes
   f. Monitoring vital signs
   g. Assisting the ECT psychiatrist and anesthesia provider in duties such as coordinating treatment logistics
3. Additional duties of the ECT treatment nurse may include
   a. Conducting standardized clinical ratings
   b. Providing patient and family education
   c. Promoting positive ECT attitudes and education
   d. Assisting with informed consent procedures
   e. Training clinical staff in ECT treatment
   f. Implementing continuous quality improvement programs
   g. Providing clinical or financial case management
   h. Managing outpatient ECT programs

3.1.2.4. Recovery Nurse

1. The recovery nurse is responsible for providing constant care of the patient from the time following the ECT treatment until the patient is stable enough either to return to their hospital room or to be discharged as an outpatient.
2. Specific duties of the recovery nurse include
   a. Monitoring vital signs, pulse oximetry, and mental status during the acute postictal/postanesthetic period
   b. Documenting vital signs and other parameters that are important to patient safety and comfort
3. Additional duties of the recovery nurse include, when clinically indicated, the following:

a. Monitoring and adjusting the flow of intravenous fluids
b. Administering oxygen
c. Suctioning oropharyngeal secretions
d. Providing behavioral management of postictal disorientation and agitation
e. Assessing patient comfort and need for pain medications
f. Reacting rapidly to any significant changes in patient status by calling for assistance and beginning cardiopulmonary resuscitation if necessary

3.2. Administrative Staffing

1. Each facility offering ECT should designate a psychiatrist privileged in administering ECT to develop, update, and oversee adherence to policies and procedures regarding ECT, including those related to staffing, equipment, and supplies.
2. Each facility offering ECT should implement a quality improvement program.

CHAPTER 4

Location, Equipment, and Supplies

4.1. Characteristics of the Treatment Site

An optimal treatment site should include three separate functional areas for waiting, treatment, and recovery and ideally should not be used concomitantly for purposes other than electroconvulsive therapy (ECT) administration. Logistically, the various areas should be as close to each other as possible. However, they should be sufficiently distinct as to isolate patients in one area from patients, caregivers, and staff in other areas. The treatment site will ideally be close to inpatient psychiatric units. It should also be readily accessible to the resources needed to treat medical emergencies, including emergency equipment, supplies, and personnel. For this reason, some facilities locate the treatment site in, or adjacent to, intensive care units or outpatient or inpatient surgical areas.

Facilities administering outpatient ECT should also consider the ease of treatment site access to outpatients and availability of space for conducting pretreatment assessments. It is also helpful to have an area (or areas) where patients and those accompanying the patient can stay before and after the treatment session. It is advantageous for this area to be near the treatment area so that significant other(s) can remain with the patient before ECT and so that the treatment team can address questions or concerns.

The treatment environment should be comfortable for patients and their families. Facilities should also ensure that space, ventilation, and lighting are sufficient to conduct treatments and recovery in a safe, unencumbered, and confidential fashion. Adequate space should also be present for storing ECT-related records, equipment, and supplies.

4.2. Equipment

4.2.1. ECT Devices

In the United States, the U.S. Food and Drug Administration (FDA) has approved ECT devices for use in treating "catatonia or a severe MDE [major depressive episode] associated with major depressive disorder [MDD] or BPD [bipolar disorder] in patients aged 13 years and older who are treatment-resistant or who require a rapid response due to the severity of their psychiatric or medical condition" (U.S. Food and Drug Administration 2018b). However, this FDA classification applies to the marketing of the machines by manufacturers and does not limit the use of the machines by psychiatrists providing care within a doctor-patient relationship, including off-label use. For further discussion of the FDA indications and their relevance to the informed consent process, see Chapters 2 and 10, respectively.

An ECT treatment device must be present in the ECT treatment area. Access to a backup ECT device is useful in the event of equipment malfunction. Additional stimulus and physiological monitoring cables are also important to have so that worn cables or connectors can be replaced immediately.

Prior to the first use of an ECT device, the ECT psychiatrist should be familiar with the principles that underlie operation of the instrumentation, including electrical safety considerations, initial testing requirements, and preventive maintenance instructions. It is also important that biomedical engineering or other qualified staff ascertain and document that the stimulus output characteristics and all other controls, parameters, and features are functioning properly and are appropriately calibrated within the tolerance levels (e.g., 10%) specified by the manufacturer in the device manual. Shipping and handling of the device can result in malfunction or miscalibration, and users should not rely solely on the calibration performed by the manufacturer. As with other medical devices, a regular schedule of retesting or recalibration by biomedical engineering or otherwise qualified staff should be implemented, particularly in terms of electrical safety considerations. The intervals between retesting should meet those stipulated in device manuals or local facility requirements.

It is relatively rare to observe drift in stimulus output characteristics with standard use of an ECT device. However, if device malfunction is suspected or unusual conditions occur that may affect the integrity of the device (e.g., electrical malfunction, fire, spillage of liquid, physical damage), immediate retesting should be done before clinical use.

Electrical safety features are incorporated into available ECT devices. For example, the pretreatment static impedance test feature shows whether stimulus cables are properly connected to the ECT device and that contact with the scalp is adequate prior to stimulus delivery. Devices also emit a distinct warning signal to alert all members of the treatment team that a stimulus is being delivered. If malfunction or other untoward events become apparent while the stimulus is being delivered, releasing the treatment button will abort the stimulus delivery. If an excessively low or high load impedance is detected by the device, the stimulus delivery is aborted automatically.

Several other steps must be taken to ensure that electrical safety standards are met when administering ECT (National Fire Protection Association 2020, 2021). The ECT device comes equipped with a three-prong grounded electrical plug that must be connected to a three-prong grounded outlet approved for medical devices. ECT devices should not be plugged into a two-prong outlet or adapter because this will defeat the grounding. In addition, individuals other than the patient should not be in contact with the metal portion of the ECT electrodes during the passage of the stimulus.

Patient contact with other devices should also be avoided, except when required for physiological monitoring. Unless battery operated, any electrical device in contact with the patient should be connected to the same electrical circuit as the ECT device. In the event of questions about the configuration and properties of electrical outlets in the ECT suite, consultation with hospital engineering personnel is recommended.

4.2.2. Additional Equipment

Both the treatment and recovery areas should contain equipment to monitor patient vital signs and provide initial management of medical emergencies. In addition to a stethoscope, this equipment should include either a manual sphygmomanometer or an automatic device for blood pressure measurement. Both areas should also contain devices for electrocardiography (ECG) and oxygen saturation of hemoglobin (pulse oximetry) monitoring as well as an oxygen delivery system capable of providing intermittent positive-pressure oxygen and suction capability. Continuous monitoring for the presence of expired carbon dioxide is also necessary while the patient is anesthetized (American Society of Anesthesiologists 2020b). To maintain an adequate airway, equipment in the treatment area should include an intubation set and equipment for managing patients with difficult airways (Apfelbaum et al. 2013; Cabrera et al. 2020; Link et al. 2015). The oxygen delivery system should be capable of providing intermittent positive-pressure oxygen by endotracheal tube as well as by mask. A defibrillator should be readily accessible. Treatment area beds or stretchers should have firm mattresses and side rails and be able to elevate both the head and the feet easily.

To determine the extent of muscle blockade prior to stimulus delivery, a reflex hammer should be present. In this regard, a peripheral nerve stimulator is also helpful, especially when nondepolarizing muscle relaxants are used or the extent of muscle relaxation is uncertain, as well as in patients who are at heightened risk for musculoskeletal complications (see Chapter 12). In determining seizure adequacy and detecting prolonged seizures, ictal electroencephalography (EEG) is essential (see Chapter 15). The treatment area should also have a sphygmomanometer or other means of monitoring ictal motor duration (see Chapter 15).

4.3. Medications

Essential medications for administering ECT include anesthetic and muscle-relaxing agents (see Chapter 12). The primary anesthetic agent is generally methohexital or propofol, with succinylcholine used as a muscle relaxant. It is often useful to have alternative anesthetic agents available (e.g., etomidate, ketamine). Specific clinical situations may require alternative or supplementary nondepolarizing muscle-relaxing agents. Typically, rocuronium is used and requires reversal with sugammadex (see Chapter 12). To potentiate ictal responses, particularly in patients who are treated with a benzodiazepine, some practitioners coadminister flumazenil with ECT (see Chapters 13 and 21). To terminate prolonged or spontaneous seizures (see Chapter 21) and/or treat postictal delirium (see Chapter 19), agents such as diazepam, midazolam, or lorazepam should be on hand. Alternatively, the primary anesthetic can be used. Although a benzodiazepine (specifically, intramuscular midazolam, intravenous lorazepam, or intravenous diazepam) is the initial therapy of choice for status epilepticus, a secondary treatment should also be available for use (e.g., fosphenytoin or, alternatively, phenytoin; valproic acid; levetiracetam) (Glauser et al. 2016).

To minimize the cardiovascular impact of ECT, several other medications are commonly given and should be available at the treatment site. For example, anticholinergic agents (e.g., atropine, glycopyrrolate) are used to diminish secretions or decrease the risk of vagally mediated bradyarrhythmias (see Chapters 12 and 19). Several agents, including adrenergic blockers and vasodilators, have been of value in minimizing the sympathetic effects of ECT. Medications for treating cardiovascular emergencies such as arrhythmias, uncontrolled hypertension, hypotension, or cardiac arrest should also be available. These drugs include pressor agents, antiarrhythmic agents, and specific agents used in advanced cardiovascular life support protocols (Link et al. 2015; Panchal et al. 2018). For initial management of severe bronchospasm or anaphylactic shock, other medications that must be available immediately include epinephrine and β-adrenergic agonists (e.g., albuterol) for administration via nebulizer (Lieberman et al. 2015).

Nausea, headache, and muscle soreness may occur after ECT (see Chapter 19). To manage these side effects, antinausea agents and non-narcotic analgesics should be present at the treatment site. Less often, a narcotic analgesic (e.g., codeine) may be indicated. Nonparticulate antacids or selective histamine type 2 blocking agents are sometimes given before ECT to decrease gastric acidity and minimize risk if aspiration were to occur (see Chapter 9, sections 9.2.7 and 9.4).

Medications should be stored securely; controlled drugs must also be inventoried and verified according to hospital policy and other applicable regulations.

4.4. Supplies

The treatment site should have the supplies needed to induce anesthesia, provide ventilation, monitor physiological functions (including seizure activity), perform resuscitation, and maintain any indicated infection control precautions. Sufficient quantities of supplies should be present to handle all anticipated needs.

Whenever possible, items that come into contact with body fluids should be disposable. Items such as bite blocks may be designated for use by an individual patient and stored in a labeled plastic bag after sterilization. All procedures for sterilization and disinfection of reusable items should conform to relevant standards (Centers for Disease Control and Prevention 2022).

Recommendations

4.1. Characteristics of the Treatment Site

1. The treatment site should consist of a well-lit and well-ventilated treatment area and separate recovery and waiting areas.
2. The treatment site should have ready access to the resources needed to treat medical emergencies, including emergency equipment, supplies, and personnel.
3. Adequate space should be available within the treatment site for ECT-related equipment, supplies, and records.
4. It is desirable for waiting patients to be isolated from auditory and visual contact with treatment and recovery areas.
5. Facilities administering outpatient ECT should consider the ease of treatment site access; provide space for conducting pretreatment assessments; and have an area (or areas), preferably near the treatment area, where the patient and persons accompanying the patient can stay before and after the treatment session.

4.2. Equipment

4.2.1. ECT Devices

1. An ECT treatment device, which includes EEG monitoring capability, must be present in the ECT treatment area.
2. Access to a backup ECT device and availability of additional stimulus and physiological monitoring cables are useful in the event of equipment malfunction.
3. Device manufacturers should provide a description of testing procedures and suggested preventive maintenance instructions.
4. Before initial use of a new device, qualified personnel should perform and document electrical safety testing procedures, including calibration of the device output characteristics; operation of controls, parameters, and features; and adherence to other pertinent standards or local requirements regarding medical devices involving patient contact.
5. Facilities should establish a policy regarding the frequency with which ECT devices undergo assessment of proper function and calibration, with retesting being suggested at least annually.

6. If device malfunction is suspected, the device should be retested or removed for servicing and any worn cables and connectors should be replaced.
7. ECT devices should be connected to the same electrical supply circuit as all other electrical devices in contact with the patient, including monitoring equipment.
8. Electrical grounding of devices should not be bypassed (e.g., by using a two-prong outlet or adapter).
9. Individuals other than the patient should not be in contact with the metal portion of the ECT electrodes during the passage of the stimulus.
10. In the event of questions about the configuration and properties of electrical outlets in the ECT suite, consultation with hospital engineering personnel is recommended.

4.2.2. Additional Equipment

1. Equipment should be available in both the treatment and recovery areas to provide suction; deliver intermittent positive-pressure oxygen; and monitor vital signs, cardiac rhythm, and hemoglobin oxygen saturation.
2. Additional equipment should be present in the treatment area for intubation, seizure induction, physiological response monitoring, monitoring for the presence of expired carbon dioxide, and initial management of medical emergencies.
3. The recovery area should contain ECG monitoring and pulse oximetry devices.
4. The treatment area should contain the following equipment:

   a. Stretcher or bed with a firm mattress, side rails, and the capacity to elevate both the head and the feet
   b. Automatic blood pressure monitoring device or manual sphygmomanometer
   c. Stethoscope
   d. ECG monitoring equipment
   e. Sphygmomanometer cuff or other method to monitor ictal motor duration
   f. Pulse oximeter
   g. Oxygen delivery system capable of providing intermittent positive-pressure oxygen by mask or endotracheal tube

h. System for monitoring for the presence of expired carbon dioxide while the patient is anesthetized
i. Suction apparatus
j. Intubation set, including laryngoscopes with several blades (Miller 3 and 4, Macintosh 3 and 4), as well as equipment for managing difficult airways
k. Reflex hammer
l. A defibrillator should be readily accessible
m. Access to a backup ECT treatment device and additional stimulus and physiological monitoring cables is encouraged
n. Availability of a peripheral nerve stimulator is encouraged

4.3. Medications

1. The treatment site should contain pharmacological agents that are sufficient to induce anesthesia and muscle relaxation; modulate the parasympathetic and sympathetic effects of the ECT seizure; and provide first-line management of uncontrolled hypertension, hypotension, cardiac arrhythmias, cardiopulmonary arrest, anaphylaxis, prolonged seizures, or status epilepticus.
2. Specific medications that should be present include

   a. A primary anesthetic agent (such as methohexital sodium)
   b. A primary muscle relaxant (such as succinylcholine)
   c. An anticholinergic agent (such as glycopyrrolate and/or atropine sulfate)
   d. Agents for first-line management of arrhythmias, hypertension and hypotension, and cardiac arrest, such as

      i. β-Adrenergic blocking agents such as labetalol and esmolol
      ii. α-Adrenergic blocking agents such as prazosin and clonidine
      iii. Pressor agents such as epinephrine, dopamine, norepinephrine, and phenylephrine
      iv. Vasodilators such as hydralazine, phentolamine, and nitroglycerin (tablets, paste, and/or sublingual spray)
      v. Antiarrhythmics such as bretylium, digoxin, lidocaine, verapamil, and procainamide
      vi. Other agents for cardiopulmonary resuscitation

   e. Agents for the initial management of severe bronchospasm or anaphylactic shock, such as epinephrine and β-adrenergic agonists (e.g., albuterol) for administration via nebulizer

    f. Other agents for managing status epilepticus, such as lorazepam or diazepam, fosphenytoin or phenytoin, valproic acid, and levetiracetam

    g. Antinausea agents such as ondansetron

    h. Nonnarcotic analgesics such as ibuprofen, ketorolac, and acetaminophen

    i. Suggested additional medications include

        i. Alternative anesthetic agents such as etomidate, ketamine, or propofol

        ii. Alternative or supplementary nondepolarizing relaxant agents such as rocuronium

        iii. Reversal agents for nondepolarizing relaxant agents such as sugammadex

        iv. A nonparticulate antacid such as sodium citrate

        v. Narcotic analgesics such as codeine

        vi. Narcotic antagonists such as naloxone

        vii. Miscellaneous agents such as the benzodiazepine antagonist flumazenil

3. Medications should be stored securely in a room with restricted access.
4. Controlled drugs need to be inventoried and verified according to hospital policy and other applicable regulations.

4.4. Supplies

1. The treatment site should have sufficient quantities of supplies to induce anesthesia, provide ventilation, monitor physiological functions (including seizure activity), perform resuscitation, and maintain any indicated infection control precautions.
2. Necessary supplies include

    a. Bite blocks (mouth guards)

    b. Intravenous catheters in assorted sizes

    c. Infusion sets

    d. Intravenous fluids

    e. Masks for oxygen delivery

    f. Oropharyngeal and nasopharyngeal airways

    g. Endotracheal tubes

    h. Suction catheters

    i. Syringes and syringe needles in assorted sizes

    j. Electrode gel or paste

    k. Monitoring electrode pads and leads

    l. Stimulus and monitoring cables for ECT device

    m. Recording paper for monitoring use

    n. Alcohol pads

    o. Material to prepare stimulus and monitoring electrode sites

    p. Gauze pads in assorted sizes

    q. Tape in assorted sizes

    r. Disposable gloves

    s. Containers for disposal of sharps and clinical waste

3. It is also useful to have access to heparin locks and flush solution.

4. Gowns, masks, and face shields for universal precautions and infection control for known or possible pathogens should be readily available.

5. Whenever possible, items that come into contact with body fluids should be disposable. Bite blocks and face masks may be designated for use by an individual patient and stored in a labeled plastic bag after cleaning.

6. All procedures for sterilization and disinfection of reusable items should conform to relevant standards.

CHAPTER 5

Documentation

5.1. Facility Responsibilities

The medical record represents the primary source of clinical information accumulated by the clinical team working with the patient. As such, the facility's medical director should maintain overall responsibility for ensuring the adequacy of documentation and the integrity of the medical record. Information contained in the medical record facilitates future evaluation and treatment decisions, fosters communication among members of the clinical team, and contributes to the provision of safe, effective, and efficient care. In this regard, notes in the clinical record should be concise and to the point, with detail limited to essential material. The patient's medical record also serves as a legal document that provides details of what did or did not take place during their contact with the health care facility. Finally, documentation assists with payment-related, utilization review, and quality improvement activities.

The medical record may be maintained in paper, electronic, or hybrid formats. Typically, with a hybrid format, information that is recorded on paper will be scanned and made accessible from within the electronic record. Record storage, both paper and electronic, should be secure, with retention of records for at least as long as mandated by applicable state and national regulations, as well as local policy. It is understood that patients, their authorized representatives, or other treating clinicians should have access to medical record data, when requested, as specified in federal, state, or local release-of-information policies and regulations (American Medical Association 2020; U.S. Centers for Medicare and Medicaid Services 2020; U.S. Department of Health and Human Services 2013).

5.2. Prior to an Acute ECT Course

An acute course of electroconvulsive therapy (ECT) should not begin until a pre-ECT evaluation has taken place, with relevant risks and benefits assessed, informed consent obtained, and a treatment plan described. Documentation of this process helps ensure that it has been completed appropriately and that potential problems have been considered. If the patient has undergone laboratory testing, imaging studies, specialty consultation, or other evaluative procedures as part of the pre-ECT evaluation, these should be noted, along with any alterations in ongoing medications or recommended modifications to ECT technique that are indicated on the basis of the pre-ECT evaluation (see Chapter 8). Although the attending physician or ECT psychiatrist may record such information, it is the responsibility of the ECT psychiatrist to make sure that necessary documentation is in order prior to treatment with ECT. A checklist or summary format can be helpful.

More specifically, it is important to address the rationale for the ECT referral and to delineate relevant risk-benefit considerations for each patient. Because determination of treatment endpoint will be influenced by baseline symptoms, major target symptoms and their severity should be recorded before treatment begins. Similarly, the ongoing assessment of adverse effects requires a baseline determination of orientation and memory function (see Chapter 20).

Before ECT, in addition to a signed formal consent document, the clinical record should contain a summary of major consent-related discussions, including discussion of factors having a major impact on risk-benefit considerations (see Chapter 10). Such a summary should either note that the patient has provided consent or describe the consent procedure used when a patient who is referred for ECT lacks capacity to provide consent.

5.3. Prior to a Maintenance Series of ECT

For maintenance ECT, documentation should include the rationale for initiating such treatment as well as the relevant aspects of the informed consent process (see Chapter 10). As with an acute course of ECT, it is important to document whether specific target symptoms and adverse effects are absent or present and, if present, to document their severity and plans to address them.

5.4. During an Acute ECT Course or Maintenance Series of ECT

5.4.1. Between ECT Treatment Sessions

For acute ECT treatments, therapeutic outcome and the presence or absence of cognitive effects should be documented regularly (see Chapters 17 and 20). Whether cognitive function is assessed formally or informally, the patient's perception of cognitive changes should be ascertained and documented (see Chapter 20). For maintenance ECT, such notes can occur at less frequent intervals.

Each facility should have a policy, in accordance with regulatory and accreditation requirements, regarding the number of ECT sessions that may be given in a series of acute or maintenance ECT treatments before reassessing and documenting the need to continue the treatment course (see Chapter 18). When an ECT course is extended past the number noted in the informed consent, a new consent should be obtained and the rationale for additional ECT should be noted in the clinical record.

5.4.2. At the Time of Each ECT Treatment Session

At the time of each ECT treatment session, the ECT team should document any changes in the patient's status, including changes in medical conditions or medications that have occurred since the last treatment. The preprocedural "time-out" (see Chapter 11), and its associated documentation, includes assuring correct identification of the patient, verifying that ECT is the procedure to be performed, verifying existence of informed consent, confirming treatment number and type (acute or maintenance), and verifying stimulus electrode placement. In addition, the essential information about the ECT procedure should be documented at the time of each treatment and include the date and time of the procedure, the name of the ECT psychiatrist, the primary indication for treatment, the ECT device used, the number of stimulations given during the session, the electrical parameters for each stimulation (i.e., pulse width, pulse frequency, pulse amplitude, stimulus duration), the stimulus electrode placement, the seizure duration (and other indices of seizure adequacy, if monitored), all medications (including dosages) given in the treatment and recovery area, and the patient's vital signs (e.g., blood pressure and pulse). Such information helps the treatment team administer subsequent treatments safely and effectively, assists future caregivers in determining treatment parameters, and is useful for ongoing quality improvement. In many facilities, members of the ECT treatment team rotate on a weekly or even daily basis, rendering such data particularly important. A dedicated form or electronic template can be helpful in facilitating consistent documentation. Although recent suggestions to documentation formats have been made to foster multisite data collection (Zandi et al. 2022), these have not yet been adopted into widespread use.

As with any procedure requiring general anesthesia, the anesthesia provider should include a brief note describing the patient's condition during the perioperative period. Similarly, recovery area staff should document vital signs and orientation while the patient is under their care. Any significant adverse effects that occur during or soon after the ECT should be documented in the patient's medical record and should include the steps taken to manage the event, including administration of medications, additional procedures, specialist consultations, and recommendations for future management.

5.5. After Completion of an Acute ECT Course or Maintenance ECT Series

Just as it is important to document the rationale for beginning ECT, it is also helpful to provide a basis for the decision to end an acute course of ECT or series of maintenance treatments. Typical reasons for stopping an acute course of ECT include achievement of maximal clinical benefit, lack of therapeutic response to an adequate trial of treatments, adverse effects (including their type and severity), and patient preference. As with any patient who receives acute treatment, a plan for maintenance treatment should be documented after an acute ECT course because the risk of relapse is high (see Chapter 23). If adverse effects are present at the time of completion of the ECT course, these effects should be noted, along with the follow-up plan. For maintenance ECT, documentation of the rationale for terminating the series should be provided, as well as the plan for future treatment and monitoring of side effects, if applicable.

Recommendations

5.1. Facility Responsibilities

It is the responsibility of the facility's medical director to ensure the integrity of the medical record and adequate documentation regarding ECT.

5.2. Prior to an Acute ECT Course

The ECT psychiatrist should confirm that the following documentation is included in the patient's clinical record:

a. Reasons for ECT referral, including an assessment of anticipated benefits and risks
b. Major target symptoms and their severity
c. Mental status examination, including baseline information pertinent to later determinations of therapeutic outcome, orientation, and memory function
d. Signed consent document
e. Summary of major consent-related discussions, including factors having a major impact on risk-benefit considerations and the process used if consent was provided by someone other than the patient
f. Pertinent laboratory results, imaging studies, consultation reports, or other evaluations, as indicated
g. Discussion of any substantial alterations planned in ongoing medications or recommended ECT technique

5.3. Prior to a Maintenance Series of ECT

Before beginning a maintenance series of ECT, the ECT psychiatrist should confirm that the patient's clinical record includes documentation of the following material:

a. Rationale for maintenance ECT
b. Signed consent document
c. Summary of major consent-related discussions, including factors having a major impact on risk-benefit considerations and the process used if consent was provided by someone other than the patient

5.4. During an Acute ECT Course or Maintenance Series of ECT

5.4.1. Between ECT Treatment Sessions

1. Documentation by the attending physician or designee should be regularly entered in the patient's clinical record and should contain information about therapeutic outcomes and the presence or absence of adverse cognitive effects, including the patient's perception of cognitive changes.

2. Documented justification should be provided before exceeding a specified maximum number of treatments (set by each facility) in an acute or maintenance ECT course.

5.4.2. At the Time of Each ECT Treatment Session

1. Any changes in the patient's status, including changes in medical conditions or medications that have occurred since the last treatment, should be documented.
2. The pre-procedural time-out, and its associated documentation, includes assuring correct identification of the patient, verifying that ECT is the procedure to be performed, verifying existence of informed consent, confirming treatment number and type (acute or maintenance), and verifying stimulus electrode placement.
3. For each treatment session, at least the following information should be documented in the patient's clinical record:
   a. Date and time of the procedure
   b. Name of the ECT psychiatrist
   c. The primary indication for treatment
   d. Vital signs at baseline and during treatment and recovery periods
   e. Medication, including dosage, given before entering the treatment room, during the treatment, and while in the recovery area
   f. Number of stimulations given during the session
   g. Stimulus electrode placement for each stimulus
   h. Stimulus parameter settings for each stimulus (i.e., pulse width, pulse frequency, pulse amplitude, stimulus duration)
   i. Seizure duration for each stimulus, noting whether by motor or electroencephalographic criteria, as well as other indicators of seizure adequacy
   j. Documentation from the anesthesia provider describing the patient's condition while in treatment and recovery areas
   k. Documentation from the ECT psychiatrist or anesthesia provider addressing any significant complications, adverse effects, or alterations in risk factors as well as any steps taken to manage the event, including administration of medications, additional procedures, specialist consultations, and recommendations for future management

5.5. After Completion of an Acute ECT Course or Maintenance ECT Series

The attending physician or designee should enter the following information into the clinical record:

a. Summary of overall therapeutic outcome and adverse effects experienced as a result of the acute ECT course or maintenance ECT series

b. The rationale for the decision to stop ECT treatment

c. The plan for post-ECT clinical management, including maintenance treatment, approaches to address any remaining acute symptoms, and plans for follow-up evaluation or treatment of any adverse effects

CHAPTER 6

Education and Training

6.1. General Considerations

Since the 1930s, electroconvulsive therapy (ECT) has evolved into a highly technical and complex treatment (American Psychiatric Association 2001; Ferrier and Waite 2019; Milev et al. 2016; Weiss et al. 2019). Major technical advances directed toward maximizing the efficacy of ECT and minimizing its risks have occurred in instrumentation, choice of stimulus waveform, stimulus dosing, stimulus electrode placement, pharmacological modification of the treatment, and physiological monitoring.

Surveys of psychiatry residents after training in ECT have supported the value of formal ECT education (Blaj et al. 2007; Raysin et al. 2018). Nonetheless, ECT training in residency programs in the United States (Dinwiddie and Spitz 2010) and other countries (Patry et al. 2013; Sienaert et al. 2006; Yuzda et al. 2002) shows considerable variation, and surveys of ECT practice outside the United States have emphasized problems with inadequate training (Patry et al. 2013; Sienaert et al. 2006; Yuzda et al. 2002). Consequently, enhancements in education are needed to ensure that future generations of practitioners are able to deliver ECT in a safe and effective fashion (Blaj et al. 2007; Fink and Kellner 2007; Kellner 2001; Sienaert et al. 2006; Weiss et al. 2019).

The practice of ECT is multidisciplinary and involves professionals trained in psychiatry, anesthesiology, and psychiatric–mental health nursing. In addition, physicians other than psychiatrists and ECT practitioners are often asked to consult on patients being evaluated for ECT or to care for patients who are either receiving or have recently received this treatment. Reports have also indicated the need for increased exposure to ECT in anesthesiology (Haddad and Benbow 1993), nursing (Arkan and Üstün 2008; Munday et al. 2003), and social work (Katz 1992) training programs.

6.2. Medical School Training

Didactic coverage of ECT should be included as part of psychiatric education in medical school (Andrews and Hasking 2004; Chakrabarti et al. 2003; Ithman et al. 2018; Warnell et al. 2005). Medical students should also be encouraged to observe ECT practice either directly or on video (Li et al. 2013). Didactic instruction should provide an overview of the history (including social contexts), indications, risks, mechanisms of action, and technique of ECT.

6.3. Psychiatry Residency Programs

6.3.1. General Issues

As the leader of the treatment team, a psychiatrist must have comprehensive knowledge of ECT-related topics, whether administering ECT or not. The recommendations for didactic and practical training in ECT that are described in subsequent sections constitute minimal requirements, and residency programs are encouraged to exceed these levels. Clinical conferences, ECT rounds, and elective opportunities for advanced training in ECT represent particularly useful ways of improving the overall learning experience.

It is understood that some residency training programs may not have sufficient resources or sufficiently qualified faculty to meet all of these requirements, particularly in those settings in which the practice of ECT is minimal or absent. Residents in such programs should be told explicitly that supplementation of their training experience will be required before they can administer ECT on an unsupervised basis. Nevertheless, attempts should be made to cover as much of the curriculum as possible, making use of assigned readings, videorecorded material, simulations, and outside speakers. Efforts should also be made to ensure the presence of direct supervision in ECT by the most highly qualified individuals available, even if such personnel must be secured from outside the department. Alternatively, the department may send residents for practical training in other educational institutions that provide such opportunities.

6.3.2. Didactic Instruction

The type and amount of didactic instruction on ECT provided in psychiatry residency training programs varies considerably. Whereas some programs provide formal lecture or seminar presentations, others incorporate ECT-related material into curricula for other aspects of psychiatry, such as psychopharmacology or mood disorders.

The Accreditation Council for Graduate Medical Education in concert with the American Board of Psychiatry and Neurology have proposed that by the end of training, residents will understand the indications for and uses of ECT and neuromodulation therapies (Accreditation Council for Graduate Medical Education 2022). Expert consensus has envisioned alternative, expanded, and more detailed training objectives for "foundational, competent, and proficient" competency levels within residency (Al-Qadhi et al. 2020; Brown 2019).

Ideally, the didactic curriculum required for residents in a program should cover all major aspects of the ECT procedure, including mechanisms of action, selection of patients (including consideration of special populations), selection of the setting for treatment, risks and adverse effects, pre-ECT evaluation, informed consent, ECT device features, methods of administration and monitoring, evaluation of therapeutic outcome, management of patients after completion of an ECT course (including the potential role of maintenance treatment with pharmacotherapy and/or ECT), documentation, risk management, and legal considerations. In areas marked by controversy, alternative viewpoints should be presented. The amount of time necessary to cover this material will vary, but a minimum of 4 hours is probably necessary to give a good overview. The ECT didactic curriculum should also include sufficient opportunities for interchange between faculty and trainees so that questions can be answered and views clarified.

Programs that are unable to provide 4 hours of ECT didactics should take explicit steps to ensure that remaining topics are covered within the context of practical experience in ECT. Videos are often a useful supplement to didactic instruction (Kellner 2001). The teaching program can also be supported by simulation exercises that are part of the educational models (Raysin et al. 2018).

6.3.3. Practical Training

With a highly technical and sophisticated medical procedure such as ECT, didactic teaching is clearly insufficient to achieve requisite expertise and must be supplemented by an intensive, well-supervised practical training experience. The amount of practical experience in ECT necessary to allow development of adequate skills will vary from resident to resident as well as from program to program. Wide variations in trainee confidence in administering ECT can be addressed by a standardized training program (Scott and Semple 2018). At a minimum, a resident should participate in the administration of at least 10 ECT treatments involving at least three distinct patients with direct supervision by a psychiatrist privileged in ECT. These minimal requirements represent a trade-off between what is optimally desirable and what is feasible in many training programs.

In addition to the actual administration of ECT, residents should gain experience in the clinical management of patients undergoing ECT. This experience should include the pre-ECT evaluation; informed consent; choice of type, number, and frequency of ECT treatments; and post-ECT management. At a minimum, each resident should actively participate in the care of at least three patients being treated with ECT. Practical experience in evaluation and case management of ECT patients is particularly important because the number of psychiatrists providing such care is much larger than the number who directly administer ECT.

Simulation technology, including team-based simulations, provides wider opportunities for practical training, particularly for programs outside major centers of ECT practice. In addition, there is preliminary evidence that use of simulations further enhances actual supervised performance of ECT (Rabheru et al. 2013; Raysin et al. 2018). The use of teaching materials such as assigned readings can also augment the educational impact of practical training in ECT and should be encouraged.

6.3.4. Advanced Training in ECT

Residency programs should offer advanced elective training opportunities directed toward providing the knowledge base and experience necessary for eventual privileging in ECT (see Chapter 7). Such training should include both didactic and practical components. Residents who wish to obtain a more intensive learning experience in ECT should be encouraged to pursue these advanced electives in ECT as well as membership at the training level in professional organizations such as the International Society for ECT and Neurostimulation.

6.3.5. Program Responsibilities in Evaluation of ECT-Related Curriculum and Resident Performance

Department chairs, residency training directors, and departmental faculty should recognize that all psychiatric residents should meet certain minimal ECT training requirements for clinical competency in psychiatry. To accomplish ECT training goals for psychiatric residency programs, it is important that department chairs and residency training directors set a priority on developing adequate curricula for education and training in ECT, including designating qualified faculty and allocating adequate time in the curriculum. Department chairs and psychiatric residency training directors and committees should also provide specific guidance for psychiatry residents' training in ECT, in collaboration with the individual(s) or committee overseeing the practice of ECT within the department. These individuals should also monitor and correct any identified deficiencies in ECT-related components of the curriculum by evaluating the performance of residents and faculty.

Because residents may eventually be applying for privileges to perform ECT (see Chapter 7), residency programs should keep records to establish adherence to the training recommendations of sections 6.3.2 and 6.3.3. Such records should document the specific ECT-related educational and training experiences offered by the program as well as resident performance in these curricular components. Taking appropriate measures to ensure confidentiality, psychiatry residents should be encouraged to keep records of both the number of ECT treatments in which they participated and the number of patients who received ECT while under their care. Tracking such information is useful in helping to satisfy ECT privileging requirements and is in line with training and documentation policies already implemented for some medical and surgical procedures.

6.4. Geriatric Psychiatry Training Programs

Because of the important role of ECT in the treatment of geriatric patients, formal training in ECT should be part of geriatric psychiatry training programs. Minimum didactic requirements should include all topics noted in section 6.3.2 for psychiatry residents as well as specific coverage of the use of ECT in geriatric patients (see Chapter 9). Likewise, practical training in ECT should include clinical exposure to the use of ECT with geriatric patients. Programs are encouraged to devote a sufficient portion of the geriatric psychiatry training experience to ECT to ensure that graduates are clinically competent in this area.

6.5. Anesthesiology Residency Programs

Anesthesiology residency programs should incorporate specific training in ECT into their curricula. It should not be assumed that general education and training in anesthesia will suffice (Haddad and Benbow 1993). It is particularly important that differences between ECT anesthesia practices and standard anesthesia practices be covered in depth. The physiological effects associated with seizure induction, for example, represent a routine part of the ECT procedure and not a cause for alarm or emergency corrective action. In addition, because of concerns about anticonvulsant effects, the dosages of anesthetic agents used for ECT are generally lower than those used with other procedures. Compared with other procedures that require general anesthesia, the depth of anesthesia is typically lighter with ECT. Finally, because ECT treatments are delivered as a series, practitioners should not approach each successive treatment as a totally new anesthetic situation.

Training in ECT for anesthesiology residents should be provided by qualified individuals and should include faculty involved in the ECT training of psychiatric residents. In terms of the didactic exposure, a concise but comprehensive perspective should be provided, including a discussion of ECT's role in contemporary psychiatric practice. Again, areas in which ECT anesthesia differs from standard anesthetic practice should be given particular attention (e.g., anesthetic choice, dosing, impact of seizure induction on physiological parameters). Other areas of specific anesthetic interest that should be covered in depth include indications for and potential risks of ECT, elements of the pre-ECT evaluation, provision of oxygenation, ventilation requirements (including the effects of hyperventilation on the ictal response), use of physiological monitoring during and following ECT, effects of the postictal state on recovery from anesthesia, and electrical safety considerations. It is also essential to provide information on the type, dosing, and pertinent interactions of medications commonly used before, during, and immediately after the ECT procedure. Major adverse effects that may occur in the treatment and recovery areas should also be enumerated and their management discussed.

Optimally, practical training in ECT is also suggested. Just as it is important that psychiatric residents receive adequate supervision in ECT, anesthesiology residents should also be supervised by qualified individuals during their practical training experience. As with the training of psychiatric residents, simulation technology, including team-based simulations, provides wider opportunities for practical training, particularly for programs outside major centers of ECT practice.

6.6. Nursing Schools

Because psychiatric–mental health nursing personnel are important members of the ECT treatment team, education in ECT should be provided as part of the nursing school experience (Arkan and Üstün 2008; Munday et al. 2003). In terms of didactic instruction, a general overview of ECT should be provided, supplemented by an in-depth focus on areas in which nursing personnel are likely to play a major role (see Chapter 3). These include the history of ECT; indications for and potential risks of ECT; pre-ECT evaluation; informed consent procedures; ECT technique; nursing participation in ECT treatment; and postanesthesia recovery, including management of emergencies. As with all aspects of ECT training, instruction should be provided by qualified individuals involved in actual clinical administration of ECT. Opportunity for observation of ECT administration is useful, either directly or through use of videorecorded material. Postgraduate training for psychiatric–mental health nursing administrators should include additional instruction and training in ECT. For nurse anesthesia programs, the curricula should incorporate the material for anesthesiology residents as described in section 6.5.

6.7. Board Examinations

As one means of helping to ensure adequate training, board examinations, regardless of professional discipline, can require exposure to education or training in ECT. At a minimum, specialty boards in psychiatry, geriatric psychiatry, and anesthesiology, as well as credentialing in psychiatric–mental health nursing, should incorporate a representative number of questions on ECT into their examinations. For medical students, the National Board of Medical Examiners should include a reasonable coverage of ECT-related topics in their examinations.

6.8. Continuing Education Programs

Continuing education opportunities allow practitioners to keep their knowledge and skills up to date and provide a means to help those with educational and training deficiencies gain clinical privileges for ECT

(Duffy and Conradt 1989; Fink 1987; Gass 1998; Jacobsma 1991; Katz 1992). Participation in such programs is particularly important for psychiatrists but can also be useful for anesthesiologists and nurses. Attendance at continuing education programs can and should be an important factor in maintaining ECT privileges (see Chapter 7).

Although a number of excellent continuing education programs have been offered, there is clearly room for more, particularly with respect to practical education and training. Relevant professional organizations, academic departments, and facilities offering ECT are encouraged to develop clinically oriented continuing education programs on ECT, including provision of continuing medical education (CME) credit, as well as research-focused lectures and symposia on ECT-related topics. Symposia, courses, seminars, and fellowship opportunities in ECT at the local, regional, and national levels should be publicized widely. Annual meetings of the American Psychiatric Association, American Association for Geriatric Psychiatry, Society of Biological Psychiatry, and American Psychiatric Nurses Association routinely include ECT topics. The annual meeting of the International Society for ECT and Neurostimulation provides a program focused primarily on ECT and other neurostimulation techniques, with updates on ECT research and clinical practice, including ECT nursing best practice.

Several practical courses and visiting fellowships, typically several days to 1 week in duration, are offered at locations around the United States. These opportunities are primarily for psychiatrists, although some are oriented toward nurses. From time to time, other experienced clinicians offer individual preceptorships of various durations at their facilities.

Medical and nursing schools as well as hospitals and clinics that provide ECT are encouraged to have a variety of reference materials applicable to ECT available to support lifelong learning. Such reference materials can include but should not be limited to videos, books, professional journals (including *The Journal of ECT*), copies of relevant published reviews, and clinical and research reports.

Recommendations

6.1. General Considerations

A comprehensive educational and training experience is necessary for professionals in psychiatry, anesthesiology, and psychiatric–mental health nursing to develop the knowledge and skills for providing ECT safely and effectively.

6.2. Medical School Training

1. Psychiatric instructional programs for medical students should include didactic exposure to the role of ECT in the treatment of severe mental disorders, including an overview of the history (including social contexts), indications, risks, mechanisms of action, and technique of ECT.
2. Didactic experience should be supplemented by observation of ECT practice, either directly or through the use of videos.

6.3. Psychiatry Residency Programs

6.3.1. General Issues

1. Psychiatric residency programs should provide comprehensive training in ECT to all residents.
2. ECT training should be provided by qualified and privileged individuals. Departments without such personnel should use consultants, appropriate community practitioners, or training at other educational institutions.
3. Videorecorded materials, simulation exercises (including team-based simulations), and use of assigned readings can augment didactic and practical instruction.
4. Clinical conferences, ECT rounds, and elective opportunities for advanced training in ECT can also improve the overall learning experience.

6.3.2. Didactic Instruction

Formal didactic education should include at least 4 hours of lecture and discussion and should cover the following topics:

1. Indications for ECT
2. Elements of the pre-ECT evaluation, including factors that are relevant to potential risks of ECT
3. Other factors related to the selection of treatment for an individual patient
4. Selection of a setting for treatment (e.g., inpatient, outpatient)
5. Informed consent content and process

6. ECT devices, including electrical safety considerations
7. Technique of ECT administration, including determination of the number and frequency of treatments, use of anesthetic and relaxant agents, oxygenation and airway maintenance, stimulus electrode placement, stimulus parameters and dosing, and management of missed and otherwise inadequate seizures
8. Monitoring during ECT, including blood pressure, oxygen saturation of hemoglobin (pulse oximetry), presence of expired carbon dioxide, electrocardiography, electroencephalography, and motor evidence of a seizure
9. Management of adverse effects during ECT, including anticipated medical emergencies
10. Evaluation of clinical outcomes, including therapeutic benefits, cognitive side effects, and other side effects of treatment
11. Management of patients after completion of an ECT course, including the potential roles of pharmacotherapy, maintenance ECT, and other neurostimulation therapies
12. Legal, risk management, and documentation considerations
13. Mechanisms of action of ECT

6.3.3. Practical Training

1. Staff members who are privileged in ECT administration should supervise psychiatry residents involved in the delivery of ECT and management of patients receiving ECT.
2. Under the direct supervision of a privileged ECT psychiatrist, each resident should actively participate in at least 10 ECT treatments involving at least three separate patients.
3. Each resident should actively participate in the care of at least three patients during the ECT workup, course of treatments, and post-ECT management.

6.3.4. Advanced Training in ECT

Elective opportunities for advanced training in ECT should be available.

6.3.5. Program Responsibilities in Evaluation of ECT-Related Curriculum and Resident Performance

1. Department chairs and psychiatric residency training directors and committees should provide specific guidance for psychiatry resi-

dents' training in ECT, in collaboration with the individual(s) or committee overseeing the practice of ECT within the department.
2. These individuals should also monitor and provide timely correction of any identified deficiencies in ECT-related components of the curriculum by evaluating the performance of residents and faculty.
3. To establish adherence to the above training recommendations and support subsequent applications for privileges, the residency training program should maintain documentation of specific ECT-related educational and training experiences as well as resident performance in these curricular components.
4. Taking appropriate measures to ensure confidentiality, psychiatry residents should be encouraged to keep records of both the number of ECT treatments in which they participated and the number of patients who received ECT while under their care.

6.4. Geriatric Psychiatry Training Programs

1. Formal training in ECT should be part of geriatric psychiatry training programs.
2. Minimum didactic requirements should include all topics noted above for psychiatry residents, specific coverage of the use of ECT in geriatric patients, and clinical exposure to the use of ECT with geriatric patients.

6.5. Anesthesiology Residency Programs

1. Anesthesiology residency programs should provide didactic instruction in ECT that is taught by appropriately qualified personnel. Optimally, practical training in ECT is also suggested.
2. Departments of anesthesiology are encouraged to involve individuals responsible for the education of psychiatry residents in ECT in the planning and delivery of this training experience.
3. Didactic instruction should include material on the following:
   a. Indications for and potential risks of ECT
   b. Elements of the pre-ECT evaluation
   c. Type, dosing, and pertinent interactions of medications commonly used before, during, and immediately after the ECT procedure
   d. Provision of oxygenation

e. Ventilation requirements, including effects of hyperventilation on the ictal response
f. Depth of anesthesia, which is lighter than most other procedures that require general anesthesia
g. Physiological monitoring
h. Electrical safety considerations
i. Effects of the postictal state on recovery from anesthesia
j. Potential adverse reactions and their management during treatment and recovery periods
k. Ways in which ECT anesthesia differs from standard anesthesia practice (e.g., anesthetic choice, dosing, impact of seizure induction on physiological parameters)

6.6. Nursing Schools

1. Nursing schools are encouraged to provide formal didactic instruction on ECT, including
   a. The history of ECT
   b. Indications for and potential risks of ECT
   c. Pre-ECT evaluation
   d. Informed consent procedures
   e. ECT technique
   f. Nursing participation in ECT treatment and postanesthetic recovery (including management of emergency situations)

2. Nursing educators are encouraged to incorporate observation of ECT into their psychiatric–mental health nursing training experience, either directly or through the use of videorecorded material.
3. Postgraduate training for psychiatric–mental health nursing administrators should include additional instruction and training in ECT.
4. Nurse anesthesia training programs should cover the material described above for anesthesiology residents.

6.7. Board Examinations

1. Training in ECT, as described above, should be considered among the requirements for specialty board eligibility.
2. Specialty board examinations for psychiatry, geriatric psychiatry, anesthesiology, and psychiatric–mental health nursing should include questions about ECT.

3. For medical students, the National Board of Medical Examiners should include ECT-related topics in their examinations.

6.8. Continuing Education Programs

1. Continuing education and training opportunities in ECT should be
   · available for practitioners in all pertinent clinical disciplines to maintain their knowledge and practical expertise in ECT and to allow those with insufficient training to develop a more adequate background in this area.
2. Attendance at continuing education programs should be a factor in ECT privileging.
3. Relevant professional organizations, academic departments, and facilities offering ECT are encouraged to develop clinically oriented continuing education programs on ECT, including provision of CME credit, as well as research-focused lectures and symposia on ECT-related topics.
4. When feasible, continuing education programs on ECT should include hands-on experience in addition to didactic material.
5. Medical and nursing schools as well as hospitals and clinics that provide ECT are encouraged to have a variety of reference materials applicable to ECT available to support lifelong learning.

CHAPTER 7

Privileging

Often, privileging covers the practice of an entire discipline, such as psychiatry or anesthesiology. In recent years, however, because of the growing level of technical sophistication involved in clinical practice, as well as a heightened sensitivity to quality of care, there has been a trend toward greater specificity in privileging. Because of the extent of knowledge and skill required to administer electroconvulsive therapy (ECT), general privileging in psychiatry will not suffice, and specific clinical privileges to administer ECT should be required.

Throughout this report, it has been made clear that provision of safe and effective ECT requires the involvement of competent staff (see Chapter 3). The determination of clinical competency of practitioners is usually handled by certification or privileging. Although certificate-granting courses in ECT are now available for practitioners, no national accrediting body presently provides assurance of clinical competence in ECT (Fink and Kellner 1998; Jaffe 2005). Accordingly, clinical competency of practitioners is presently ensured through local privileging. In practice, clinical privileges for a given specialty, subspecialty, or procedure are typically granted by a designated committee of the facility's medical staff, which, in turn, reports to the facility director. Specific educational, training, experience, and skill criteria for such privileging are set by the facility's organized medical staff. The materials provided by the applicant in this process constitute their credentials. To maintain privileges, staff members must usually reapply at regular intervals. Through such a peer review process, each facility ensures that its clinical services are provided in as safe and effective a fashion as possible.

Privileges to administer ECT should be granted only to psychiatrists who meet formal, documented criteria set by the organized medical staff. Before an applicant administers ECT on an unsupervised basis, the facility's medical director should establish that these criteria are met. The medical director should use qualified personnel to assist with this determination, including outside consultants as appropriate. The applicant's education, training, experience (including history of past ECT privileging), and demonstrated skill should be the specific determinants in the granting of ECT privileges. The extent of training and experience required should be sufficient to at least satisfy the educational and training recommendations described in Chapter 6. Medical licensure, satisfactory completion of residency training, and board certification or eligibility should be considered in addition to ECT-related material, such as evidence of satisfactory completion of relevant residency and continuing medical education (CME) training experiences, holding of malpractice insurance covering the practice of ECT, and letters of recommendation. To help establish the presence of adequate skills in the administration of ECT, the applicant should be observed in the delivery of ECT and should demonstrate sufficient skill to satisfy the privileging authority. The individual evaluating the applicant's clinical skills should be a psychiatrist already privileged in ECT. If no such person is available in the facility, provisions should be made for the use of an outside consultant. The proceedings of all privileging actions should be documented.

In cases in which an applicant's education, training, or skill in ECT is deficient, further training should be required. This training experience should consist of didactic instruction and/or individualized reading as well as a formal or informal clinical practicum, if indicated (see Chapter 6). Decisions about the scope and depth of the training program should be guided by the type and degree of deficiencies present. Following satisfactory completion of the training program, the applicant should still be required to demonstrate proficient administration of ECT in the facility granting privileges. They should become familiar with the facility's policies and procedures for ECT as well as the layout of the ECT treatment suite and the use of applicable ECT devices, seizure monitoring equipment, and supplies.

Each facility granting privileges for ECT should also devise policies and procedures to maintain such privileges. This practice is required to ensure that a sustained level of clinical competence is achieved. The plan for maintaining privileging should make use of ongoing quality improvement programs as well as the monitoring of individual practice patterns, especially the number of treatments administered yearly. Any evidence of deficiencies in practice should be corrected. This plan should also include a requirement for CME in ECT-related areas. Reapplication for clinical privileges should be made at least every 2 years or as otherwise specified by regulation or by general local policies covering clinical privileging. The plan should include a provision for reassessment of clinical skills for individuals whose practice of ECT has been inactive for a considerable time, for example, 1 year.

Problems occur when a facility is so small that it does not have an organized medical staff or when the facility does not have sufficient expertise to adequately evaluate candidates for ECT privileges. In such situations, the existence of concurrent clinical privileges obtained from a separate facility may be an acceptable substitute, although an attempt should be made to institute policies and procedures for formal in-house privileging as soon as possible, involving the use of outside consultants as deemed necessary. Ongoing monitoring of adherence to these policies and procedures should be undertaken by means of a quality improvement program or equivalent process, with corrective action taken as indicated.

Recommendations

1. Clinical competency of practitioners is presently ensured through local privileging of the hospital medical staff. Privileges to administer ECT should be granted only to psychiatrists who meet formal, documented criteria set by the organized medical staff. Before an applicant administers ECT on an unsupervised basis, the facility's medical director should establish that these criteria are met.
2. The extent of training and experience required should be sufficient to at least satisfy the educational and training recommendations described in Chapter 6.
3. Each facility granting privileges for ECT should also devise policies and procedures to maintain such privileges.

CHAPTER 8

Pre-ECT Evaluation of the Patient

8.1. Typical Elements of the Pre-ECT Evaluation

The decision to start a course of electroconvulsive therapy (ECT) is based on the type and severity of the patient's psychiatric illness, the patient's treatment history, and a risk-benefit analysis of available psychiatric therapies. Consequently, information on each of these factors must be obtained as part of the pre-ECT evaluation. Although some components of the evaluation depend on the patient's clinical presentation and history, each facility should have a minimal set of procedures that are to be undertaken for all patients (Coffey 2003).

Although no data exist on the optimal time interval between the pre-ECT evaluation and the first treatment, the evaluation should be performed as close as possible to the initiation of treatment. Still, the pre-ECT evaluation may have to be spread over a number of days because of the need for specialty consultations, laboratory testing, and meetings with the patient and significant others and other factors. The treatment team should be aware of pertinent changes in the patient's condition over this time interval and should initiate further evaluation as indicated.

To ensure that an appropriate indication for ECT exists, the pre-ECT evaluation should include a psychiatric history, including past response to ECT and other treatments, and a mental status examination, including baseline measures of treatment outcome and cognition (see Chapters 17 and 20, respectively). It is also important to identify preexisting medical conditions that may influence the risk associated with treatment (Tess and Smetana 2009). Thus, the pre-ECT evaluation should include a careful medical history and examination, focusing particularly on neurological, cardiovascular, and pulmonary systems, as well as on effects of previous anesthesia. An attending psychiatrist who has privileges to administer ECT should perform an evaluation prior to ECT.

Findings should be documented in the medical record and should summarize the indications for and risks of ECT. Documentation may also suggest additional evaluative procedures, alterations in ongoing medications (see Chapter 13), or modifications that may be needed in ECT technique (see Chapter 14).

The anesthesia provider should also perform a thorough evaluation prior to treatment (Tess and Smetana 2009), including an interview with the patient, review of the patient's medical history, and review of any laboratory data. In addition, the anesthesiologist should conduct a physical examination, including assessment of the patient's airway to identify potential sources of difficulty if intubation becomes necessary. Assessment by the anesthesiologist (or a dentist, if indicated) should include an inquiry about dental problems and inspection of the mouth, looking for loose or missing teeth and noting the presence of dentures or other appliances (see Chapter 12, section 12.1.3).

Medical consultation can be helpful in managing physical health conditions, understanding the patient's medical status, and clarifying the patient's medical stability prior to administration of ECT treatments. However, to simply ask for "clearance" for ECT assumes that such consultants have the special experience or training required to assess all risks and benefits of ECT compared with treatment alternatives. Instead, requests for consultation should be accompanied by a clear question for the consultant. The ECT team is also encouraged to establish an ongoing relationship with a cardiologist, a neurologist, and perhaps a pulmonologist so that these specialists are knowledgeable about ECT procedures and can provide appropriately focused input when patients need further evaluation.

Laboratory testing, imaging studies, and other evaluations are used to confirm the presence and severity of medical risk factors identified by the medical history and examination. Some facilities do not specify any specific routine laboratory testing, whereas others have protocols involving specification of testing on the basis of age or certain medical risk factors such as cardiovascular or pulmonary history (Mankad et al. 2010). Young, physically healthy patients may not require laboratory evaluation, although it is common to perform a screening battery of tests, which often includes a complete blood count, measurement of serum potassium and sodium levels, and an electrocardiogram (ECG). A pregnancy test should be considered in individuals with childbearing potential. Although ECT is generally safe for both the fetus and the pregnant individual, some medications used during the procedure (e.g., benzodiazepines) may pose risks to the fetus and may need to be avoided, particularly in the first trimester (see Chapter 9, section 9.4.1). Because the risk of musculoskeletal injuries with ECT has been largely obviated by the use of muscular relaxation, spinal X-rays are no longer routinely necessary; they may, however, be useful in patients with clinically significant preexisting disease affecting the spine. Similarly, an electroencephalogram, brain computed tomography scan, or brain magnetic resonance imaging scan should be considered if the patient's physical examination or other data suggest that a structural brain abnormality may be present.

8.2. Circumstances in Which Additional Evaluation May Be Indicated

There are specific patient populations that may need additional screening (see Chapters 9 and 12); an algorithm for this screening is described by Sundsted et al. 2014. For example, pregnant patients should be evaluated by their obstetrician, with a discussion of the risks and benefits of ECT (see Chapter 9, section 9.4.1). The fetal heart rate should be monitored before and after the treatment if the fetal heart rate can be detected (usually by 8–12 weeks and certainly by 14 weeks).

Patients with cardiovascular, cerebrovascular, and pulmonary disease may also need further evaluation, particularly if they have an unstable medical condition. In addition, patients with diabetes are at higher risk for cardiac disease and should be evaluated carefully prior to ECT.

In patients with coronary artery disease, the workup needs to include basic laboratory studies and an ECG. The history should focus on acute decompensation, with indicators such as poorly controlled hypertension, heart failure, chest pain, shortness of breath, orthopnea, and new onset arrhythmias or edema.

In general, ECT can be administered safely in patients who have well-compensated heart failure, myocardial infarctions older than 6 months, or mild to moderate aortic stenosis (Mueller et al. 2007; Sundsted et al. 2014). Further evaluation, including a cardiology consultation, is warranted in patients with unstable cardiac conditions, and an echocardiogram should be considered in patients with decompensated heart failure, valvular heart disease, or a new-onset heart murmur (Sundsted et al. 2014). Because of the potential for conversion to a normal sinus rhythm with the ECT stimulus delivery, patients with atrial fibrillation should be assessed to determine that their heart rate is adequately controlled, that they are on a stable dose of anticoagulant therapy, and that they have a therapeutic international normalized ratio (INR) if they are treated with warfarin (Petrides and Fink 1996a; Rasmussen et al. 2002).

Several large case series have shown that ECT can be provided safely to patients with implanted cardiac pacemakers (Dolenc et al. 2004a; MacPherson et al. 2006). In fact, implanted cardiac pacemakers generally have a protective effect during ECT because they improve control of cardiac rate and rhythm (Alexopoulos and Frances 1980; Morgan 1987; Pearlman 1986). Patients with a pacemaker should have the pacemaker interrogated to ensure that it is functioning properly, but it does not have to be converted to a fixed pacing mode (Dolenc et al. 2004a; Giltay et al. 2005; MacPherson et al. 2006). With appropriate pretreatment screening and posttreatment monitoring, ECT can also be administered in patients with implanted cardiac defibrillators (Dolenc et al. 2004a; Goldberg and Badger 1993; Pornnoppadol and Isenberg 1998), although a cardiac electrophysiologist should be consulted to determine whether the unit's defibrillator function should be inhibited at the time of each treatment.

Patients with unrepaired abdominal aortic aneurysms (AAAs) should have a screening ultrasound prior to ECT and are at risk of rupture, particularly if the aneurysm is larger than 5.5 cm in women and 5.0 cm in men (Sundsted et al. 2014). There are several case reports of patients with AAAs being treated safely with ECT (Mueller et al. 2009; Porquez et al. 2003).

Patients with previous or current evidence of cerebrovascular disease, including focal findings or papilledema on neurological examination, should be screened with neuroimaging and, when clinically indicated, a neurological consultation. Patients can be treated safely with ECT following a stroke, particularly if the stroke occurred more than 30 days before the planned treatment, there is no evidence of a mass effect or brain edema on brain imaging, blood pressure is tightly controlled, and the stroke is ischemic (Sundsted et al. 2014). However, hemorrhagic strokes may be subject to rebleeding (Weintraub and Lippmann 2000). The same principles can be applied to patients with brain tumors or masses. The patient should have neuroimaging and, when clinically indicated, a neurology consultation prior to treatment (Rasmussen et al. 2002; Sundsted et al. 2014) but can be treated safely if asymptomatic and medically stable (e.g., well-controlled blood pressure). Routine neuroimaging will sometimes detect cerebral aneurysms or angiomas. In this circumstance, a neurosurgery consultation may be helpful before ECT, but these patients can also be treated safely with ECT with careful blood pressure control (Kang and Passmore 2004; Sundsted et al. 2014).

Patients with pulmonary disease, including chronic obstructive pulmonary disease (COPD) and asthma, should be stable without labored breathing, significant wheezing, or decreased oxygen saturation. In such patients, ECT can proceed with minimal risk of complications if they use their inhaler on the morning of ECT or receive a nebulizer treatment if they are symptomatic (Mueller et al. 2006; Schak et al. 2008). Pulmonary embolism has rarely been reported after ECT, although patients receiving ECT are at risk for venous thromboembolism and pulmonary embolism due to prolonged inactivity, particularly in the context of obesity and diabetes (Mamah et al. 2005).

Patients with chronic renal disease are at risk for bone fractures due to decreased bone density (Ott 2009). They are also at risk for high serum potassium levels, which can be further increased by succinylcholine. Consequently, serum potassium should be monitored carefully during ECT and within 24 hours of hemodialysis. Adequate ventilation should occur prior to the seizure to ensure that the patient does not develop respiratory acidosis (Sundsted et al. 2014).

8.3. Determining Whether ECT Should Be Administered on an Inpatient or Outpatient Basis

The decision to treat on an inpatient or outpatient basis is an important component of the pre-ECT evaluation. This choice depends on a number of criteria, including patient preference. The decision should be viewed as a dynamic, ongoing process throughout the ECT course, and any indicated changes should be made on the basis of the patient's clinical status. Certain situations (e.g., resolution of psychosis, significant reduction in suicide risk) may indicate a need to switch from an inpatient to an outpatient setting, and others (e.g., worsening symptoms, lack of post-ECT supervision) will suggest a need to switch in the opposite direction . In making this decision, the same indications, relative contraindications, consent requirements, and components of the pre-ECT evaluation hold for both inpatient and outpatient ECT.

8.3.1. General Considerations for Inpatient Treatment

The inpatient setting should be used whenever the patient's psychiatric condition precludes safe and effective management on an outpatient basis. For example, patients at high risk of suicide should not be treated as outpatients until such risk is sufficiently diminished that they can be discharged from the inpatient setting (Jacobs and Brewer 2006). Psychotic ideation, inanition, or severe preexisting cognitive impairment may also raise questions about the patient's capacity to receive outpatient ECT (Fink et al. 1996).

Patients should receive ECT while hospitalized if they are at high risk of serious medical complications or anesthetic difficulties as suggested by meeting criteria for categories 4 or 5 of the American Society of Anesthesiologists (ASA) Physical Status Classification System based on medical condition and history prior to treatment (American Society of Anesthesiologists 2020a); see Table 8–1. In addition, facilities should have appropriate medical capabilities to address potential emergencies related to medical or anesthetic complications (Tess and Smetana 2009).

For patients in ASA category 3 (e.g., severe systemic disease such as poorly controlled hypertension or diabetes) or with other conditions that could complicate anesthetic management, decisions about the setting of ECT should be made on an individual basis depending on factors such as the type and extent of risk (Fink et al. 1996; Ross and Tucker 1990). For patients at significant anesthetic risk, consideration should also be given to the location of the treatment area (e.g., general hospital, freestanding psychiatric facility).

It may also be prudent to initiate ECT treatments on an inpatient basis when the degree of anesthetic risk or the extent of the patient's ability to adhere to the outpatient behavioral requirements are difficult to assess prior to an acute ECT course (Fink et al. 1996; Lisanby 2007). Examples include individuals who are at substantially increased risk to develop a post-ECT delirium (e.g., those with preexisting neurological impairment, significant ECT-induced cognitive impairment during previous courses of treatment; see Chapter 20) or patients with other medical conditions that significantly increase potential risks of ECT (see

Table 8–1. *American Society of Anesthesiologists (ASA) Physical Status Classification System*

ASA Physical Status Classification	Definition	Adult examples
ASA I	A normal healthy patient	Healthy, nonsmoking, no or minimal alcohol use
ASA II	A patient with mild systemic disease	Mild diseases only without substantive functional limitations Current smoker, social alcohol drinker, pregnancy, obesity (30<BMI<40), well-controlled DM or HTN, mild lung disease
ASA III	A patient with severe systemic disease	Substantive functional limitations One or more moderate to severe diseases Poorly controlled DM or HTN, COPD, morbid obesity (BMI≥40), active hepatitis, alcohol dependence or abuse, implanted pacemaker, moderate reduction of ejection fraction, ESRD undergoing regularly scheduled dialysis, history (>3 months) of MI, CVA, TIA, or CAD or stents
ASA IV	A patient with severe systemic disease that is a constant threat to life	Recent (<3 months) MI, CVA, TIA, or CAD or stents, ongoing cardiac ischemia or severe valve dysfunction, severe reduction of ejection fraction, shock, sepsis, DIC, ARD, or ESRD not undergoing regularly scheduled dialysis

Table 8–1.   *American Society of Anesthesiologists (ASA) Physical Status Classification System (continued)*

ASA Physical Status Classification	Definition	Adult examples
ASA V	A moribund patient who is not expected to survive without the operation	Ruptured abdominal or thoracic aneurysm, massive trauma, intracranial bleed with mass effect, ischemic bowel in the face of significant cardiac pathology or multiple organ or system dysfunction
ASA VI	A declared brain-dead patient whose organs are being removed for donor purposes	

Note. ARD=acute renal disease; BMI=body mass index; CAD=coronary artery disease; COPD=chronic obstructive pulmonary disease; CVA=cerebrovascular accident; DIC=disseminated intravascular coagulation; DM=diabetes mellitus; ESRD=end-stage renal disease; HTN=hypertension; MI=myocardial infarction; TIA=transient ischemic attack.

Source.   Excerpted from Statement on ASA Physical Status Classification System 2020 of the American Society of Anesthesiologist. A copy of the full text can be obtained from ASA, 1061 American Lane, Schaumburg, Illinois 60173.

Chapter 9). Once it can be shown that these risks are sufficiently low to allow safe outpatient management, a change in the treatment setting can be considered.

8.3.2. General Considerations for Outpatient Treatment

Administration of ECT on an outpatient basis is appropriate when the type and seriousness of the patient's psychiatric illness is appropriate to manage on an outpatient basis and when anticipated risks associated with ECT are detectable and manageable either during the ECT session or with outpatient follow-up care (Reti et al. 2012). The patient must also be willing and able, with the assistance of specified significant others or caregivers, to adhere to behavioral requirements over the course of the treatment. The availability of one or more significant others or caregivers can also help assure patient safety and adherence to the treatment plan.

8.3.3. Relevant Behavioral Restrictions for Determining the Setting of Care

Before beginning ECT and as part of the informed consent process (see Chapter 10), each patient, significant other, or caregiver should be instructed by the treatment team about the type and duration of behavioral limitations that must be followed. The use of a supplementary written instruction sheet is encouraged when providing instruction about behavioral limitations during the ECT course. When patients are receiving outpatient ECT, reinstruction should be provided verbally after each treatment and supplemented by a standardized information sheet given on discharge from the facility.

Activities that are likely to be substantially impaired by the anticipated adverse cognitive effects of ECT should generally be avoided, during and shortly after an acute ECT course, particularly if they involve a significant level of risk and especially on the day of each treatment. At a minimum, patients receiving an acute course of ECT should be specifically instructed to refrain from making major life decisions, including those related to matters of business, personal finances, and interpersonal relations, until the ECT course is completed and residual cognitive side effects have cleared. Patients should also be strongly cautioned that ECT may impair driving ability. Patients should be told not to operate motor vehicles during an acute ECT course and, at a minimum, on the day of the treatment with maintenance ECT. Additional restrictions may be needed during the maintenance course based on the patient's risk factors (e.g., age, neurological comorbidities) and the severity and duration of ECT-associated cognitive and functional side effects. For patients receiving maintenance ECT at short (e.g., weekly) intervals, some restrictions on activities may be warranted. In contrast, with longer intervals between treatments, fewer limitations in activities may be needed because adverse cognitive effects may not persist beyond the day of treatment.

Other behavioral restrictions are relevant to decisions about whether ECT is appropriate to administer on an outpatient basis. Because a patient's condition may change with time, adherence to behavioral requirements should be assessed before each treatment, and suitability for continued outpatient ECT should be reevaluated regularly. Such behavioral requirements include the ability to avoid oral intake for several hours before each ECT, to follow specific directions regarding medication adjustments in conjunction with each treatment, and to advise the attending physician and ECT treatment team about adverse effects of ECT as well as any changes in psychiatric symptoms, medications, or medical conditions.

To help with adherence to these requirements, outpatients should have a responsible person available to assist the patient and provide input to the treatment team. The absence of such an individual will make outpatient ECT difficult unless these "caretaking" functions can be provided by temporary transfer to a structured environment (such as a skilled nursing facility or day hospital program) for the duration of the acute ECT course. When travel hardship is substantial, inpatient treatment may be necessary.

Recommendations

8.1. Typical Elements of the Pre-ECT Evaluation

1. Prior to the initiation of ECT, an attending psychiatrist who has privileges to administer ECT should perform an evaluation and summarize the findings in the medical record, including indications for and risks of ECT and a risk-benefit analysis of other available psychiatric therapies.
2. Specific elements of the pre-ECT evaluation should include
    a. A psychiatric history, including the type and severity of the patient's psychiatric illness and past response to ECT and other treatments
    b. A mental status examination, including baseline measures of treatment outcome and cognition
    c. A medical history to identify preexisting medical conditions that may influence the risk associated with treatment or may require alterations in ongoing medications or modifications that may be needed in ECT technique
    d. Other evaluative procedures, if clinically indicated, such as laboratory testing, imaging studies, or specialty consultations
    e. Alterations in ongoing medications, or necessary modifications in ECT technique

3. Prior to the initiation of ECT, an anesthesiologist or other anesthesia provider should perform a thorough evaluation, including an interview with the patient, review of the patient's medical history, review of any laboratory data, and a physical examination, including assessment of the patient's mouth and airway.

8.2. Circumstances in Which Additional Evaluation May Be Indicated

Additional evaluation, which may include specialty consultation, is typically indicated prior to ECT for pregnant patients and for patients with any of the following conditions:

1. Significant cardiovascular disease (e.g., poorly controlled hypertension; coronary artery disease; myocardial infarction; heart failure; unrepaired AAAs; valvular heart disease; chest pain; shortness of breath; orthopnea; atrial fibrillation; implanted pacemaker or cardioverter defibrillator; new onset arrhythmias, edema, or heart murmur)
2. Previous or current evidence of cerebrovascular disease (e.g., ischemic or hemorrhagic stroke, cerebral aneurysms, cerebral angiomas, papilledema, focal findings on neurological examination)
3. Pulmonary disease (e.g., COPD, asthma)
4. Chronic renal disease

8.3. Determining Whether ECT Should Be Administered on an Inpatient or Outpatient Basis

8.3.1. General Considerations for Inpatient Treatment

1. ECT should be administered on an inpatient basis whenever the patient's psychiatric condition precludes safe and effective management on an outpatient basis, such as when a patient has high suicide risk, psychosis, inanition, or substantial cognitive impairment or is otherwise severely incapacitated.
2. Inpatient ECT should be provided to patients who are at high risk for serious complications on the basis of significant medical conditions or an ASA Physical Status Classification of 4 or 5.
3. Initiation of ECT on an inpatient basis may also be indicated when the type and extent of anesthetic or medical risk are unclear (e.g., ASA Physical Status Classification of 3), when patients are at signif-

icant risk of post-ECT delirium, or when the patient's ability to adhere to outpatient behavioral requirements is difficult to assess prior to an acute ECT course.

8.3.2. General Considerations for Outpatient Treatment

Outpatient administration of ECT is appropriate when

1. The type and seriousness of the patient's psychiatric illness is appropriate to manage on an outpatient basis.
2. Anticipated risks associated with ECT are detectable and manageable either during the ECT session or with outpatient follow-up care.
3. The patient is willing and able, with the assistance of specified significant others or caregivers, to adhere to behavioral requirements over the course of the treatment.

8.3.3. Relevant Behavioral Restrictions for Determining the Setting of Care

1. Before beginning ECT and as part of the informed consent process, each patient, significant other, or caregiver should be instructed by the treatment team about the type and duration of behavioral limitations that must be followed.
2. Outpatients should have a responsible person available to provide assistance to the patient and input to the treatment team.
3. A supplementary written information sheet and verbal review of behavioral restrictions should be given to outpatients on discharge from the facility after each treatment and are encouraged to be provided to inpatients.
4. At a minimum, patients receiving an acute course of ECT should be specifically instructed to refrain from making major life decisions that could be impaired by the anticipated adverse cognitive effects of ECT.
5. Patients should be told not to operate motor vehicles during an acute ECT course and, at a minimum, on the day of the treatment for the maintenance course.
6. Patients and significant others should be instructed to inform the attending physician or the ECT treatment team of any adverse effects of ECT or changes in psychiatric symptoms or medical conditions that have occurred since the prior treatment.

CHAPTER 9

Use of Electroconvulsive Therapy in Special Populations

9.1. General Considerations

Special populations include patients with complex medical comorbidities (e.g., cardiac, pulmonary, neurological comorbidities) as well as children, adolescents, geriatric patients, and pregnant patients who may require additional screening prior to electroconvulsive therapy (ECT) and monitoring during the ECT course. Although the overall risks of ECT have been shown to be low in population-based samples (Blumberger et al. 2017), an individual patient may need additional screening to ensure that treatment proceeds without significant complications (see Chapter 8).

The primary criteria for determining if ECT should be administered remains the same (see Chapter 2), with an assessment of the relative risks and benefits of ECT performed for each patient. This analysis should include 1) consideration of the severity and duration of the psychiatric illness and its threat to life, 2) the likelihood of therapeutic success with ECT, 3) the medical risks of ECT and the degree to which these risks can be diminished, and 4) the benefits and risks of alternative treatments and of no treatment. After such an analysis, a choice can be made regarding the optimal intervention for an individual patient, discussed in the informed consent process (see Chapter 10) and documented. This risk-benefit analysis is performed by the ECT psychiatrist and the mental health team caring for the patient, if different from the ECT psychiatrist.

9.2. ECT in Patients With Comorbid Medical Disorders

Concomitant medical conditions may have an impact on both the likelihood of response and the risks of ECT. For example, the medical risk of ECT is increased for patients with hypertension, coronary artery disease, heart failure, implanted cardiac devices, atrial fibrillation, chronic obstructive pulmonary disease (COPD), or asthma (Tess and Smetana 2009). In addition, effective management of medical conditions is often more difficult in patients with psychiatric disorders because of factors such as diminished adherence to medical treatment (Chang et al. 2021; Koenig and Kuchibhatla 1998; Sternhell and Corr 2002). In contrast, the presence of severe cardiac disease, for example, may make it more difficult to maintain a patient on an antidepressant and increase the urgency in treating their depression. Furthermore, effective psychiatric treatment often improves medical outcomes (Huffman et al. 2014; Thompson et al. 1998), and in patients with major depression, ECT may reduce short- and long-term mortality (Avery and Winokur 1976; Philibert et al. 1995; Watts et al. 2021).

To some extent, medical adverse events can be anticipated. The organ systems of most importance when considering the medical risks of ECT are the cardiovascular, central nervous, and pulmonary systems. Individuals who experienced medical complications with earlier courses of anesthesia or ECT are also likely to be at increased risk (Zielinski et al. 1993). In addition, in patients referred for ECT, it is especially important to understand the interactions among coexisting medical conditions, physiological events associated with anesthetic induction, electrical stimulation of the brain, and induced seizure activity.

The pre-ECT evaluation (see Chapter 8) is designed to identify coexisting medical illnesses and their impact on the risks and benefits of ECT and to suggest ways to minimize adverse effects. Careful medical evaluation is an essential component of this process and may include consultations with internists, cardiologists, neurologists, and other specialists (see Chapter 8). Additional laboratory evaluations will often be a part of this information-gathering process. This material facilitates the treatment team's ability to arrive at a medically sound decision about whether ECT should be recommended. If so, the pre-ECT evaluation will assist in optimizing the patient's medical condition prior to ECT and determine whether any procedural modifications or medication adjustments are indicated (see Chapter 8). Multiple reviews and expert consensus documents have focused on the appropriate medical evaluation and accommodations for patients with significant cardiovascular (Applegate 1997; Dolinski and Zvara 1997; Duma et al. 2019; Hermida et al. 2022; Rayburn 1997; Rice et al. 1994), pulmonary (Mueller et al. 2006; Schak et al. 2008), and neurological (Agüera-Ortiz et al. 2021; Folkerts 1995; Kennedy et al. 2003; Krystal and Coffey 1997; Lambrecq et al. 2012; Rosenquist et al. 2018; van Waarde et al. 2001) disease.

Despite careful pre-ECT evaluation, medical complications may arise that have not been anticipated. ECT facilities should be appropriately equipped and staffed with personnel to manage potential clinical emergencies (see Chapters 3, 4, 6, 7, and 12). Additional information related to mortality and adverse events during ECT is provided in Chapter 19.

9.2.1. Cardiovascular Disorders

In general, patients with cardiovascular disease can be safely managed during ECT (Abrams 1991, 1997; Applegate 1997; Dolinski and Zvara 1997; Hermida et al. 2022; Kufner et al. 2022; Nordenskjöld et al. 2022; Rayburn 1997; Weiner et al. 2000; Zwil and Pelchat 1994). The pre-ECT evaluation (see Chapter 8) should include a review of the patient's medications, including medications such as antihypertensives, β-blockers, diuretics, and antiarrhythmics that are prescribed to manage cardiovascular conditions. Typically, patients should be told to take these medications with a sip of water as prescribed on the morning before the treatment; however, if patients are on high doses of a diuretic, dose reduction or changes in dose timing may be needed to minimize the risk of hypovolemia and hypotension while taking nothing by mouth (NPO). Additionally, because of its pronounced anticonvulsant effects, lidocaine should be avoided prior to and during the induced seizure (DeToledo et al. 2002).

If cardiovascular disease is present, optimization prior to ECT should be attempted, keeping in mind any risks that may be associated with delaying the start of ECT. In addition, the ECT practitioner should be mindful of conditions that contribute to significantly higher risk of adverse cardiovascular events so that cardiology consultation can be obtained prior to initiating treatment.

In general, for noncardiac surgical procedures, risk is elevated in the presence of an acute coronary syndrome (unstable angina or myocardial infarction), acute decompensated heart failure, severe symptomatic aortic stenosis, or tachyarrhythmias or bradyarrhythmias associated with hypotension or requiring urgent medical attention (Fleisher et al. 2014; Ganesh et al. 2021; Smilowitz and Berger 2020). Other factors that are associated with a higher risk of cardiovascular events in noncardiac surgical procedures include heart failure, arrhythmias, valvular heart disease, systemic or pulmonary hypertension, or a history of ischemic heart disease or coronary stenting (Fleisher et al. 2014; Ganesh et al. 2021; Smilowitz and Berger 2020). Chronic kidney disease and diabetes also confer an increase in risk (Smilowitz and Berger 2020).

Although ECT is a low-risk procedure compared with many noncardiac surgical procedures, risks associated with ECT treatment may be increased by certain cardiovascular conditions, such as uncontrolled hypertension, recent myocardial infarction (MI) (<60 days), unstable angina, decompensated heart failure, severe aortic stenosis, uncontrolled atrial fibrillation, unrepaired abdominal aortic aneurysms >5.0 cm, or tachyarrhythmias or bradyarrhythmias associated with hypotension or requiring urgent medical attention (Sundsted et al. 2014; Tess and Smetana 2009). In addition, the type and severity of preexisting cardiac disease affect the likelihood, type, and severity of cardiac complications during ECT (Bryson et al. 2013; Cristancho et al. 2008; Huuhka et al. 2003; Prudic et al. 1987; Rice et al. 1994; Zielinski et al. 1993).

The cardiovascular risks of ECT derive primarily from the marked changes in heart rate and blood pressure that typically occur during and immediately after the electrical stimulus and induced seizure (Dolinski and Zvara 1997; Fuenmayor et al. 1997; Messina et al. 1992; Webb et al. 1990; Zielinski et al. 1993). Although ECT does cause elevations in blood pressure during treatment, a study of patients who were free from systemic disease demonstrated this elevation to be transient and not associated with any serious adverse events (Takada et al. 2005). Similar results were reported in a retrospective study that included patients with and without hypertension, who showed no statistically significant change in measures of blood pressure before and after ECT (Albin et al. 2007). Nevertheless, in patients with aortic or other vascular aneurysms, transient elevations in blood pressure could contribute to an increased risk of rupture, and more aggressive blood pressure management may be indicated (Caliyurt et al. 2003; Mueller et al. 2009).

Recent MI is believed to represent a risk for reinfarction during ECT (Applegate 1997). In the absence of relevant supporting data with ECT, this concept of *recency* is difficult to define. However, in patients undergoing noncardiac surgical procedures, a delay of at least 60 days after MI significantly reduces the risk of postoperative reinfarction, with additional decreases in risk at 90 and 120 days (Fleisher et al. 2014; Ganesh et al. 2021). These risks are also influenced by other factors, such as whether heart failure or a reduced ejection fraction are present, whether coronary artery bypass graft surgery or stent placement occurred after the MI, the type of stent (if any), and the complexity and risk of the planned procedure (Fleisher et al. 2014; Ganesh et al. 2021). With ECT, the risks of providing treatment following a recent MI or other cardiovascular event must also be balanced against the risk of not treating a life-threatening psychiatric condition (Kaster et al. 2021; Nordenskjöld et al. 2022; Rönnqvist et al. 2021). As an example, in one published case report, ECT was administered safely and effectively 10 days after a non–ST elevation MI, but the patient had a preserved ejection fraction, had no ischemia on a stress echocardiogram, and was experiencing life-threatening depression with catatonic features (Magid et al. 2005).

Information about use of ECT in individuals with heart failure is limited but suggests that ECT can be done safely with appropriate pre-ECT optimization and anesthetic management. A review of the early literature (Rayburn 1997) described several examples of individuals with heart failure who experienced complications with ECT, but a substantial percentage of other individuals with cardiac issues did not. Unfortunately, these early reports did not provide a detailed description of the patient's underlying cardiac disease or whether approaches were taken to minimize risk. A subsequent retrospective study described 35 individuals who received a total of 513 ECT treatments and who had had a history of heart failure with reduced left ventricular systolic function (Rivera et al. 2011). Input from anesthesiology and cardiology consultants was used to guide the pre-ECT evaluation and optimize the treatment approach. In addition, patients were not exhibiting symptoms of heart failure at the time of treatment. For patients who experienced marked hypertension or tachycardia, prophylactic treatment with a β-blocking agent was used at subsequent treatments to blunt this sympathetically mediated response. All patients had a good response of their depressive symptoms, and no major complications were noted, although several individuals experienced a brief arrhythmia.

Some evidence suggests that patients may be susceptible to arrhythmias during ECT. In a meta-analysis of cardiac events with ECT, the estimated incidence of arrhythmias was 14.82–25.83 per 1,000 patients and 0.87–4.66 per 1,000 ECT treatments, depending on the meta-analytical statistical model that was used (Duma et al. 2019). Patients with an increased baseline QTc interval appear to have an increased rate of arrhythmias with ECT (Pullen et al. 2011). Thus, evaluating the patient's medication regimen for medication interactions or specific medications that could prolong QTc intervals may be useful as part of the pre-ECT evaluation (Pullen et al. 2011).

Other studies have examined whether ECT or ECT-related arrhythmias are associated with increases in QT dispersion (i.e., the difference between the maximum and minimum QT interval on a 12-lead electrocardiogram). Two small studies suggest that baseline values for QT dispersion are increased in patients presenting for ECT and that additional increases occur during ECT treatment (Tezuka et al. 2010; Yamaguchi et al. 2011), which may be more prominent in geriatric patients (Yamaguchi et al. 2011). An additional study suggested that QT dispersion may predict the occurrence of arrhythmias with ECT (Rasmussen et al. 2007b). However, concerns have been raised about the utility and reliability of QT dispersion, although it has been used to stratify arrhythmia risk in patients with underlying cardiac disease (Bazoukis et al. 2019; Malik and Batchvarov 2000; Verrier et al. 2021). Thus, the implications of QT dispersion for predicting risk of arrhythmia with ECT are unclear.

Atrial fibrillation is a common arrhythmia in community samples (Björck et al. 2013; Essa et al. 2021). When atrial fibrillation is present in a patient who is referred for ECT, heart rate should be well controlled. In addition, because the autonomic effects of ECT may convert atrial fibrillation to a sinus rhythm, some practitioners recommend routine anticoagulation of patients with this condition to diminish the risk of embolism from atrial mural thrombi (Harsch 1991; Petrides and Fink 1996a). Anticoagulation is generally felt to be safe in patients receiving ECT (see section 9.2.9); however, decisions about anticoagulation should occur in consultation with a cardiologist. Furthermore, at least 4 weeks may be needed between initiating anticoagulation and receipt of ECT unless a transesophageal echocardiogram excludes the presence of an atrial thrombus.

If cardiac function is normal, patients who have undergone cardiac transplant do not appear to have specific cardiac risks during ECT (Bloch et al. 1992; Kellner et al. 1991a; Lee et al. 2001; Pargger et al. 1995).

9.2.2. Pulmonary Disorders

Severe pulmonary conditions may lead to difficulties in airway management during and after the ECT procedure (Smetana 1999). Consultation with anesthesiology or other specialists is often indicated to optimize management as well as to identify medication adjustments that may be needed during treatment (see Chapters 8 and 12). Patients with COPD should receive pretreatment with any prescribed bronchodilators or inhalers as well as preoxygenation on the morning of each ECT treatment (Schak et al. 2008; Wingate and Hansen-Flaschen 1997). Although practice guidelines no longer recommend use of theophylline in the routine treatment of COPD (Qaseem et al. 2011), it is important to note that prolonged seizures have occurred in patients who have received ECT while taking theophylline (Abrams 2002; Devanand et al. 1988a, 1998; Fink and Sackeim 1998; Peters et al. 1984; Rasmussen and Zorumski 1993; Schak et al. 2008). Thus, if theophylline is used, it should be discontinued or levels should be kept as low as clinically feasible to minimize this risk (Devanand et al. 1988a; Fink and Sackeim 1998; Peters et al. 1984; Rasmussen and Zorumski 1993). Checking levels at the time of treatment can help guide future dose adjustments.

ECT can be safely administered to asthmatic patients, although a minority of patients may experience an exacerbation of their symptoms, which can be managed with standard asthma medications (Mueller et al. 2006). Patients with a history of asthma should have bronchodilators available for use both before and after each ECT treatment.

Several case reports suggest that with additional treatment precautions, ECT can be safely administered shortly after the occurrence of a pulmonary embolism. However, prior to and during the ECT course, specific attention should be paid to cardiac function, evidence of residual deep vein thrombosis (e.g., ultrasound findings, clinical signs such as redness and swelling of the affected limb), and adequacy of anticoagulation (Buday et al. 2020b; Dean and Coconcea 2016; Singh and Wahi 2008; Suzuki et al. 2008; Tsao and Nusbaum 2007).

Use of ECT in individuals with other pulmonary conditions has been reported less often, but one case report has described the uncomplicated use of ECT in a patient with cystic fibrosis (Fogg-Waberski et al. 2006). There is also a case report of the successful management of catatonia using ECT in a patient with idiopathic pulmonary arterial hypertension (Hobo et al. 2016).

One case report described the administration of ECT to an individual with life-threatening catatonia in the context of coronavirus disease 2019 (COVID-19) infection with pulmonary involvement on imaging requiring supplemental oxygen (Braithwaite et al. 2020). Multiple other reports have also been published of individuals receiving ECT subsequent to COVID-19 infection, although it was not clear whether residual pulmonary disease was present (Austgen et al. 2022; Boland and Dratcu 2020; Chacko et al. 2020; Hassani et al. 2020; Kashaninasab et al. 2020; Reinfeld and Yacoub 2021). In two reports, patients developed a pulmonary embolism, with the coagulation abnormalities associated with COVID-19 infection viewed as a possible contributor (Hillow et al. 2021; McCarron et al. 2020). Thus, for individuals being treated with ECT who have a past COVID-19 infection, attention should be given to any residual pulmonary issues and to the potential for coagulation abnormalities, including pulmonary emboli. For patients with active COVID-19 infection, use of appropriate personal protective equipment and infection control precautions is crucial (see Chapter 12).

9.2.3. Neurological Disorders

9.2.3.1. Intracerebral Mass Lesions

Traditionally, there have been significant concerns about administering ECT in a patient with an intracerebral mass such as a brain tumor or hematoma (Maltbie et al. 1980). Most reports of dire outcomes in patients with brain masses are from a period when ECT techniques and brain imaging studies were far less sophisticated. In general, the size and acuity of space-occupying cerebral lesions is associated with the magnitude of risk. Consequently, clinical judgment must be exercised in determining the risk-benefit ratio for each individual. For example, there are now multiple case reports of successful and uncomplicated ECT in the presence of meningiomas (Buday et al. 2020a; Frajo-Apor et al. 2017; Fried and Mann 1988; Greenberg et al. 1988; Hsiao and Evans 1984; Kellner and Rames 1990; Kohler and Burock 2001; Malek-Ahmadi and Sedler 1989; McKinney et al. 1998; Nakatake et al. 2010; Teraishi et al. 2012; Thukral-Mahajan et al. 2017; Zwil et al. 1990). Only rarely would one need to avoid ECT in a patient with a small, slow-growing meningioma. On the other hand, it would also be rare to treat a patient with a large brain tumor, increased intracranial pressure, or other signs of a mass effect (Buday et al. 2020a; Patkar et al. 2000; Salaris et al. 2000). Patients with signs of increased intracranial pressure (e.g., significant headache, papilledema, focal neurological deficits) or who have brain edema, mass-related displacement, or cerebrovascular fragility on imaging studies are at increased risk of acute neurological decompensation (Buday et al. 2020a; Krystal and Coffey 1997). Nevertheless, there are case reports of patients with increased intracranial pressure or a mass effect who have safely undergone a course of ECT (Patkar et al. 2000; Rasmussen et al. 2007d; Youssef et al. 2021a). If the relative benefits of ECT are judged to outweigh these risks, hyperventilation at the time of ECT and treatment with antihypertensive agents, steroids, and diuretics can be used to help mitigate treatment-related risks.

9.2.3.2. Cerebrovascular Disease

Patients with preexisting cerebrovascular disease are commonly referred for ECT. Published case reports have documented the safe use of

ECT for patients with cerebrovascular disease (Adam and Crowe 2003; Harmandayan et al. 2012; Kang and Passmore 2004; Malek-Ahmadi and Hanretta 2002; Rodenbach et al. 2019; van Herck et al. 2009; Weintraub and Lippmann 2000), and the risk of an intracerebral infarct or bleed is believed to be small in patients with stable lesions (Farah et al. 1996; Weisberg et al. 1991). In a study of 174,534 patients enrolled in the Danish National Patient Registry between 2005 and 2016, the association between ECT and a subsequent stroke was examined (Rozing et al. 2019). In 5,781 patients without previous stroke who received ECT, there was no increase in the occurrence of strokes. Furthermore, there was no recurrence of stroke in the 228 patients who had a history of stroke and received ECT. Another cohort study, conducted using the National Health Insurance Research Database of Taiwan, identified 6,264 patients who had received ECT between 2002 and 2007 and compared them with a group of 18,664 mentally ill patients who were matched by age, sex, and diagnosis but had not received ECT (Hsieh et al. 2019). After controlling for stroke risk factors such as age, diabetes, hypertension, coronary heart disease, and sociodemographic status, the cohort that received ECT was found to have a lower incidence of subsequent stroke than the comparison cohort. Thus, the findings from both of these studies suggest that ECT is not associated with an elevated risk of incident or recurrent stroke.

Concern is greater for individuals with very recent strokes or cerebral aneurysms (Bruce et al. 2006; Sundsted et al. 2014). Consequently, when ECT is given to patients at risk for a cerebrovascular bleed, the acute ECT-related hypertensive surge is generally blunted with antihypertensive medications (Bader et al. 1995; Kolano et al. 1997; Krystal and Coffey 1997; Mehdi and Devanand 2021; Najjar and Guttmacher 1998; Viguera et al. 1998; Wechsler et al. 2021) (see Chapter 12). However, care must be taken to avoid excessive hypotension. A case report has shown that with careful monitoring, select patients with increased intracranial pressure can receive ECT with minimal complications (Adam and Crowe 2003). In fact, a study examining the transcranial Doppler pulsatility index as an indicator of increased intracranial pressure found no increases associated with the ECT stimulus or the induced seizure (Derikx et al. 2012).

Patients with clinically silent cerebrovascular disease, as evidenced by subcortical hyperintensities on magnetic resonance imaging (MRI) scans, do not appear to be at increased risk with ECT (Coffey 1996; Coffey et al.

1987a). Nevertheless, the likelihood of ECT-induced delirium may be increased in some patients who have had strokes (Martin et al. 1992) or hyperintensities in the basal gangliaon MRI scans (Figiel et al. 1991), and clinical response may be somewhat reduced (Steffens et al. 2001).

9.2.3.3. Seizure Disorders

Patients with epilepsy may be at slightly increased risk for prolonged or spontaneous seizures during or after ECT (Chathanchirayil and Bhat 2012; Devinsky and Duchowny 1983). However, because of its anticonvulsant effects, ECT may be associated with improved seizure control in some patients (Conway et al. 2018; Griesemer et al. 1997; Kalinowsky and Kennedy 1943; Koong and Chen 2010; Krystal and Coffey 1997; Lambrecq et al. 2012; Regenold et al. 1998; Sackeim et al. 1983; Schnur et al. 1989; Shah et al. 2012; Shin et al. 2011). In addition, ECT has been used to treat patients with status epilepticus that has been refractory to other interventions (García-López et al. 2020; Katzell et al. 2023; Lisanby et al. 2001a; Pinchotti et al. 2018; San-Juan et al. 2019; Schneegans et al. 2019; Singla et al. 2022; Tan et al. 2020; Woodward et al. 2023).

Treatment with an anticonvulsant medication may raise the seizure threshold, making it difficult to induce a seizure with ECT, or may affect seizure expression, resulting in reduced clinical efficacy of ECT. Nevertheless, the use of anticonvulsants does not represent a contraindication to ECT treatment (Cinderella et al. 2022) (see Chapters 8 and 13). Instead, the indication for anticonvulsant treatment should be confirmed, and dosage should be kept as low as clinically feasible during the ECT series. A retrospective chart review of epileptic patients who received ECT indicated that most patients experienced a moderate to marked reduction in psychiatric symptoms without needing adjustment in their anticonvulsant medication dosage (Lunde et al. 2006). In addition, in patients treated with an anticonvulsant medication, the use of a stimulus dose titration procedure at the time of the first treatment is particularly desirable because it allows the most accurate assessment of the patient's actual seizure threshold (see Chapter 14).

The relationship between ECT and the subsequent development of epilepsy is unclear, but the risk appears to be low. In one retrospective review of 619 patients, no reports of spontaneous seizures occurred; however, patients at high risk of spontaneous seizures prior to ECT were excluded from the study (Ray 2013). In the Danish National Patient Registry, researchers examined records of 169,457 patients with mood disorders to determine whether ECT was associated with an increased risk of epilepsy (Bøg et al. 2018). In patients younger than age 40 years, ECT had a positive association with a subsequent diagnosis of epilepsy after adjustment for covariables (hazard ratio [HR]=1.84; 95% CI=1.24–2.74). In patients ages 41–60 years, ECT was not associated with epilepsy, whereas for those older than age 60 years, ECT was associated with a lower rate of epilepsy (HR=0.57; 95% CI=0.37–0.89). However, the authors cautioned that some of the associations may have been subject to confounding risk factors related to ECT.

Several case reports have described epileptiform activity or new onset of seizures in individuals who have received ECT. A case series of five patients who received maintenance ECT for at least 8 months found temporal epileptiform abnormalities on electroencephalograms (EEGs) despite normal neuroimaging findings and no history of epilepsy (Bryson et al. 2016). Three of these patients showed clinical symptoms consistent with seizure activity, but the EEGs normalized in all of the patients after ECT was discontinued. An additional case report described a 73-year-old patient with psychosis who had received 173 ECT treatments over 5 years and had the new onset of a spontaneous tonic-clonic seizure (Selvadurai et al. 2016). On the basis of these reports, clinicians should be observant for any clinical evidence of seizure activity in patients receiving ECT, although the evidence for kindling phenomena or spontaneous seizures associated with ECT is very limited.

9.2.3.4. Traumatic Brain Injury

Case reports suggest that patients with a history of brain trauma respond to ECT (Hořínková et al. 2017; Kant et al. 1999; Martino et al. 2008) and that ECT can be used safely in patients with skull defects or metallic implants (Amanullah et al. 2012; Francois et al. 2014; Gahr et al. 2014; Glezer et al. 2009; Katz et al. 2017; Ling et al. 2010; Madan and Anderson 2001). Such objects should be detected during the pre-ECT evaluation, and if an intracerebral shunt is present, its patency should be assessed (Coffey et al. 1987b; Gardno and Simpson 1991; Karthik et al. 2022; Sharma et al. 2005). To avoid stimulation over any skull defects, a modified stimulus electrode placement should be used (Crow et al. 1996; Everman et al. 1999; Hartmann and Saldivia 1990; Kant et al. 1999; Wijeratne and Shome 1999). Modifications to anesthetic technique or use of antihypertensive agents may also be warranted to blunt the cardiovascular response to ECT (see Chapter 12).

9.2.3.5. Dementia

Patients with a concomitant diagnosis of dementia would be expected to have an increased risk of transient cognitive worsening with ECT (Bachu et al. 2023; Beale et al. 1997a; Goetz and Price 1993; Krystal and Coffey 1997; Mulsant et al. 1991; Price and McAllister 1989; see Chapter 20). However, in patients with dementia, ECT can be both safe and effective in the treatment of mood disorders (Fruitman and Francois 2022; Hausner et al. 2011) as well as in reducing agitation and aggression (Acharya et al. 2015; Bachu et al. 2023; Chan et al. 2022; Ujkaj et al. 2012). ECT is also effective in the treatment of the dementia syndrome of depression or "reversible dementia" (Alexopoulos et al. 1993; Bright-Long and Fink 1993) and can have a positive therapeutic effect with manageable cognitive side effects (Nelson and Rosenberg 1991; Price and McAllister 1989).

9.2.3.6. Parkinson's Disease

Although ECT can treat depression, psychosis, and motor symptoms in patients with Parkinson's disease (Agüera-Ortiz et al. 2021; Andersen et al. 1987; Borisovskaya et al. 2016; Faber and Trimble 1991; Ffytche et al. 2017; Grover et al. 2018; Kellner et al. 1994a; Kennedy et al. 2003; Murayama et al. 2021; Narang et al. 2015; Popeo and Kellner 2009; Takamiya et al. 2021; Ueda et al. 2010; Usui et al. 2011; Wilkins et al. 2008), dopaminergic medications in combination with dopaminergic changes produced by ECT may also result in psychosis or dyskinesia (Cumper et al. 2014). These effects may be addressed by reducing doses of concomitant dopaminergic medications, particularly L-dopa, or simply holding morning doses of dopaminergic medications until after the ECT treatment (McGarvey et al. 1993; Nymeyer and Grossberg 1997; Rudorfer et al. 1992; Zervas and Fink 1992). Some reports have also indicated that patients with Parkinson's disease may have an increased incidence of delirium or greater cognitive dysfunction after ECT (Figiel et al. 1991; Kellner et al. 1994a; Tsujii et al. 2019). This potential complication may be minimized by the use of right unilateral (RUL) ECT, ultrabrief pulse width ECT, and a less frequent schedule of treatments (Tsujii et al. 2019; Williams et al. 2017).

9.2.3.7. Huntington's Disease

Huntington's disease is inherited in an autosomal-dominant fashion and is caused by a CAG triplet repeat expansion in the *HTT* gene, which encodes the huntingtin protein (Ross and Tabrizi 2011). The molecular pathogenesis of Huntington's disease is not fully delineated, but a key neurological finding is cortical atrophy and degeneration of the corpus striatum. Although patients with Huntington's disease typically present with prominent choreiform movements and cognitive decline that starts in the fourth or fifth decade, these patients also have high rates of depression, suicide, psychosis, and agitation. Case reports suggest that psychiatric symptoms in Huntington's disease can show a good response to ECT and that ECT is generally well tolerated (Adrissi et al. 2019; Beale et al. 1997a; Cusin et al. 2013; Petit et al. 2016; Shah et al. 2017). However, a minority of patients developed delirium or worsening of their movement disorder (Abeysundera et al. 2019; Ranen et al. 1994), perhaps due to alterations in dopaminergic systems, with ECT superimposed on a hyperdopaminergic state in the mesolimbic system in patients with Huntington's disease (Petit et al. 2016).

9.2.3.8. Myasthenia Gravis

Myasthenia gravis is an autoimmune disease that results in weakness in the skeletal muscles due to antibodies that target the postsynaptic membranes of the neuromuscular junction, primarily the nicotinic acetylcholine receptors. Myasthenia gravis is associated with resistance to and slow recovery from depolarizing muscle relaxants such as succinylcholine (Pande and Grunhaus 1990; Wainwright and Brodrick 1987; Warren et al. 2018). Patients with myasthenia gravis may have a decreased number of acetylcholine receptors at the neuromuscular junction (Calarge and Crowe 2004) and they are often taking medications that interfere with the breakdown of succinylcholine (e.g., the acetylcholinesterase inhibitor pyridostigmine). Use of a nondepolarizing muscle-relaxing agent, such as rocuronium, is a good alternative to succinylcholine. Furthermore, rocuronium can be reversed with sugammadex, which does not affect the release or breakdown of acetylcholine, unlike traditional reversal agents such as neostigmine (Warren et al. 2018). Increased sensitivity to succinylcholine may also be seen in patients with upper motor neuron disease, such as quadriplegia and amyotrophic lateral sclerosis (Janis et al. 1995).

9.2.3.9. Multiple Sclerosis

Patients with multiple sclerosis generally tolerate ECT without experiencing major adverse effects (Coffey et al. 1987d; Fitzsimons et al. 2007; Krystal and Coffey 1997; Rasmussen and Keegan 2007; Steen et al. 2015;

Yahya and Khawaja 2021), but there are potential risks associated with neuromuscular blocking anesthetic agents (Yahya and Khawaja 2021). Patients with active cerebral demyelination may experience deterioration in neurological function (Mattingly et al. 1992; Steen et al. 2015). Input from neurological and radiological consultants can help determine the most appropriate imaging approach to identify patients at risk for neurological complications (Wattjes et al. 2021).

9.2.4. Endocrine Disorders

ECT may necessitate changes in management of diabetes, particularly in patients whose blood sugars are hard to control (Finestone and Weiner 1984; Reddy and Nobler 1996; Weiner and Sibert 1996; Williams et al. 1992). Medical or endocrinological consultation should be considered, particularly for individuals whose diabetes is unstable or insulin dependent. The clinician evaluating a diabetic patient should also be aware of the patient's increased risk for other medical complications, including cardiac complications.

ECT itself appears to have minimal effects on blood glucose. In a study of 18 patients with type 2 diabetes mellitus, none had a significant rise or drop in blood glucose 20 minutes after ECT (Rasmussen et al. 2006). The average rise was only 9% (Rasmussen et al. 2006), which was comparable to that seen in nondiabetic patients (Rasmussen and Ryan 2005). Another retrospective study found no changes in daily insulin requirements in a group of 19 patients with insulin-requiring type 2 diabetes (Netzel et al. 2002). Nevertheless, blood glucose should be monitored closely during the ECT course, taking care to avoid hypoglycemia (<80 mg/dL), because of increased glucose needs in the brain during seizures and hyperglycemia, because of alterations in seizure threshold and risk of dehydration. In addition, adjustments to doses of insulin and antidiabetic medications may also be needed on days of ECT treatments when patients are not taking food or fluids by mouth (Sundsted et al. 2014; Tess and Smetana 2009). Point-of-care blood glucose testing within the hour before each treatment can allow for detection and treatment of hypoglycemic states. Infusion of intravenous glucose solutions is indicated in such situations and also may be helpful before ECT in some patients with brittle, insulin-dependent diabetes.

Clinically significant hyperthyroidism is likely to increase the risk of thyroid storm at the time of ECT, but several case reports describe safe and effective use of ECT in patients with hyperthyroidism (Farah and McCall 1995; Nibuya et al. 2002; Saito et al. 2012). Treatment of hyperthyroid states should be optimized with the assistance of specialty consultation, and β-blocking agents should be used at the time of ECT unless otherwise contraindicated. However, mild subclinical elevations in thyroid function on test results, which may occur in conjunction with episodes of mood disorder, do not appear to affect the risk of ECT. ECT has been performed without complications in individuals with hypothyroidism (Garrett 1985), hypoparathyroidism (Cunningham and Anderson 1995), and pseudohypoparathyroidism (McCall et al. 1989), although case reports primarily have described individuals with relatively stable endocrine function.

The presence of a pheochromocytoma is associated with a significant risk for hypertension with ECT (Carr and Woods 1985; Simon and Evans 1986; Weiner et al. 2000). If ECT is essential before definitive treatment of the pheochromocytoma can occur, this risk can be minimized through the use of α- or β-blocking agents (Carr and Woods 1985; Simon and Evans 1986; Weiner et al. 2000).

Case reports have described the successful treatment of psychiatric symptoms due to Cushing's disease with few complications (Ries and Bokan 1979; van Rooijen et al. 2016). Because ECT is associated with transient adrenocortical stimulation, patients with Addison's disease and other patients with steroid dependence may require an increased dose of steroids before each treatment (Heijnen et al. 2013; Triplett et al. 2020).

9.2.5. Electrolyte Abnormalities

Abnormalities in serum sodium and potassium are of particular importance in patients who are receiving ECT. When possible, such abnormalities should be corrected prior to ECT treatment because they may increase ECT risk or require alterations in ECT technique. Hypokalemia may be associated with prolonged paralysis and apnea after ECT, whereas spontaneous seizures can occur with significant hyponatremia, particularly if it is severe or acute (Finlayson et al. 1989; Greer and Stewart 1993). Even subclinical changes in the level of sodium can change the quality of ECT-induced seizures (Belz et al. 2020). Hyperkalemia and hypernatremia may occur in patients who are dehydrated, particularly those who have decreased their fluid intake because of their psychiatric disorder and those who are restricted from eating or drinking prior to ECT (Mashimo et al. 1996). Patients with hyperkalemia are at increased risk of cardiotoxic effects because of the transient rise in serum potassium with succinylcholine (Bali 1975; Hudcova and Schumann 2006). If serum potassium cannot be normalized prior to treatment, a switch to a nondepolarizing muscle relaxant should be made. Heightened release of potassium can occur with succinylcholine administration in patients with diffuse muscle membrane dysfunction, such as extensive severe muscular rigidity, prolonged immobility due to conditions such as catatonia, or widespread acute third-degree burns (Dwersteg and Avery 1987; Hudcova and Schumann 2006; Mashimo et al. 1997; Zisselman and Jaffe 2010). Use of a nondepolarizing muscle relaxant is also warranted in patients with these conditions.

9.2.6. Renal and Bladder Disorders

Chronic kidney disease is associated with an increased risk of electrolyte imbalance and seizures (Sundsted et al. 2014; Títoff et al. 2019). Patients who are receiving hemodialysis are particularly prone to hyperkalemia and other electrolyte abnormalities. In addition to ongoing monitoring of electrolyte levels, ECT treatments should be scheduled on the day after dialysis when possible (McGrane et al. 2022; Pearlman et al. 1988; Watanabe et al. 2023; Wille 2007; Williams and Ostroff 2005). Adequate muscle relaxation should be assured at the time of ECT because patients with chronic kidney disease have decreased bone density and may be at a heightened risk of fracture with the ECT-induced seizure (Sundsted et al. 2014). In patients with a renal transplant, one case report suggests that ECT can be given with appropriate monitoring of medications and renal function (Malaty et al. 2020).

Urinary retention can be the result of psychiatric medications, psychiatric conditions (e.g., catatonia), concomitant medical problems (e.g., prostatic hypertrophy), or medications given during the ECT procedure (e.g., atropine). There are two reported instances of bladder rupture during ECT. The first report was from 1984 in a 74-year-old patient who had modified ECT and a history of difficulty with urinary retention (Irving and Drayson 1984). The second report was in a patient receiving unmodified ECT who had powerful abdominal muscle contractions (O'Brien and Morgan 1991). The risk of bladder rupture seems unlikely, although in severe cases of urinary retention, placement of a foley catheter or straight catheterization before ECT should be considered when the bladder has not been adequately emptied.

9.2.7. Gastrointestinal Disorders

Esophageal reflux with or without hiatal hernia is a common clinical problem and is associated with an increased risk of aspiration during procedures involving general anesthesia (Weiner et al. 2000). Esophageal reflux is particularly common in patients with gastroparesis, morbid obesity, and pregnancy (most notably in the third trimester). Histamine-2 antagonists such as ranitidine (150 mg) given orally the night before and the morning of a treatment will diminish gastric acidity. Metoclopramide, a dopamine receptor antagonist that promotes gastric emptying, is particularly useful in patients with gastroparesis. Another agent that may be used is sodium citrate, which neutralizes gastric contents.

With patients at moderate to high risk of reflux, some anesthesia providers use cricoid pressure during the period of anesthesia, although the effectiveness of this technique is unclear (Brimacombe and Berry 1997). Because of the potential for complications with multiple intubations over an ECT course, endotracheal intubation should be reserved for situations in which the risk of aspiration is high (see Chapter 8 and section 9.4.1 in this chapter).

9.2.8. Skeletal Disorders

Bone fractures occur very rarely with modern ECT techniques. Data from state-mandated reporting programs showed a risk of fracture of 3.56 per 1,000,000 treatments and 2.38 per 100,000 patients treated with ECT (Luccarelli et al. 2020c). Nevertheless, patients with joint or bone disease, including moderate to severe osteoporosis, often need an increased dose of muscle relaxant to assure adequate muscle relaxation with ECT and minimize fracture risk (Coffey et al. 1986; Dighe-Deo and Shah 1998; Hanretta and Malek-Ahmadi 1995; Kellner et al. 1991b; Mashimo et al. 1995; Milstein et al. 1992; Weller and Kornhuber 1992); see Chapter 12. Patients who have recently undergone orthopedic procedures, including spinal surgery, require similar dose adjustments (Musgrave et al. 2020). When indicated by medical history or examination, radiological evaluation prior to ECT can help establish the extent and severity of such conditions. At the time of ECT, a peripheral nerve stimulator can be used to confirm muscle relaxation prior to stimulus delivery (Beale et al. 1994a) (see Chapter 12).

9.2.9. Hematological Disorders

Coagulation abnormalities, due to hematological disorders or treatment with anticoagulants, raise concerns about cerebral hemorrhage due to postictal hypertension with ECT. Several case reports have suggested that patients with hemophilia can safely receive ECT with careful monitoring and administration of factor XIII to reduce bleeding risks (Glaub et al. 1996; Saito et al. 2014). Thrombocytopenia is associated with an increased risk of spontaneous bleeding, although case reports show that ECT can be done safely in this patient population (Gonzalez-Arriaza et al. 2001; Kardener 1968) as well as in patients with thrombocythemia (Hamilton and Walter-Ryan 1986).

In patients with thrombophlebitis and other hypercoagulable states who are receiving ECT, heparin or warfarin have typically been used as anticoagulants (Weiner et al. 2000). With warfarin, an international ratio (INR) in the range of 2–3 is generally viewed as safe for patients to undergo ECT (Mehta et al. 2004; Petrides and Fink 1996a).

An alternative to use of heparin or warfarin is one of the direct oral anticoagulants (DOACs), including dabigatran, which is a direct thrombin inhibitor, and apixaban, rivaroxaban, and edoxaban, which are factor Xa inhibitors (Centanni et al. 2021). DOACs appear to have a lower risk of spontaneous major bleeding and intracranial hemorrhages compared with warfarin and do not require blood monitoring for INR levels or other coagulation measures, but they have no standardized approach for measuring the degree of anticoagulation or potential toxicity (Chai-Adisaksopha et al. 2014). A retrospective cohort study in a medically complex sample of patients receiving ECT showed that few major adverse events were associated with anticoagulation with either a DOAC or warfarin (Centanni et al. 2021).

Patients with sickle cell disease have also tolerated ECT according to several reported cases (Dhossche et al. 2009; Ghignone et al. 2015; LaGrone 1990), but use of the cuff technique is contraindicated to avoid stasis and induction of red blood cell sickling in the cuffed extremity.

Patients with acute hepatic porphyria, such as acute intermittent porphyria, are intolerant to barbiturates and must be switched to an alternative anesthetic agent (Shaw and McKeith 1998). Prolonged fasting and dehydration should be avoided, and acute attacks of porphyria require input from a porphyria specialist (Wilson-Baig et al. 2021).

9.2.10. Ophthalmological Disorders

Administration of ECT is associated with a brief increase in intraocular pressure, presumably by multiple mechanisms (Edwards et al. 1990; Van Den Berg and Honjol 1998; Wachtel et al. 2014). Although this effect is theoretically a concern, case reports support the safety of ECT after intraocular lens implantation due to cataracts (Aneja et al. 2013;

Dubuc et al. 2022; Saad et al. 2000; Sienaert and Vanholst 2013) and in patients with open-angle glaucoma (Amritwar et al. 2016; Aneja et al. 2013; Good et al. 2004; Song et al. 2004; Van Den Berg and Honjol 1998). Most practitioners administer antiglaucoma medications before each treatment for patients who take them on a routine basis. Long-acting anticholinesterase ophthalmic solutions, such as demecarium and echothiophate, could prolong succinylcholine-induced apnea (Chessen et al. 1974; Messer et al. 1992; Packman et al. 1978). These medications can be replaced by alternative agents for an appropriate time period prior to ECT, or a nondepolarizing muscle relaxant can be substituted for succinylcholine (Messer et al. 1992; Packman et al. 1978). A single case report described use of ECT in a patient with a titanium-based uveoscleral stent for glaucoma (Rasheed et al. 2022). Closed- or narrow-angle glaucoma is a medical emergency and represents a greater risk with ECT, although no reports have been made of such patients being referred for ECT.

Retinal detachment has been considered a substantial risk with ECT. Case reports have described successful use of ECT after surgery for retinal reattachment (Friedlander and Francois 2020; Wachtel et al. 2014). It should be noted, however, that ECT was associated with bilateral posterior detachment of the vitreous humor in two patients (Martínez-Amorós et al. 2009; Taye et al. 2018), with ECT stopped in one patient and continued in the other. Given the potential complications, including blindness, ophthalmological consultation and careful consideration of benefits and risks of treatment are needed before deciding to administer ECT in patients with a history of retinal detachment.

9.2.11. Other Medical Conditions

In patients with neoplastic disease, modifications in ECT technique are needed only if a mass effect is present in the brain, if associated hematological changes affect coagulation, if affected organ systems raise the risk associated with transient ECT-induced autonomic changes, or if the patient's antineoplastic agents adversely interact with medications used at the time of ECT (Beale et al. 1997b; Magen and D'Mello 1995).

Case reports suggest that patients with HIV can be safely treated with ECT (Ferrando and Nims 2006; Kessing et al. 1994; Schaerf et al. 1989). There are no clear data on the development of CNS disease in patients with blood-borne infections who are being treated with ECT. Nevertheless, there is a theoretical possibility that such infections could enter the CNS with the transient opening in the blood-brain barrier associated with the ECT-induced increase in blood pressure (Andrade and Bolwig 2014; Bolwig et al. 1977; Zimmermann et al. 2012).

9.3. ECT in Patients With Implanted Medical Devices

Implanted medical devices can also contribute to risk when providing ECT. As one example, the presence of a cochlear implant has been described as a relative contraindication to ECT because of possible damage to the device during the ECT stimulus (Malek-Ahmadi and Hanretta 2003). The FDA states that patients may not be able to have ECT with cochlear implants (U.S. Food and Drug Administration 2021). Manufacturers also describe ECT as contraindicated in patients with cochlear implants (Cochlear 2022). However, a review of the available literature, which consisted of four case reports and a cadaveric study, suggested that it may be possible to administer ECT in patients with cochlear implants (Albertsen and Lauridsen 2022; Cooper et al. 2019; Jiam et al. 2021; Labadie et al. 2010; McRackan et al. 2014). Some clinicians have recommended that risks might be decreased by using contralateral or bifrontal ECT to minimize the proximity of the cochlear implant to the ECT stimulus electrodes (Reveles Jensen et al. 2020). Prior to administering ECT, the potential benefits and risks of ECT should also be discussed in consultation with an otolaryngologist and with the patient as part of the informed consent process (see Chapter 10).

Vagus nerve stimulation (VNS) involves the implantation of a pulse generator that connects to the vagus nerve and provides brief intermittent amounts of electrical stimulation for the treatment of refractory depression and refractory seizures (see Chapter 24). Patients with a VNS device can be safely treated with ECT (Baweja and Singareddy 2013; Katzell et al. 2023; Sharma et al. 2009); however, it is recommended that the device be deactivated prior to each treatment (Burke and Husain 2006). Following ECT, the device should be interrogated to ensure proper functioning and then reset to the patient's usual stimulation parameters.

Data regarding the use of ECT on patients with an implanted deep brain stimulation (DBS) electrode is currently limited. Case reports suggest that ECT can be administered to patients undergoing DBS (Bailine et al. 2008; Bukowski et al. 2022; Chou et al. 2005; Moscarillo and Annunziata 2000; Nasr et al. 2011; Vila-Rodriguez et al. 2014; Volkaerts et al. 2020); however, additional research is still needed to establish the safety and efficacy of ECT in this group of patients. One case report describes the administration of ECT shortly after removal of a DBS electrode (Reinfeld et al. 2023).

Patients with implanted cardiac pacemakers (Dolenc et al. 2004a; MacPherson et al. 2006; Purohith et al. 2023) and implanted cardiac defibrillators (Dolenc et al. 2004a; Goldberg and Badger 1993; Pornnoppadol and Isenberg 1998) can safely receive ECT with appropriate pretreatment screening and posttreatment monitoring. In fact, implanted cardiac pacemakers generally have a protective effect during ECT because they improve control of cardiac rate and rhythm (Alexopoulos and Frances 1980; Morgan 1987; Pearlman 1986). Conversion of a demand pacemaker to a fixed pacing mode is not typically needed (Dolenc et al. 2004a; Giltay et al. 2005; MacPherson et al. 2006), although the pacemaker should be interrogated to ensure that it is functioning properly. For patients with implanted cardiac defibrillators, a cardiac electrophysiologist should be consulted to determine whether the unit's defibrillator function should be inhibited at the time of each treatment (Dolenc et al. 2004a; Goldberg and Badger 1993; Pornnoppadol and Isenberg 1998; Streckenbach et al. 2020), although in such circumstances, the pacemaker function should remain operative.

Other implanted devices (e.g., spinal stimulators) are generally considered to be safe for use in patients receiving ECT (Chen et al. 2020; Conklin and Nussbaum 2021; Mingo and Kominsky 2018); however, to avoid unintended changes to device settings, such devices should be disabled or turned off at the time of ECT.

9.4. ECT During Pregnancy and the Puerperium

9.4.1. Pregnancy

When ECT is clinically indicated for the management of a specific disorder, information from hundreds of case reports supports its use in all three trimesters of pregnancy as a treatment with high efficacy and relatively low risk (Anderson and Reti 2009; Calaway et al. 2016; Coshal et al. 2019; Ray-Griffith et al. 2016; Rose et al. 2020; Sinha et al. 2017; Ward et al. 2018; Yonkers et al. 2004). In addition, a report from the American Psychiatric Association and the American College of Obstetricians and Gynecologists on the treatment of depression during pregnancy emphasizes the effectiveness and safety of ECT (Yonkers et al. 2009). Nevertheless, facilities intending to use ECT during pregnancy should have resources available to deal with obstetric and neonatal emergencies

(American College of Obstetricians and Gynecologists 2019; Practice Guidelines for Obstetric Anesthesia 2016; Rabie et al. 2021; Rose et al. 2020; Ward et al. 2018).

Prior to ECT, an obstetrician should be consulted to clarify the risks to the patient and fetus and to suggest any indicated treatment modifications (Rose et al. 2020). Special emphasis should be placed on assessing risk factors for spontaneous abortion, preterm labor, placental abruption, uteroplacental insufficiency, and fetal arrhythmias (Anderson and Reti 2009; Coshal et al. 2019; Sinha et al. 2017; Ward et al. 2018). Potential risks of medications should be reviewed in terms of teratogenic effects, neonatal toxicity, and maternal side effects. It should also be noted that lack of effective treatment could adversely affect the health and welfare of both the patient and the fetus (Cohen et al. 2006; Jarde et al. 2016; Marcus 2009; Suri et al. 2014; Viguera et al. 2000). Discussions of these issues should be included as part of the informed consent process (see Chapter 10).

From the standpoints of teratogenicity and neonatal toxicity, ECT is considered relatively safe. Estimations of the strength of the electric field that could reach the fetus suggest that levels would be below international thresholds and unlikely to produce any impact on the fetal brain (Kibret et al. 2018). Brief exposures to anesthetic agents are not likely to be problematic even in the first trimester of pregnancy because at ordinary therapeutic doses, teratogenesis is largely a function of exposure duration (U.S. Department of Health and Human Services 2005).

In terms of medications used during ECT, succinylcholine has a relatively low ratio of placental transfer (Briggs et al. 2022; Guay et al. 1998). Thus, although data are limited, the medication is not expected to have an effect on the fetus (Briggs et al. 2022; Guay et al. 1998). In the Collaborative Perinatal Project, no fetal abnormalities were noted in the 26 women who received succinylcholine in the first trimester (Heinonen et al. 1977). Data on vecuronium and rocuronium in pregnancy are limited, particularly during the first trimester (Briggs et al. 2022). At later times during pregnancy, vecuronium appears to have little, if any, risk to the fetus or neonate, but fewer data are available for rocuronium (Briggs et al. 2022). If a nondepolarizing muscle-relaxing agent is indicated, however, the Society for Obstetric Anesthesia and Perinatology recommends avoiding use of sugammadex in early pregnancy and avoiding sugammadex or using it with caution near term because of possible effects on progesterone (Society for Obstetric Anesthesia and Perinatology 2019).

For anesthetic agents, the FDA has issued a safety announcement warning that "repeated or lengthy use of general anesthetic and sedation drugs during surgeries or procedures…in pregnant patients during their third trimester may affect the development of children's brains" (U.S. Food and Drug Administration 2016, 2017). However, the American College of Obstetricians and Gynecologists' Committee on Obstetric Practice and the American Society of Anesthesiologists noted that "There is no evidence that in utero human exposure to anesthetic or sedative drugs has any effect on the developing fetal brain; and there are no animal data to support an effect with limited exposures less than 3 hours in duration" (American College of Obstetricians and Gynecologists 2019). On this basis, the risk of brief periods of anesthesia with ECT appears to be low but warrants consideration in discussing the potential benefits and risks of treatment as part of informed consent (see Chapter 10).

In terms of teratogenic risks, study has been limited (Briggs et al. 2022), although data from the Collaborative Perinatal Project do not suggest any increase in teratogenesis for methohexital (Friedman 1988; Heinonen et al. 1977). Placental transfer of barbiturates does occur (Briggs et al. 2022), and if methohexital is given just prior to delivery, it may be associated with a dose-related increase in neonatal sedation, respiratory depression, and slowing of fetal heart rate (Holdcroft et al. 1974; Ward et al. 2018). Data on etomidate are also limited, but etomidate does not appear to confer an increased risk of fetal or neonatal harm near term (Briggs et al. 2022). Two small studies suggested that etomidate used at the time of cesarean section was associated with transient reductions in cortisol (Crozier et al. 1993; Reddy et al. 1988), but the implications of this finding for etomidate use with ECT are unclear. Data on propofol are similarly sparse, but propofol crosses rapidly into the placenta, with umbilical blood concentrations that are approximately 70% of maternal blood concentrations (Briggs et al. 2022). In research done at the time of cesarean section, most studies showed no effect of propofol on the neonate on time to sustained spontaneous respiration, infant Apgar scores, or neurological or neurobehavioral ratings at bolus doses of 2.5 mg/kg; however, there are some reports of lower Apgar scores and neurobehavioral depression, particularly with higher continuous doses of propofol such as 9 mg/kg/hr (Briggs et al. 2022).

Anticholinergic agents are not routinely used during pregnancy because they may augment aspiration risk by decreasing the tone of the lower esophageal sphincter (Ward et al. 2018). If an anticholinergic agent is indicated in the pregnant patient, glycopyrrolate is usually preferable because its placental transfer rate is more limited than that of atropine (Abboud et al. 1983; Ali-Melkkilä et al. 1990; Briggs et al. 2022; Proakis and Harris 1978).

Because of the increased risks of gastric reflux and possible aspiration during pregnancy, premedication with a non-particulate antacid such as sodium citrate is suggested, particularly after the first trimester, to reduce the risk of developing aspiration pneumonitis. Aspiration-related risks can also be reduced by administering agents that enhance gastric motility, such as metoclopramide, or histamine type 2 (H_2) antagonists (American Society of Anesthesiologists 2017). Of the available H_2 antagonists, famotidine has been used during pregnancy without apparent teratogenicity or neonatal toxicity (American Society of Anesthesiologists 2017; Briggs et al. 2022; Koren and Zemlickis 1991; Magee et al. 1996; Ward et al. 2018). Cimetidine has also been used during pregnancy but may be less preferred because of reports of antiandrogenic effects in adult humans and fetal rats (Briggs et al. 2022).

At the time of ECT, patients should be well oxygenated to maximize delivery of oxygen to the fetus (Ward et al. 2018). However, hyperventilation should be avoided because this may diminish fetal oxygenation by decreasing placental blood flow and by reducing the dissociation of oxygen from hemoglobin (Tomimatsu et al. 2013; Ward et al. 2018). Before each treatment, intravenous hydration with a balanced salt solution is also important to assure adequate blood volume for the patient and the fetus (Ward et al. 2018).

After 20 weeks of gestation, a wedge should be placed under the patient's right hip to provide left uterine displacement and minimize restrictions on blood return from a compressed vena cava (Ward et al. 2018). Some studies suggest that a tilt of 30° is optimal (Auron et al. 2021; Lee and Landau 2017), but such measurements are challenging in clinical settings. Instead, fetal heart rate monitoring is typically used to assure that placental perfusion is adequate.

Decisions on the use of fetal monitoring and its type should be individualized on the basis of gestational age (American College of Obstetricians and Gynecologists 2019). In addition, if the fetus is likely to be viable ex utero, determination of a monitoring approach and the need for steroids or other prophylactic medications will depend on the wishes of the patient for management if fetal distress occurs preterm.

Typically, when gestational age is more than 14–16 weeks, fetal heart rate should be measured by Doppler ultrasound before and after each treatment (American College of Obstetricians and Gynecologists 2019; Ward et al. 2018). Beyond 23 weeks, simultaneous electronic fetal heart rate and contraction monitoring is typically performed before and after each treatment (American College of Obstetricians and Gynecologists 2019). Some obstetricians suggest continuous fetal heart rate monitoring and simultaneous contraction activity monitoring throughout any procedure involving anesthesia for nonobstetrical surgery (Auron et al. 2021), and such an approach has also been used in patients receiving ECT during pregnancy (Rabie et al. 2021). In selected circumstances, additional monitoring may be indicated to optimize the well-being of the fetus (American College of Obstetricians and Gynecologists 2019; Ward et al. 2018). Near term, the treatment location should assure ready access to facilities and equipment for handling obstetric and neonatal emergencies.

Some anesthesiologists consider intubation with ECT during pregnancy (Ward et al. 2018). Although the ECT literature has typically mentioned the possibility of intubation beyond 24 weeks of gestation and particularly near term, decisions should be made on the basis of individual patient characteristics. Some patients may benefit from intubation earlier in pregnancy, whereas others can be appropriately treated without intubation late in pregnancy. In all instances, the risks of aspiration should be weighed against the risks of repeated intubations, both of which are greater in the pregnant patient. In the context of ECT, most experience involves endotracheal intubation, but use of a laryngeal mask airway can also be considered (Brown et al. 2003).

For post-ECT headache and muscle soreness during pregnancy, acetaminophen is the treatment of choice (Briggs et al. 2022). Particularly in the third trimester of pregnancy, aspirin and nonsteroidal anti-inflammatory agents should not be administered because they may contribute to altered hemostasis in the patient and fetus and to early constriction or closure of the fetal ductus arteriosus (Briggs et al. 2022).

Metoclopramide can be used for symptomatic treatment of nausea (Briggs et al. 2022). Doxylamine-pyridoxine and ondansetron have also been used to treat nausea and vomiting in the context of hyperemesis gravidarum (McParlin et al. 2016) and may also be appropriate for treating these symptoms in the context of ECT. However, there is conflicting evidence as to whether ondansetron use in the first trimester might increase the possibility of oral clefts or cardiac abnormalities (Damkier et al. 2021; Huybrechts et al. 2018; Kaplan et al. 2019; Picot et al. 2020). Consequently, some sources suggest that doxylamine-pyridoxine should be the treatment of choice for nausea and vomiting in pregnancy and that ondansetron use should be avoided, particularly in the first trimester (Briggs et al. 2022).

9.4.2. Puerperium

Evidence from case reports suggests that ECT is highly effective for treatment of postpartum depressive or manic episodes, with or without psychosis, as well as in treatment of catatonia (Babu et al. 2013; Focht and Kellner 2012; Forray and Ostroff 2007; Gonzales et al. 2014; Gressier et al. 2015; Haxton et al. 2016; Herzog and Detre 1976; Katona 1982; Nahar et al. 2017; Protheroe 1969; Reed et al. 1999; Robinson and Stewart 1986; Rundgren et al. 2018). Rates of response appear to be at least as high as and perhaps higher than when ECT is used outside the perinatal period.

When a course of acute or maintenance ECT is administered in the postpartum period, breastfeeding need not be interrupted because it has clear benefits for the infant as well as for the patient. Nevertheless, the informed consent process should discuss the potential effects on the breastfed infant of medications given during ECT (see Chapter 10). In addition, exposure of breastfeeding infants to medications may be lessened if the patient delays the feeding for several hours after an ECT treatment.

Anesthetic agents administered with ECT pose little risk to the nursing infant. Infant exposure to succinylcholine is minimal, and absorption of succinylcholine from the gastrointestinal tract is poor (Lee and Rubin 1993). For methohexital, the relative infant exposure from breast milk has been estimated to be less than 1% of the administered dose (Borgatta et al. 1997). Limited information is available on etomidate, but one study showed negligible concentrations persisting in breast milk 120 minutes after a single dose of the medication (Esener et al. 1992). Amounts of propofol in breast milk also appear to be small and unlikely to have an effect on the infant (Nitsun et al. 2006).

Other medications administered during ECT may also be excreted into breast milk. Consequently, the indications for such medications and their potential effects on the nursing infant should be evaluated prior to administration. The small concentrations of atropine that appear in breast milk are generally safe for the suckling infant (American Academy of Pediatrics Committee on Drugs 2001), but some infants have exhibited sensitivity to the toxic effects of anticholinergic medications (Dillon et al. 1997). No data are available on glycopyrrolate levels in breast milk (Briggs et al. 2022).

H_2 receptor antagonists are excreted into breast milk but at levels that are less than those achieved when these medications are used for therapeutic purposes in newborns (National Library of Medicine 2020b, 2020c). Acetaminophen or nonsteroidal anti-inflammatory medications, such as ibuprofen, may be used to treat headache or muscle soreness after ECT (National Library of Medicine 2018a, 2018b). Use of aspirin is not recommended because it has been associated with adverse effects in nursing infants (American Academy of Pediatrics Committee on Drugs 2001; Briggs et al. 2022). Furthermore, it is not clear whether aspirin contributes to risk of Reye syndrome in an infant (National Library of Medicine 2020a).

9.5. Children and Adolescents

Although the extremely low rate of ECT use in younger populations (Trivedi et al. 2021) has precluded clinical trials, there is accumulating evidence from case reports (Castaneda-Ramirez et al. 2023; Døssing and Pagsberg 2021; Ghaziuddin et al. 2004; Puffer et al. 2016; Rey and Walter 1997; Stein et al. 2020) and a national registry study (Rask et al. 2023) that ECT is a safe and effective treatment modality for children and adolescents whose symptoms have not responded to treatment or who require an urgent definitive response. The low utilization rate of ECT in children and adolescents in the United States is associated with multiple factors, including regulatory issues (Livingston et al. 2018), lack of knowledge of child and adolescent psychiatrists about the use of ECT (Ghaziuddin et al. 2001; Walter et al. 1997), and concerns that sequelae of induced seizures may be greater in a developing nervous system than in adults (Døssing and Pagsberg 2021). However, the absence of severe or developmentally disruptive adverse cognitive effects in younger individuals in long-term follow-up studies has significantly reduced these earlier concerns (Cohen et al. 2000; de la Serna et al. 2011; Mitchell et al. 2018). In addition, medical risks associated with ECT are low unless the patient is medically unstable prior to referral (Stein et al. 2020). At the present time, in terms of state regulations, ECT is subject to age-related constraints in multiple states and is prohibited in California for patients younger than age 12 years and in Texas and Colorado for those younger than 16 years (Livingston et al. 2018). Nationally, the FDA has recommended ECT only for those age 13 or older (U.S. Food and Drug Administration 2018b); however, in contrast to prohibitive state regulations mentioned above and analogous to the use of medications, off-label ECT use is allowable for all ages if otherwise justified.

Literature reviews of acute ECT efficacy (Døssing and Pagsberg 2021) have reported similar rates of improvement as in adult populations (see Chapter 2) when ECT is administered to children and adolescents with mood disorders (Cohen et al. 1997; Luccarelli et al. 2021c; Walter and Rey 1997), schizophrenia (Zhang et al. 2012), and catatonia (Consoli et al. 2010; Dhossche and Withane 2019; Ghaziuddin et al. 2017; Raffin et al. 2015). A registry-based study of ECT in Sweden compared individuals younger than age 18 to adults and found that a significant proportion of those younger than 18 responded to ECT (57% response, 30% remission, $n=95$), although they were more severely ill, on average, than adult patients (Rask et al. 2023). Patients younger than age 18 with depression and psychosis showed particularly robust responses to treatment (90% with response, 60% with remission, $n=10$; Rask et al. 2023). In addition, a growing number of case reports and series have demonstrated the value of ECT for autoimmune encephalitis with behavioral and autonomic dysfunction (Mooneyham et al. 2021; Tanguturi et al. 2019; Warren et al. 2019), neuroleptic malignant syndrome (Ghaziuddin et al. 2017), severely debilitating self-injurious behavior associated with autism (Rootes-Murdy et al. 2019; Wachtel 2019), and status epilepticus (Nath et al. 2021) in children and adolescents. Little has been written about the use of maintenance ECT with children and adolescents, although there is some evidence from case series that it appears to be effective and well tolerated (Ghaziuddin et al. 2011).

Each institution should have policies for the use of ECT in minors. These policies should be compatible with applicable state and federal regulations and should include discussion of informed consent, particularly with regard to the circumstances under which individuals should be considered adults for the purposes of consent for medical procedures (see Chapter 10). If ECT is provided to children younger than age 13 years, it should be only with the concurrence of two consultants experienced in treating psychiatric disorders of this age group. These consultants should deliver their opinion only after interviewing the patient and family or other collateral sources, reviewing the clinical record, and discussing the child with the patient's attending physician.

Given a more substantial literature documenting the safety and efficacy of ECT in adolescents (Ghaziuddin et al. 2004), one consultant should suffice for this age group. The consent process, including discussion of the risks and benefits of ECT, should involve the parents or guardians of the child (Taieb et al. 2001). When clinically appropriate or if required by local regulations, assent of the child or adolescent should also be obtained (see Chapter 10).

Stimulus dosing must take into account the fact that seizure thresholds in children and adolescents are likely to be considerably lower than those in adults (Ghaziuddin et al. 2004). Use of empirical dose titration with low initial dosage settings is particularly encouraged in this age group (see Chapter 14). In addition, there is evidence that children and adolescents may have longer seizures than do adults, including more frequent prolonged seizures (Ghaziuddin et al. 2020). For this reason, the treatment team should be prepared to intervene to terminate the seizure with an appropriate medication if the seizure duration is prolonged (see Chapter 21).

For additional information on the use of ECT in adolescents, the reader is referred to the practice parameter of the American Academy of Child and Adolescent Psychiatry (Ghaziuddin et al. 2004) as well as their more recent treatment guidelines on the management of adolescents with specific disorders (Birmaher et al. 2007; McClellan et al. 2007, 2013). Reviews discussing relevant age-appropriate measures for assessing treatment outcome are also available (Stallwood et al. 2021; Stockings et al. 2015).

9.6. Geriatric Patients

ECT has a special role in the treatment of late-life depression and other psychiatric conditions in geriatric patients (Kerner and Prudic 2014; McDonald 2016; Meyer et al. 2020; Weiner et al. 2023), who as a group constitute a relatively high proportion of the patients who receive ECT. In states requiring mandatory reporting of all ECT treatments, the proportion of ECT provided to individuals age 65 years or older ranged from 22%· in Vermont (2009–2018) to 30.8% in California (2008–2017) (Luccarelli et al. 2020b). In comparison with a depressed cohort not receiving ECT, a recent Swedish National Registry study (Stenmark et al. 2021) reported a higher median age with the ECT group (59 years vs. 45 years).

Although age per se does not constitute a particular indication for ECT in major depressive disorder or other diagnostic groups, geriatric patients may have an increased likelihood of factors leading to referral for ECT (see Chapter 2). Such factors include intolerance or resistance to antidepressant medications as well as urgent need for a rapid, definitive response (e.g., presence of severe inanition, refusal to eat, psychosis) (Haq et al. 2015; Heijnen et al. 2019). Such findings are consistent with evidence that the acute efficacy of ECT for treatment of major depression is at least as great with geriatric patients as with younger age groups (O'Connor et al. 2001; van Diermen et al. 2018), as is improvement in quality of life (Güney et al. 2020; McCall et al. 2018). In this regard, a recent study of ultrabrief RUL ECT in a geriatric cohort reported acute response and remission rates of 70% and 62% using conservative outcome measures (Kellner et al. 2016b). In addition to acute efficacy, maintenance ECT in geriatric patients also has beneficial effects on both relapse (Kellner et al. 2016a; Rapinesi et al. 2013) and rehospitalization rate (O'Connor et al. 2010; Shelef et al. 2015; Stenmark et al. 2021).

Administration of ECT in geriatric patients presents certain age-related issues. Seizure threshold rises with increasing age, and effective seizures may be more difficult to induce (Boylan et al. 2000; Gálvez et al. 2015; Sackeim et al. 1987b) (see also Chapter 14, section 14.7). In addition, because of altered metabolism in geriatric patients, dosages of medications used with ECT may need to be adjusted.

The risk of adverse medical effects is also greater with ECT in geriatric patients, although evidence suggests that this increased risk relates to greater medical comorbidity with age rather than to age per se (Kaster et al. 2021). In addition, the morbidity and mortality of not intervening with ECT often outweighs the risks involved with ECT administration, particularly in severely medically compromised geriatric patients who have not responded to other treatments. There is also evidence that successful treatment with ECT in depressed geriatric patients results in lower long-term morbidity and mortality rates (Philibert et al. 1995; Rhee et al. 2021).

Given the increased likelihood of preexisting cognitive impairment with aging, concerns have been raised that geriatric patients have a greater risk for acute treatment-related cognitive impairment with ECT, particularly in regard to memory function (Kumar et al. 2016; Tielkes et al. 2008). However, more recent evidence that controls for baseline cognitive impairment suggests that ECT is relatively well tolerated (Copersino et al. 2022; Dominiak et al. 2021b; Luccarelli et al. 2022), particularly with the use of ultrabrief pulse widths and RUL electrode placement (Lisanby et al. 2020). For that matter, ECT appears to be well tolerated even in geriatric patients with coexisting mild cognitive impairment (Hausner et al. 2011). In addition, ECT does not appear to increase long-term risk of developing dementia (Hjerrild et al. 2021).

Recommendations

9.1. General Considerations

1. An assessment of the relative risks and benefits of ECT should be undertaken for each patient that includes the following:
   a. Consideration of the severity and duration of the psychiatric illness and its threat to life
   b. Likelihood of therapeutic success with ECT
   c. Medical risks of ECT and the degree to which these risks can be diminished
   d. The benefits and risks of alternative treatments and of no treatment

2. After assessing the relative risks and benefits of ECT as compared with other options, a choice of treatment is made, discussed as part of the informed consent process, and documented in the medical record.

9.2. ECT in Patients With Comorbid Medical Disorders

1. The risks of medical adverse events should be minimized by modifying ECT procedures or by optimizing the patient's medical condition prior to ECT, keeping in mind any risks that may be associated with delaying the start of ECT.

2. ECT facilities should be appropriately equipped and staffed with personnel to manage potential clinical emergencies.

9.2.1. Cardiovascular Disorders

1. Unless there is clear evidence to the contrary, current medications likely to diminish cardiovascular risk with ECT (e.g., antihypertensives, β-blocking agents, diuretics, antiarrhythmics) should be continued. If the medication is prescribed for morning administration, it can be taken on the morning of ECT with a sip of water.

2. Because of its pronounced anticonvulsant effects, lidocaine should be avoided prior to and during the induced seizure unless a potentially life-threatening complication is present.

3. Cardiovascular risks of ECT derive primarily from the marked changes in heart rate and blood pressure that typically occur during and immediately after the electrical stimulus and induced seizure.
4. The type and severity of preexisting cardiac disease affects the likelihood, type, and severity of cardiac complications during ECT.
5. Cardiovascular conditions that may be associated with an increase in risk and that warrant careful evaluation as part of the pre-ECT assessment include arrhythmias, systemic or pulmonary hypertension, valvular heart disease, coronary artery disease, heart failure, a reduced ejection fraction, vascular aneurysms, or a history of coronary artery stenting or coronary artery bypass graft surgery.
6. A significant increase in risk may be present in patients with uncontrolled hypertension, recent MI (<60 days), unstable angina, decompensated heart failure, severe aortic stenosis, uncontrolled atrial fibrillation, unrepaired abdominal aortic aneurysms >5.0 cm, or tachyarrhythmias or bradyarrhythmias associated with hypotension or requiring urgent medical attention.
7. When atrial fibrillation is present in a patient who is referred for ECT, heart rate should be well controlled.
8. Because ECT may convert atrial fibrillation to a sinus rhythm, anticoagulation may be indicated to diminish risk of embolism from atrial mural thrombi; however, decisions related to anticoagulation should occur in consultation with a cardiologist.

9.2.2. Pulmonary Disorders

1. Consultation with anesthesiology or other staff regarding management (e.g., pre-ECT use of bronchodilators, attention to pretreatment oxygenation) is often indicated in patients with significant pulmonary disease.
2. Patients with COPD should receive pretreatment with any prescribed bronchodilators or inhalers as well as preoxygenation on the morning of each ECT treatment.
3. Caution is recommended when administering ECT to patients taking theophylline, which has been associated with prolonged seizures.
4. ECT can be safely administered to asthmatic patients; however, these patients should have bronchodilators available for use both before and after each ECT treatment.

5. ECT can be safely administered shortly after the occurrence of pulmonary embolism, with attention before and during the ECT course to cardiac function, anticoagulation status, and evidence of residual deep vein thrombosis either clinically or by ultrasound.

6. For patients with active COVID-19 infection or other respiratory infections, appropriate personal protective equipment and infection control precautions are crucial in addition to monitoring of the patient's pulmonary status.

9.2.3. Neurological Disorders

1. The size and acuity of space-occupying cerebral lesions is associated with the magnitude of risk.

2. Patients with signs of increased intracranial pressure (e.g., significant headache, papilledema, focal neurological deficits) or who have brain edema, mass-related displacement, or cerebrovascular fragility on imaging studies are at increased risk of acute neurological decompensation and should be evaluated carefully prior to ECT.

3. Risk mitigation strategies in individuals with an increased intracranial pressure or other risk factors for herniation may include hyperventilation at the time of ECT and treatment with antihypertensive agents, diuretics, and steroids to reduce the acute ECT-related hypertensive surge and intracerebral edema.

4. When ECT is determined to be indicated in individuals at risk for a cerebrovascular bleed (e.g., very recent hemorrhagic strokes, cerebral aneurysms), the acute ECT-related hypertensive surge should be pharmacologically blunted, whereas in patients with ischemic cerebrovascular disease, aggressive antihypertensive therapy is generally not needed and may be associated with a risk of hypotensive morbidity.

5. The use of anticonvulsant medication during ECT can complicate treatment; therefore, the indication for anticonvulsant treatment should be confirmed and the dosage of the anticonvulsant should be kept as low as clinically feasible during the ECT course.

6. The evidence for spontaneous seizure activity or a form of kindling associated with ECT is very limited, although clinicians should be observant for any clinical evidence of seizure activity in patients receiving ECT.

7. Patients with intracerebral shunts should have shunt patency assessed prior to ECT.

8. The presence of any skull defects or metallic implants should be noted, and stimulation over a skull defect or metallic implant should be avoided if possible.

9. Patients with traumatic brain injuries or neurodegenerative conditions (e.g., Parkinson's disease, Huntington's disease, dementia) may have an increased risk of developing cognitive side effects during a course of ECT.

10. Patients with Parkinson's disease may develop psychosis or dyskinesia from the combination of dopaminergic medication use and dopaminergic changes produced by ECT; thus, it may be necessary to hold morning doses or reduce doses of dopaminergic medications, particularly L-dopa.

11. Patients with myasthenia gravis or who have upper motor neuron diseases may have altered sensitivity to or slower recovery from depolarizing muscle relaxants such as succinylcholine; a nondepolarizing muscle-relaxing agent (e.g., rocuronium) may be preferable.

12. Patients with multiple sclerosis may benefit from neurological and radiological consultation to determine the optimal imaging approach to identify patients with active cerebral demyelination who are at increased risk of neurological complications with ECT.

9.2.4. Endocrine Disorders

1. Patients with difficult-to-control diabetes or who are treated with insulin may benefit from medical or endocrinological consultation to assist with recommendations about the following:

   a. Monitoring of blood glucose, including assessment within the hour before each treatment

   b. Dosing of antidiabetic agents to account for the fasting period prior to each ECT treatment

2. Treatment of clinically significant hyperthyroidism should be optimized with the assistance of specialty consultation, and β-blocking agents should be used at the time of ECT unless otherwise contraindicated.

3. In a patient with a pheochromocytoma who requires ECT prior to definitive treatment, the risk of hypertension can be minimized

through the use of α-blockers, β-blockers, and blockers of tyrosine hydroxylase.

4. Patients with Addison's disease or steroid dependence may require an additional or increased dose of steroids before each treatment.

9.2.5. Electrolyte Abnormalities

1. Abnormalities in serum sodium and potassium should be corrected, insofar as possible, prior to ECT treatment because they may require alterations in ECT technique or increase ECT risk:

   a. Hypokalemia may be associated with prolonged paralysis and apnea after ECT

   b. Hyponatremia, particularly when severe or acute, can lead to spontaneous seizures

   c. Hyperkalemia can be associated with cardiac effects, particularly because potassium levels may increase further with succinylcholine administration

2. A switch to a nondepolarizing muscle relaxant should be considered for patients with hyperkalemia as well as in those who may experience heightened potassium release with succinylcholine due to diffuse muscle membrane dysfunction (e.g., extensive severe muscular rigidity, prolonged immobility due to conditions such as catatonia or widespread acute third-degree burns).

9.2.6. Renal and Bladder Disorders

1. Chronic kidney disease is associated with electrolyte abnormalities, particularly in patients who are receiving hemodialysis, and ongoing electrolyte monitoring is essential.

2. ECT treatments should be scheduled on the day after hemodialysis when possible.

3. Patients with chronic kidney disease have decreased bone density and may be at a heightened risk of fracture if muscle relaxation is not assured at the time of ECT.

9.2.7. Gastrointestinal Disorders

1. Esophageal reflux is associated with an increased risk of aspiration with anesthesia and is particularly common in patients with gastropa-

resis, morbid obesity, and pregnancy (most notably in the third trimester).

2. The risks associated with possible aspiration can be decreased by the following:

   a. H_2 antagonists such as ranitidine (150 mg) given orally the night before and the morning of a treatment to diminish gastric acidity
   b. Metoclopramide, a dopamine receptor antagonist that promotes gastric emptying, which is particularly useful in patients with gastroparesis
   c. Sodium citrate, which neutralizes gastric contents

3. Endotracheal intubation has a risk of complications, particularly when it occurs multiple times during an ECT course; it should be reserved for patients whose risk of aspiration is high.

9.2.8. Skeletal Disorders

1. An increased dosage of muscle relaxant may be needed in patients with recent orthopedic procedures and in those with joint or bone disease, including moderate to severe osteoporosis.
2. Use of a peripheral nerve stimulator at the time of ECT can help confirm muscle relaxation prior to stimulus delivery.

9.2.9. Hematological Disorders

1. Patients with hematological disorders that have an increased risk of spontaneous bleeding (e.g., hemophilia, thrombocytopenia) can receive ECT with careful monitoring and targeted therapy (e.g., factor XIII for hemophilia) as clinically indicated.
2. Patients with thrombophlebitis and other hypercoagulable states can receive ECT while receiving therapeutic doses of heparin, DOACs, or warfarin (e.g., with INR of 2–3).
3. Patients with sickle cell disease can receive ECT, but use of the cuff technique is contraindicated to avoid stasis and induced red blood cell sickling in the cuffed extremity.
4. Patients with acute hepatic porphyria, such as acute intermittent porphyria, must be switched to a nonbarbiturate anesthetic agent and should avoid prolonged fasting and dehydration.

9.2.10. Ophthalmological Disorders

1. With the exception of long-acting anticholinesterase ophthalmic solutions (e.g., demecarium, echothiophate) that could prolong succinylcholine-induced apnea, patients with glaucoma can have their regular antiglaucoma medications administered before ECT.
2. Patients treated with long-acting anticholinesterase ophthalmic solutions can have these medications replaced by alternative antiglaucoma agents for an appropriate time period prior to ECT, or a nondepolarizing muscle relaxant (e.g., rocuronium) can be used in lieu of succinylcholine for muscle relaxation.
3. Ophthalmological consultation and careful consideration of benefits and risks of treatment are needed before deciding to administer ECT in patients with a history of retinal detachment.

9.2.11. Other Medical Conditions

In patients with neoplastic disease, modifications in ECT technique may be needed (e.g., for CNS masses, significant coagulation or organ system abnormalities, interactions between medications given with ECT and antineoplastic medications).

9.3. ECT in Patients With Implanted Medical Devices

1. The risks and benefits of ECT should be considered carefully before instituting ECT in patients with cochlear implants. Although FDA and manufacturers' warnings caution that ECT is contraindicated in patients with cochlear implants because of the potential damage to the implant, limited evidence suggests that ECT can be done safely in patients with cochlear implants and that risks can be minimized by obtaining otolaryngological consultation and applying the ECT electrodes as far from the site of the implant as possible.
2. Patients with a VNS device can be safely treated with ECT; however, it is recommended that the device be deactivated prior to each treatment, interrogated to ensure proper functioning after each treatment, and then reset to the patient's usual stimulation parameters.
3. Limited information is available about use of ECT in patients with a deep brain stimulator, although case reports suggest that safe treatment with ECT is possible.

4. Patients who have an implanted cardiac device have an increased chance of medical complications during ECT due to underlying cardiac conditions and should have additional pre-ECT screening, cardiology consultation, and post-ECT monitoring.
5. Conversion of a demand pacemaker to a fixed pacing mode is typically not needed; however, the pacemaker should be interrogated to ensure that it is functioning properly.
6. Implanted cardiac defibrillators are not generally problematic with ECT, and the pacemaker function should remain operative; nevertheless, a cardiac electrophysiologist should be consulted to determine whether the unit's defibrillator function should be inhibited at the time of each treatment.
7. Other implanted devices (e.g., spinal stimulators) are generally considered to be safe for use in patients receiving ECT; however, to avoid unintended changes to device settings, such devices should be disabled or turned off at the time of ECT.

9.4. ECT During Pregnancy and the Puerperium

9.4.1. Pregnancy

1. ECT may be used in all three trimesters of pregnancy when it is clinically indicated for the management of a specific disorder.
2. In pregnant patients, obstetrical consultation should be obtained prior to ECT to suggest any indicated treatment modifications and to clarify the risks to the patient and fetus (e.g., spontaneous abortion; preterm labor; placental abruption; uteroplacental insufficiency; fetal arrhythmias; potential side effects, including teratogenic effects and neonatal toxicity).
3. At facilities administering ECT to pregnant individuals, resources for managing obstetric and neonatal emergencies should be readily accessible.
4. The risks to the fetus of ECT anesthetic agents are likely to be low, but potential teratogenic effects and neonatal toxicities should be discussed in the informed consent process.
5. The informed consent process should also note that lack of effective treatment could adversely affect the health and welfare of both the patient and the fetus.
6. Pregnant patients should be well oxygenated but not hyperventilated during ECT.

7. The risk of aspiration is increased in pregnant patients, and modifications in the ECT procedure (e.g., withholding anticholinergic agents; using endotracheal intubation; administering nonparticulate antacids, gastrointestinal motility enhancing agents, or H_2 blockers) can be considered to alter this risk.

8. Intravenous hydration with a non-glucose-containing solution is suggested before each ECT treatment.

9. After 20 weeks of gestation, uterine blood flow should be optimized by placing a wedge under the patient's right hip to provide left uterine displacement and minimize restrictions on blood return from a compressed vena cava, with monitoring of fetal heart rate to assure that placental perfusion is adequate.

10. Decisions on the use of fetal monitoring and its type should be individualized on the basis of gestational age.

11. If the fetus is likely to be viable ex utero, determination of a monitoring approach and the need for steroids or other prophylactic medications will depend on the wishes of the patient for management if fetal distress occurs preterm.

12. Typically, when gestational age is more than 14–16 weeks, fetal heart rate should be measured by Doppler ultrasound before and after each treatment.

13. Beyond 23 weeks, simultaneous electronic fetal heart rate and contraction monitoring is typically performed before and after each treatment.

14. Some obstetricians suggest continuous fetal heart rate monitoring and simultaneous contraction activity monitoring.

15. In selected circumstances, additional monitoring may be indicated at the time of ECT.

16. Near term, the treatment location should assure ready access to facilities and equipment for handling obstetric and neonatal emergencies.

17. For symptomatic treatment of nausea, headache, or muscle soreness, medications should be chosen that are appropriate for use during pregnancy.

9.4.2. Puerperium

1. ECT is a highly effective treatment for postpartum depressive or manic episodes, with or without psychosis, as well as in treatment of catatonia.

2. Breastfeeding does not usually need to be interrupted during an acute or maintenance course of ECT; however, the informed consent process should include a discussion of the potential risks to the infant of breastfeeding during the ECT course.
3. The indications for medications administered with ECT and their potential effects on the nursing infant should be evaluated before the medications are given.
4. Anesthetic agents administered with ECT generally pose little risk to the nursing infant, but other medications given during ECT may be excreted into breast milk.
5. Infant medication exposure from breastfeeding may be lessened by delaying feeding for several hours after an ECT treatment.

9.5. Children and Adolescents

1. In children and adolescents, ECT should be reserved for instances in which other viable treatments have not been effective or in which an urgent definitive response is needed.
2. Diagnostic indications for ECT in children and adolescents are the same as those described for adults in Chapter 2 and can include patients with treatment-resistant autoimmune encephalitis with behavioral and autonomic dysfunction, severely debilitating self-injurious behavior associated with autism, and status epilepticus.
3. Before ECT is administered to children younger than age 13, concurrence with the recommendation for ECT should be provided by two consultants who are experienced in the treatment of children. For adolescents, concurrence needs to be provided by only a single consultant.
4. Stimulus dosing should take into account that seizure thresholds are likely to be lower in children and adolescents than in adults.
5. Practitioners should be aware that ECT seizures are often longer than in adults and that the likelihood of prolonged seizures is greater.
6. Each facility offering ECT for children or adolescents should have policies, including policies on informed consent, that address the use of ECT in this patient population.

9.6. Geriatric Patients

1. ECT may be used with geriatric patients, regardless of age.
2. All somatic treatments, including ECT, are associated with increased risk in geriatric patients because of greater medical comorbidity

with increasing age. However, any such increase in risk should be considered in the context of the risks associated with the underlying illness and of other treatment options.

3. Doses of anticholinergic, anesthetic, and relaxant agents may need to be modified on the basis of the physiological changes associated with aging.

4. ECT stimulus dosing should take into account the fact that seizure threshold generally increases with age.

5. Decisions about ECT technique should be guided by the possibility that ECT-induced cognitive dysfunction may be greater in geriatric patients, particularly if preexisting cognitive or neurological impairment is present.

CHAPTER 10

Consent for Electroconvulsive Therapy

10.1. General

The formal legal doctrine of informed consent has evolved over decades from "the core notion that decisions regarding medical care are to be made in a collaborative manner between patient and physician" (Appelbaum et al. 1987, p. 12) to informed consent being based on the disclosure of applicable information to a patient possessing capacity who is permitted to make a voluntary decision regarding a proposed treatment (Appelbaum 2007). In this regard, the conceptual requirements for informed consent proposed by the 1978 and the 2001 American Psychiatric Association Task Force on ECT are still applicable: 1) the provision of adequate information, 2) a patient (or legally ascertained surrogate consenter) who is capable of understanding and acting reasonably on such information, and 3) the opportunity to consent in the absence of coercion. The physician's role in these informed consent interactions also includes involving the consenter in the decision-making process and remaining sensitive to the consenter's thoughts and feelings about the informed consent process. Because consent for electroconvulsive therapy (ECT) is an ongoing process, the physician also needs to keep the consenter abreast of any new information that may modify decisions about treatment. Accordingly, a collaborative interaction between the consenter and the physician is a key component of the informed consent process.

Specific recommendations concerning consent for ECT often reflect a trade-off between preserving patient autonomy and ensuring that patients are not deprived of the opportunity to receive effective treatment (Ottosson 1992). Regulations should not unduly obstruct the patient's access to treatment, and judicial and legislative efforts should be made to correct overregulation (Taub 1987; Winslade et al. 1984). Unnecessary suffering, increased physical morbidity, and even fatalities may result from prolonged delays in provision of ECT to minors and patients who lack the capacity to give consent (Johnson 1993; Miller et al. 1986; Mills and Avery 1978; Roy-Byrne and Gerner 1981; Tenenbaum 1983; Walter-Ryan 1985). In this regard, ECT should not be considered different from other medical or surgical procedures with comparable risks and benefits. A substantial body of literature has described general aspects of informed consent as they relate to ECT (Hersh 2013; Parry 1986; Roth 1986; Taub 1987; Winslade 1988) as well as issues of capacity for consent and use of ECT in legally determined incompetent or involuntarily hospitalized patients (Appelbaum et al. 1987; Bean et al. 1996; Boronow et al. 1997; Culver et al. 1980; Gutheil and Bursztajn 1986; Levine et al. 1991; Mahler et al. 1986; Martin and Bean 1992; Martin and Glancy 1994; Reiter-Theil 1992; Roth et al. 1977; Roy-Byrne and Gerner 1981; Salzman 1977; Wettstein and Roth 1988; Zisselman and Jaffe 2010). Special issues of consent arise for individuals who are incarcerated in jails and prisons, but literature on this topic is limited (Williams and Arvidson 2021).

10.2. When and by Whom Should Consent Be Obtained?

Because informed consent for ECT is mandated both ethically and by regulation, it is incumbent on facilities using ECT to implement and monitor adherence to reasonable and appropriate consenting policies and procedures. Ideally, the consent process involves discussions with the consenter about general aspects of ECT and information unique to the patient, as well as the signing of the informed consent document. The information essential to consent to ECT should be provided by a psychiatrist with clinical ECT privileges (ECT psychiatrist) acting individually or in concert with other professional staff. Consent for anesthesia is often separately obtained by an anesthesia provider, as with many other procedures involving general anesthesia, although it has been combined with the ECT consent process in some settings.

As with consent for medical and surgical procedures, the patient should provide informed consent unless they lack capacity or unless otherwise specified by law. The involvement of significant others in the consent process should be encouraged (Consensus Conference 1985) but is not required (Tenenbaum 1983).

ECT is unusual but not unique among medical procedures because it involves a series of repetitive treatments spaced over an appreciable time period (typically 2–4 weeks for an acute ECT course). Because it is the series of treatments, rather than any single treatment, that confers both the benefits and the adverse effects of ECT, consent for an acute ECT series should apply to the treatment course as a whole (unless otherwise required by law). However, consent should be repeated if an unusually large number of treatments (typically more than 15 or as locally determined) are required to manage an acute episode of illness (see section 10.3).

In addition, because an acute ECT course generally extends over multiple weeks, informed consent should be viewed as a process that continues across this period. Local standards and approaches may vary in the way the consent process is implemented. Information conveyed in the original consent may need to be repeated because patient recall of consent is commonly faulty even for medical and surgical procedures (Hutson and Blaha 1991; Ladenheim et al. 1992; Meisel and Roth 1983; Roth et al. 1982; Swan and Borshoff 1994). For patients receiving ECT, recall may be further diminished by both the underlying illness and the treatment itself (Semkovska and McLoughlin 2010; Squire 1986; Sternberg and Jarvik 1976). In addition, the consenter should be given ongoing feedback about clinical progress and side effects as well as any factors that may substantially influence these outcomes. Any questions or concerns that arise during the ECT course should be addressed (American Psychiatric Association Council on Psychiatry and Law 1997). If the consenter expresses reluctance about receiving ECT, reasons for this reluctance should be explored and addressed, if possible. The consenter should also be reminded of the right to accept or refuse further treatment.

Maintenance ECT differs from an acute course of ECT in that 1) its purpose is to prolong remission and/or minimize risk of relapse, 2) the patient's clinical condition is improved compared with that preceding the acute ECT course, and 3) it is characterized by both a greater intertreatment interval and a less well defined endpoint. Given these distinctions from an acute ECT course, a new informed consent process should be initiated, including the signing of a separate consent form. Because maintenance ECT is provided to individuals who are clinically improved and already knowledgeable about the treatment, informed consent should be obtained initially and renewed on the basis of the number of treatments or a specified duration of time as dictated by local or state requirements. A new consent is also indicated if there are changes in the patient's psychiatric or medical status that would significantly influence the benefits and risks of treatment.

10.3. Information to Be Conveyed

Use of a formal consent document for ECT ensures the provision of essential information to the consenter. Earlier task force recommendations (American Psychiatric Association 1978, 1990, 2001), other professional guidelines, and regulatory requirements (Mills and Avery 1978; Taub 1987; Tenenbaum 1983; U.S. Food and Drug Administration 2018b; Winslade 1988; Winslade et al. 1984) have encouraged the use of comprehensive written information about ECT as part of the consent process. It is advisable that the generic portions of this material—those not specific to the individual patient—be either contained within the formal consent document or included as a patient information supplement. In either case, informational material should be given to the consenter to keep. In patients who consent to surgical procedures, patient information supplements have been shown to significantly enhance recall of information provided prior to surgery (Askew et al. 1990).

Informational material provided as part of the consent process should be sufficient in scope and depth to allow a reasonable person to understand and evaluate the risks and benefits of ECT compared with other treatment alternatives. Because individuals vary considerably in education and cognitive status, efforts should be made to tailor information to the consenter's ability to comprehend such material. In this regard, the practitioner should be aware that too much technical detail can be as counterproductive as too little detail. Sample consent forms are included in the Appendix. If these documents are used, appropriate modifications should be made to reflect local requirements. In addition, clinicians should be sure that warnings shared by the manufacturer are included in the written consent form and in the discussion of risks and benefits with patients. It is also suggested that reproductions be in large type to ensure readability by patients with poor visual acuity. In addition, appropriate interpreter services should be made available for individuals whose primary language is not English.

To rely entirely on such generic materials as the sole informational component of the informed consent process is ill advised. Although patients with psychiatric disorders do not perform worse than patients undergoing medical or surgical procedures (Meisel and Roth 1983), many patients understand less than half of what is contained in a typical medical consent form, even with considerable attention to readability (Roth et al. 1982). To further enhance the understanding of ECT, many practitioners now augment written content with visual materials (e.g., digital video files) designed to cover the topic of ECT from the layman's perspective (Battersby et al. 1993; Baxter et al. 1986; Dillon 1995; Guze et al. 1988; Tsai et al. 2020; Westreich et al. 1995). Potential visual materials should, to the extent possible, be reviewed with respect to the current accuracy of material conveyed therein. Major discrepancies from other material provided in the consent process should be conveyed to the consenter.

An essential feature of the consent process is a discussion between the consenter and the ECT psychiatrist (American Psychiatric Association Council on Psychiatry and Law 1997). The consent process generally includes coverage of the topics listed below. As previously noted, it is advisable that the consent form and/or patient information sheet contain the generic portions of this material (i.e., those portions not specific to the individual patient), including

- Who is recommending ECT and for what reason.
- A brief rationale for the use of ECT if it is being recommended for a condition that would be considered off-label in terms of the most recent U.S. Food and Drug Administration (FDA) medical device classification.[1]
- A description of applicable treatment alternatives for the patient.
- A description of the ECT procedure, including the times when treatments are typically given (e.g., Monday, Wednesday, Friday mornings) and the location of treatment (i.e., where treatments will take place).
- A discussion of the relative merits and risks of different types of stimulus electrode placement and dosage, as well as rationale regarding clinical choice of technique for the planned ECT series.

---

[1] At the time of this writing, off-label situations include use of ECT for conditions other than unipolar or bipolar major depression, absence of treatment resistance or need for rapid response, patient younger than age 13, or maintenance ECT continuing longer than 3 months following initiation of an acute ECT course (U.S. Food and Drug Administration 2018b).

- The typical range for number of treatments to be administered as well as a statement that consent will be repeated if an unusually large number of treatments (typically more than 15 or as locally determined) are required to manage an acute episode of illness.

- A statement that there is no guarantee that ECT will be effective, that the patient should not expect improvement in comorbid mental illness, and that there is a small chance that such conditions might even worsen.

- A statement that there is generally a substantial risk of relapse after an acute ECT course and that maintenance treatment of some type is nearly always indicated.

- The likelihood (e.g., extremely rare, rare, uncommon, or common) and anticipated severity of major risks associated with the procedure, including mortality, adverse effects on cardiovascular and central nervous systems (including both transient and persistent cognitive adverse effects), and common minor side effects. It also should be noted that the very rare possibility of other serious medical complications cannot be ruled out.

- An acknowledgment that consent for ECT also entails consent for appropriate emergency treatment in the event that this is clinically indicated. In this regard, such consent implies the need for a temporary suspension of do not resuscitate (DNR) orders (as is typically the case with other medical or surgical procedures involving general anesthesia).

- A description of behavioral restrictions, including limitations on food and fluid intake prior to treatments, driving, and work, and other limitations that may be necessary during the pre-ECT evaluation period, the ECT course, and the recuperative interval.

- An offer to answer questions at any time regarding the recommended treatment and the name(s) of the individual(s) who can be contacted with such questions.

- A statement that consent for ECT is voluntary and can be withdrawn at any time.

In addition to summarizing the main features of the consent document, the consent discussion allows a further opportunity for the consenter to express their wishes and have questions answered. In response to a common question about effects of ECT on the brain, for example, it can be noted that the accumulated body of data has demonstrated no evidence that structural "brain damage" is a potential risk of treatment (Anderson 2018; Bassa et al. 2021; Besse et al. 2020; Devanand et al. 1994; Dwork et al. 2004, 2009; Gbyl and Videbech 2018; Kranaster et al. 2014; Palmio et al. 2010).

The consent process should also provide individual-specific information applicable to the patient for whom ECT is considered. At its culmination, this consent discussion should be briefly documented in the patient's clinical record, including noting of factors that significantly impact ECT risks. Examples of individual-specific information include the rationale for ECT, reasonable treatment alternatives, specific benefits and risks, major alterations planned in the ECT procedure, or other factors relevant to individual patients. For example, individuals with thick hair may need to style their hair differently to allow appropriate placement of ECT electrodes. Patients with significant medical conditions (see Chapter 9) or who are pregnant or breastfeeding (see Chapter 9, section 9.4) should receive individualized information on benefits, risks, and suggested treatment modifications as part of the consent process. For individuals who are pregnant, potential teratogenic effects and neonatal toxicities of ECT anesthetic agents should be discussed, although the risks to the fetus are likely to be low. The informed consent process should also note that lack of effective treatment could adversely affect the health and welfare of both the patient and the fetus. In addition, major systemic factors significantly impacting ECT risk, such as those that occurred during the coronavirus disease 2019 (COVID-19) pandemic, should also be included in the consent discussion (Lapid et al. 2020).

As treatment proceeds, substantial alterations in the treatment procedure or other factors having a major effect on risk-benefit considerations should be conveyed to the consenter on a timely basis. The consenter's continued agreement to proceed with ECT in such cases should be documented in the patient's clinical record. The need for ECT treatments exceeding the typical range and the switching of stimulus electrode placement represent two examples of such alterations.

10.4. Capacity to Provide Voluntary Consent

Informed consent requires that a patient be capable of understanding and acting reasonably on information provided about the procedure. For the purpose of these recommendations, the term *capacity* reflects this criterion. There is no clear consensus about what constitutes the capacity to consent. Criteria for capacity to consent have tended to be vague, although formal "tests" of capacity have been investigated, such as the MacArthur Competence Assessment Tool for Treatment (MacCAT-T; Bean et al. 1996; Grisso and Appelbaum 1995; Grisso et al. 1997; Martin and Glancy 1994). The following general principles are suggested when making a determination about an adult's capacity to provide consent. First, capacity to consent should be assumed to be present unless compelling evidence exists to the contrary. Second, the occurrence of psychotic ideation, irrational thought processes, or involuntary hospitalization do not in themselves constitute such evidence. Third, the patient should demonstrate sufficient comprehension and retention of information, as well as adequacy of judgment and decision-making, so that they can reasonably decide whether to consent for ECT.

Unless otherwise mandated by statute, a determination of capacity is generally made by the ECT psychiatrist. Should the ECT psychiatrist be uncertain as to whether capacity to consent is present, or if other questions regarding capacity arise, further background information should be obtained, and, where indicated, an institutionally delegated consultant or entity not otherwise associated with the patient's care may be asked to assist in this capacity determination.

In a study of 40 patients with intact decisional capacity and severe depression who were referred for ECT, capacity was further improved by providing education about ECT (Lapid et al. 2003). A follow-up analysis showed that geriatric patients referred for ECT had adequate decisional capacity to consent to ECT and that education enhanced their decisional capacity to a greater degree than did additional education given to younger patients (Lapid et al. 2004). Given the potential impact of severe cognitive impairment (e.g., dementia) on capacity, medical evaluation of geriatric patients referred for ECT should give careful consideration to any history or findings consistent with cognitive impairment.

Informed consent is defined as voluntary when the consenter's ability to reach a decision is free from coercion or duress. Particularly susceptible to undue influence are consenters who either are highly ambivalent or are unwilling or unable to take full responsibility for the decision, either of which can be present among patients referred for ECT.

For patients with the capacity to consent, ECT should be administered only with their agreement. To do otherwise would infringe on their right to refuse treatment. If ECT is refused or consent for ECT is withdrawn, the ECT psychiatrist and/or other members of the treatment team should inform the consenter of anticipated effects of this action on the patient's clinical course and treatment planning.

As noted earlier in this section, patients who have been involuntarily hospitalized may still have the capacity to provide consent. Several suggestions have been offered to help guarantee the right of involuntarily hospitalized patients to accept or refuse specific components of the treatment plan, including ECT. Examples of such recommendations include the use of psychiatric consultants not otherwise involved in the patient's care, appointed lay representatives, formal institutional review committees, and legal or judicial determination.

Situations in which the patient lacks capacity to consent are generally covered by state regulations that include how and from whom surrogate consent may be obtained (Livingston et al. 2018), including statutes pertinent to emergency situations in which a delay in treatment may lead to death or serious impairment in health. Patients who have previously been adjudicated legally incompetent for medical purposes usually have consent for ECT provided by a legally appointed guardian or conservator, although this may vary with jurisdiction.

In all such instances, a surrogate consenter should receive all of the information that is typically provided to a patient regarding ECT and alternative treatment options. To the extent allowable by law, consideration should be given to any opinions expressed by the patient while in a previous state of determined or presumed capacity. Opinions of the patient's major significant others should also be considered.

Provision of ECT for unemancipated minors represents a special situation as far as consent is concerned. As discussed in Chapter 9, section 9.5, ECT use in children and adolescents is uncommon but can be clinically indicated for the same diagnostic conditions as with adults whose conditions are treatment resistant or urgently require definitive effective clinical intervention. Although ECT use for individuals younger than 13 is presently off-label from an FDA perspective (U.S. Food and Drug Administration 2018b), such designation, as with other off-label situations, does not preclude use of ECT if it is clearly indicated and documented in the medical record. There is typically a legal presumption that unemancipated minors lack capacity to consent and that surrogate consent is primarily (although not exclusively) provided by a parent, unless local or state regulations mandate otherwise. However, the minor should still be involved in the consent process to the extent possible.

Recommendations

10.1. General

1. Policies and procedures should be developed that are consistent with state and local regulations, including those related to the use of ECT in children and adolescents, and that ensure proper informed consent, including when, how, and from whom consent is to be obtained and the nature and scope of information to be provided.

10.2. When and by Whom Should Consent Be Obtained?

1. Informed consent should be obtained from the patient except when the patient lacks capacity to consent.
2. Specific aspects of the informed consent process will depend on legal, regulatory, or local policy considerations.
3. Informed consent for ECT is given for a specified acute treatment course or for a defined period of maintenance ECT.
4. Informed consent for ECT, including the signing of a formal consent document, should also be obtained

   a. Before beginning an acute ECT treatment course
   b. If an unusually large number of treatments become necessary during an acute ECT treatment course
   c. Before initiating a period of maintenance ECT and renewed on the basis of the number of treatments or a specified duration of time as dictated by local or state requirements
   d. If there are changes in the patient's psychiatric or medical status that would significantly influence the benefits and risks of maintenance ECT

5. Informed consent should be obtained by the patient's ECT psychiatrist (unless otherwise specified by law).
6. When separate informed consent for ECT anesthesia is required, it should be obtained by a privileged or otherwise authorized anesthesia provider.
7. Throughout the ECT course, the consenter should receive ongoing feedback about clinical progress and side effects, and any questions or concerns should be addressed.
8. If the consenter expresses reluctance about the treatment at any time before or during the ECT course, they should be reminded of the

right to accept or refuse treatment and to withdraw consent for future treatments at any time.

10.3. Information to Be Conveyed

1. Information describing ECT should be conveyed in a written consent document; a separate consent document is often required for the provision of anesthesia.
2. The consent document and/or a summary of general information related to ECT should be given to the consenter to keep.
3. The ECT psychiatrist, treating psychiatrist, or other knowledgeable physician should also provide a verbal overview of general information on ECT as well as information specific to the individual patient.
4. Further information may also be provided by other staff members, and other supplementary patient information material (including digital video files) may be helpful.
5. All information should be provided in a form understandable to the consenter and should be sufficiently detailed to allow a reasonable person to understand the risks and benefits of ECT and to evaluate the available treatment options.
6. The consenter should have an opportunity to ask questions relevant to ECT or treatment alternatives.
7. The consenter should be informed of substantial alterations in the treatment procedure (e.g., stimulus electrode placement) or other factors that may have a major effect on risk-benefit considerations; such discussions should be documented in the clinical record along with the consenter's decision whether to proceed with treatment.
8. Specific information provided as part of the consent process should include coverage of the following topics:
    a. Who is recommending ECT and for what reason.
    b. A brief rationale for the use of ECT if it is being recommended for a condition that would be considered off-label in terms of the most recent FDA medical device classification. At the time of this writing, off-label situations include use of ECT for conditions other than unipolar or bipolar major depression, absence of treatment resistance or need for rapid response, patient younger than age 13, or maintenance ECT continuing longer than 3 months following initiation of an acute ECT course (U.S. Food and Drug Administration 2018b).

c. A description of applicable treatment alternatives.

d. A description of the ECT procedure, including the times when treatments are given and the location where treatments will occur.

e. A discussion of the relative merits and risks of the different stimulus electrode placements and dosage and rationale for such technical choices in regard to the proposed ECT course.

f. The typical range for number of treatments to be administered as well as a statement that consent will be repeated if an unusually large number of treatments (typically more than 15 or as locally determined) are required to manage an acute episode of illness.

g. A statement that there is no guarantee that ECT will be effective, that the patient should not expect improvement in comorbid mental illness, and that there is a small chance that such conditions might even worsen.

h. A statement concerning the need for maintenance treatment.

i. Discussion of warnings shared by the manufacturer if not already reviewed with the consentor.

j. A description of common minor side effects of ECT (e.g., headaches, musculoskeletal pain) and the likelihood and severity (in general terms) of major risks associated with the procedure, including mortality, cardiopulmonary dysfunction, confusion, and acute and persistent cognitive adverse effects as well as the very rare possibility of other serious medical complications.

k. A description of any other significant risk-benefit considerations that are specific to the individual being referred for ECT (e.g., medical conditions, pregnancy, breastfeeding).

l. A statement that consent for ECT also entails consent for appropriate emergency treatment if this becomes clinically necessary while the patient is not fully conscious.

m. A description of any restrictions on patient behavior, including food and liquid intake, driving, work, and other limitations likely to be necessary before, during, or after ECT.

n. An offer to answer questions at any time regarding the recommended treatment and the name(s) of the individual(s) who can be contacted with such questions.

o. A statement that consent for ECT is voluntary and can be withdrawn at any time.

10.4. Capacity to Provide Voluntary Consent

1. Use of ECT requires voluntary consent from an individual with capacity to make such a decision.
2. If ECT is refused or consent for ECT is withdrawn, the attending physician and/or treating psychiatrist should inform the consenter of anticipated effects of this action on the patient's clinical course and treatment planning.
3. Unless otherwise specified by statute, the determination of capacity to consent should generally be made by the patient's ECT psychiatrist. If the ECT psychiatrist is uncertain as to whether capacity to consent is present or if other questions regarding capacity arise, further background information and/or input from an institutionally delegated consultant or entity not otherwise associated with the patient's care may be obtained.
4. Individuals with psychiatric illness are considered to have the capacity to consent to ECT unless evidence to the contrary is compelling. The presence of psychosis, irrational thinking, or involuntary hospitalization can impair capacity but does not constitute proof that capacity is lacking.
5. For patients with the capacity to consent, ECT should be administered only in the presence of voluntary patient agreement, including signing of a formal consent document.
6. For patients lacking the capacity to provide consent, state and local laws covering consent to treatment should be followed, including statutes pertinent to emergency situations in which a delay in treatment may lead to death or serious impairment in health.
7. Surrogate decision-makers should be provided with the same information that would be given to a patient who has capacity to provide consent.
8. To the extent allowable by law, consideration should be given to any positions previously expressed by the patient when in a state of determined or presumed capacity as well as to the opinions of major significant others.
9. With unemancipated minors, state or local regulations will determine processes for surrogate consent; however, the minor should still be involved in the consent process to the extent possible.

CHAPTER 11

Preparation of the Patient for Electroconvulsive Therapy

This chapter is meant to cover aspects of patient preparation provided in the treatment suite or area on the date of the first and subsequent electroconvulsive therapy (ECT) treatments. Most of the elements of patient preparation discussed in Chapter 8 will have already been accomplished, either at the time of the ECT consultation or over the intervening time period, by the ECT program medical and/or nursing staff. In addition, it is assumed that a determination has been made as to whether ECT should be initiated on an outpatient or inpatient basis (see Chapter 8) and also that information concerning patient limitations during an ECT course has already been provided to the patient and/or surrogate consenter.

11.1. Preparation on the Day of the First Treatment

ECT nursing staff should meet with the patient and accompanying individual (if applicable) and, if not already accomplished, orient them to the ECT treatment suite or area and to the periprocedural aspects involved in receiving an ECT treatment in the particular location. This orientation should take into account whether the patient is receiving treatment as an inpatient or outpatient. The nursing staff should confirm that the pre-ECT evaluation is complete and that adequate patient educational information has been provided to the patient or surrogate consenter regarding the nature, risks, and benefits of ECT, including relevant behavioral limitations (see Chapter 10). In most cases, the anesthesia preoperative evaluation and anesthesia consent will have also been completed, although sometimes this is done the day of the first treatment. The nursing staff should also ensure that ECT or anesthesia consent forms are readily available in case they have not already been signed. In the case of surrogate consent, the staff should also ensure that relevant legal paperwork is present and that the surrogate consenter is readily available to provide legally viable consent.

The ECT psychiatrist should interview the patient and, if applicable, the surrogate consenter and should review the medical record to confirm that the pre-ECT evaluation is complete, that all relevant pre-ECT medical orders have been carried out, and that results of laboratory tests, imaging studies, and consultative reports have been reviewed. On the basis of this assessment and review, the ECT psychiatrist should determine if any significant changes have occurred since the initiation of the pre-ECT evaluation that would require further evaluation or treatment or that would indicate a need for changes or even cancellation of the procedure. Once it is determined that the procedure is still indicated, any uncompleted components of the informed consent process should be finalized, including signing of the ECT consent form by the patient or surrogate consenter, as discussed in Chapter 10. Again, in cases of surrogate consent, the relevant legal documents should be reviewed. When possible, this interview and signing of the consent form should be done in an area allowing an appropriate level of privacy.

11.2. Preparation on the Day of Each Treatment

A local protocol should be in place delineating the intake process and workflow for patients arriving in the treatment suite or area for receipt of ECT. This protocol should include all aspects of patient preparation prior to the actual treatment delivery, including patient education activities, and applies to the first treatment as well as to subsequent treatments. Information regarding this protocol should be provided both orally and in clear, understandable written format to the patient and/or caregiver, including reiteration of behavioral limitations during the ECT course. For non-English speaking patients, written instructions should be provided in the language understood by both the patient and their caregiver.

When possible, patient intake and subsequent preparatory steps should occur in an area that allows a reasonable level of privacy. Staff should ensure compliance with any local requirements related to infectious disease control, such as for coronavirus disease 2019 (COVID-19) (Bryson and Aloysi 2020; Espinoza et al. 2020).

When patients arrive for ECT, nursing staff should ascertain whether patients have adhered to restrictions on ECT-related behavioral constraints. In addition, they should be asked when they last had food or drink. Typical recommendations are for a fasting period of 6–8 hours for solid food or milk and 2 hours for clear liquids (American Society of Anesthesiologists 2017). Care should be taken to ensure that no items remain in the patient's mouth. This is particularly important for patients who chew gum or use hard candy (Kellner et al. 2015). The anesthesia provider should be made aware if patients have smoked within 2 hours of ECT. Patients with cognitive impairment or psychosis may have difficulty remembering food and water intake restrictions and may require supervision.

The nursing staff should have the patient void, check the patient's head and hair for pins and jewelry, and ensure that the patient's hair is clean, dry, and suitably styled to allow appropriate placement of ECT electrodes. Placement of unilateral electrodes can be challenging depending on hairstyle and thickness of the patient's hair. Hair spray or cream could theoretically produce shorting of the electrical current through the hair, which may singe the hair and interfere with seizure induction. Eyeglasses, contact lenses, and hearing aids should be removed prior to entry to the treatment area itself. The mouth should be checked for loose or sharp teeth or other foreign bodies. Dentures and other dental appliances should be removed unless specially indicated (e.g., to protect loose or isolated teeth). Finger rings need not be removed unless loose, although tape should be used to secure them to the finger. It is best to remove other superficially located jewelry such as necklaces and bracelets. Transdermally attached body jewelry such as rings or studs should be removed from the face, head, and hands if at all possible. All removed items, as well as other personal effects, should be saved in a secure fashion for postprocedural return or given to the patient's accompanying person. The fingernails or toenails used for pulse oximetry should be free of nail polish.

Vital signs should be recorded and current medication regimen and allergies confirmed. Medications taken the day of treatment should be confirmed, including route of administration and dosage. Any medications needing to be administered at the facility should be provided and documented. Pretreatment cognitive orientation should be assessed, and the patient should be given the opportunity to ask any questions regarding the procedure.

With outpatients, it is helpful to provide a waiting area for individuals who accompany them to the facility if operationally feasible. Optimally, this area should be convenient to the location where the patients are being prepared for treatment so that the significant other(s) can stay with the patient and help them remain comfortable during the pre-ECT period. Attention to such patient satisfaction issues facilitates the development and maintenance of a positive relationship among patients, their significant others, and the ECT team. For many patients, the prospect of receiving an ECT treatment can lead to psychological and even behavioral manifestations of anxiety, fear, or agitation, which can augment symptoms of the patient's psychiatric illness and which may or may not decrease over a course of ECT (Obbels et al. 2017). For these reasons, the ECT nurses, as well as other members of the treatment team, need to be proactively aware of the potential for such effects and to be able to rapidly address them in an empathic and caring fashion. When possible, supportive behavioral interventions, sometimes implemented with the assistance of a patient's significant other, should be used instead of pharmacological management.

Prior to entry to the actual treatment room or area, intravenous access should be established. This access often involves maintaining an intravenous line with a saline or lactated Ringer's drip, although some practitioners prefer to inject medications directly into a lockable indwelling catheter. In either case, the intravenous line should be adequate to handle emergency needs, and care should be taken to ensure that all intravenously administered medications are flushed. Intravenous access should be maintained during the posttreatment recovery period at least until the patient is conscious and vital signs are stable. For patients with difficult intravenous access, options include leaving a lockable indwelling catheter in place between treatments or using a peripherally inserted central catheter (PICC) line or portacath (Mackenzie et al. 1996).

Prior to the treatment, additional assessment of the patient and review of the record are essential. Given the relative lack of privacy as well as the level of distraction generally present in the actual treatment area, these assessments should occur in a separate allocated space if possible. Using the recovery area space itself is not desirable because it exposes alert patients to those who are emerging from the postictal, anesthetized state. As part of this process, the ECT psychiatrist should review the patient's medical record since the last treatment (or ECT consultation), including any orders that have been entered since the last ECT, as well as consultation reports, changes in documented medications, and any laboratory test or imaging results that have appeared in the medical record over the intervening time period. The ECT psychiatrist should also interview outpatients receiving ECT to determine whether any further evaluations, alterations in treatment technique, or changes in treatment frequency are needed on the basis of significant events that have occurred since the last treatment. Such events may include unexpected or severe adverse effects; modifications in medication regimen or adherence; or alterations in mental status, medical conditions, or other clinical symptoms. In addition, the ECT psychiatrist or another member of the clinical treatment team should provide an appropriate level of assessment of therapeutic and cognitive outcome (see Chapters 17 and 20). This information should be considered in decisions regarding ECT technique changes and timing of subsequent ECT treatments. Findings that may be relevant to the provision of anesthesia, such as changes in medications or medical status, should be discussed by the ECT psychiatrist and anesthesia provider. In addition, the treating anesthesia provider should be made aware of the medications administered to the patient prior to entry to the treatment room or area.

Because ECT is analogous to a surgical procedure, current practice now requires the use of a universal protocol with pre-procedure verifications and a time-out in the treatment room or area, involving all staff present. This protocol is accomplished in the treatment area itself and is considered an integral part of the ECT administration procedure (Watts 2016). At a minimum, the time-out procedure includes assuring correct identification of the patient, verifying that ECT is the procedure to be performed, verifying existence of informed consent, confirming treatment number and type (acute or maintenance), and verifying stimulus electrode placement.

Recommendations

11.1. Preparation on the Day of the First Treatment

1. Nursing staff should ensure that all aspects of pre-ECT evaluation have been completed and documented, including pre-ECT orders, laboratory tests, imaging, and requested consultations.
2. Nursing staff should ensure that consent forms are available, that any legal documentation relevant to surrogate consent is present, and that any surrogate consenter is readily available.

3. The ECT psychiatrist should review results of the pre-ECT evaluation and obtain informed consent, if not already obtained.

11.2. Preparation on the Day of Each Treatment

1. Nursing staff should follow local protocol regarding intake processes and steps for patient preparation prior to ECT treatments, including any infectious disease precautions and monitoring of patients' adherence with behavioral restrictions and limitations on oral intake.
2. Nursing staff should obtain from the patient and/or other relevant parties any recent changes in medical history, allergies, and medication use, as well as monitoring patient adherence with medications prescribed to be taken prior to ECT on the day of treatment and the preceding night.
3. Before the patient enters the treatment room or area, nursing staff should administer pre-ECT medications that have been ordered to be taken at the facility.
4. Nursing staff should assist patients with other preparations for ECT (e.g., voiding; ensuring that hair is clean and styled to permit appropriate electrode placement; removing eyeglasses, contact lenses, hearing aids, and jewelry).
5. Nursing staff, with the assistance of other staff, as needed, should address psychological and/or behavioral aspects of patient anxiety, fear, and agitation regarding the ECT procedure.
6. Nursing staff should ensure adequate IV access, with assistance from other staff as needed.
7. The ECT psychiatrist should review the medical record of patients receiving ECT for any clinically significant changes since the last treatment and should briefly assess outpatients in terms of therapeutic effects, adverse effects (including cognitive side effects), and changes in medications or medical conditions that might affect ECT risk, technique, or anesthesia.
8. On the basis of the above review and assessment, as well as the outcome of prior treatments, the ECT psychiatrist should implement any indicated changes in the treatment protocol. When applicable, such changes should be discussed with, and input obtained from, the anesthesia provider and the consenter.

9. The patient should be given the opportunity to ask any questions regarding the procedure.
10. The ECT psychiatrist, in collaboration with all other members of the treatment team, should implement a structured time-out procedure to help ensure that the treatment will be both safe and effective.

CHAPTER 12

Anesthesia

A trained anesthesia provider, either an anesthesiologist working alone or supervising a certified registered nurse anesthetist, physician assistant anesthetist, or anesthesiologist assistant, is a required member of the electroconvulsive therapy (ECT) treatment team. The primary goals of the anesthesia experience are patient safety and comfort. Encompassed in the anesthesia experience are airway management, oxygenation, induction, muscle relaxation, and cardiovascular management. Brief, light general anesthesia, with airway management by mask and bag, is typical for the vast majority of ECT patients (Bryson et al. 2017; Chawla 2020; Stripp et al. 2018). Infection control should also be incorporated into anesthetic practices with ECT, as indicated.

12.1. Airway Management

As with any procedure involving anesthesia, the anesthesia provider is responsible for airway management during the entire ECT procedure until care is turned over to the postanesthesia care unit staff. Before the first ECT treatment of each day, the anesthesia provider should verify that relevant equipment is functioning adequately and that supplies for resuscitation are available.

12.1.1. Establishing an Airway

For each patient, the ability to provide adequate ventilation should be verified before the muscle relaxant is administered. Patients who may require particular attention include those who are in the second or third trimester of pregnancy and those with morbid obesity, obstructive sleep apnea, pulmonary disease, or a history of difficult ventilation during prior anesthetics. Endotracheal intubation is only rarely indicated during ECT; situations in which intubation may be necessary are patients in the second and third trimesters of pregnancy (see Chapter 9, section 9.4.1) or who have anatomic airway anomalies. A laryngeal mask airway (LMA) may be used to facilitate airway management in some situations but does not provide the aspiration protection of an endotracheal tube.

12.1.2. Oxygenation

Oxygenation (100% O_2, positive pressure, and a respiratory rate of at least 15–20 breaths per minute) should be maintained from the onset of anesthesia until adequate spontaneous respiration resumes, except during application of the electrical stimulus. To monitor adequacy of oxygenation, oximetry should be used in all patients during the entire procedure and in the recovery period. A minimum of 2–5 minutes of preanesthetic oxygenation via nasal cannula or face mask (15–20 breaths per minute of 100% oxygen at 5 L/min) is considered routine by many practitioners (Gold et al. 1981; Valentine et al. 1990). Preoxygenation may be particularly useful for patients at risk for myocardial ischemia or rapid hemoglobin oxygen desaturation after anesthetic induction. This latter group includes morbidly obese patients (Koyama et al. 2020), patients during the third trimester of pregnancy, and patients with pulmonary disease. For patients with chronic renal failure, adequate ventilation prior to the seizure will help minimize the risk of respiratory acidosis (Sundsted et al. 2014). If a patient has had weakly expressed or short seizures, hyperventilation (40–50 breaths per minute) prior to, and during, the seizure has been shown to improve seizure quality. Hyperventilation is also associated with a lower seizure threshold (Bryson et al. 2017; Gómez-Arnau et al. 2018), longer seizures (Haeck et al. 2011; Loo et al. 2010), and decreased time to reorientation after ECT (Mayur et al. 2010).

Oxygen delivery should be resumed during the seizure (Lew et al. 1986; McCormick and Saunders 1996; Swindells and Simpson 1987) because cerebral oxygen consumption increases substantially with seizure activity (Fabbri et al. 2003; Saito et al. 1996). Care should be taken to avoid inducing electroencephalogram (EEG) artifacts while ventilating the patient. Because of the effects of the muscle relaxant and the seizure, patients remain apneic during the immediate postictal state and require airway management with oxygenation until the recovery of spontaneous respiration.

12.1.3. Protecting the Teeth and Other Oral Structures

The patient's mouth should be checked for the presence of foreign bodies and loose or sharp teeth before initiating anesthesia. Before applying the electrical stimulus, an appropriately sized, flexible, protective foam or rubber bite block should be inserted in the mouth. The tongue should be pushed inferiorly and posteriorly so that it is not between the teeth. During delivery of the electrical stimulus, the patient's chin should be manually supported, keeping the jaw tight against the bite block.

Application of the electrical stimulus directly stimulates pterygoid, masseter, and temporalis muscles and produces a clamping action of the jaw muscles, which is not blocked by the muscle relaxant (Minneman 1995; Ogami et al. 2014). Use of a flexible material that extends across the mouth and has maximal cushioning in the molar area will absorb the force of this clamping action and protect the teeth, tongue, and other oral structures (Ogami et al. 2014). Use of a plastic airway (e.g., Guedel type) as a bite block is not recommended because of the increased risk of tooth fracture or jaw injury (Abrams 2002). For patients with full dentures on top and bottom, these will typically be removed but may be left in place (e.g., to facilitate airway management). A bite block should still be inserted in either circumstance. In patients with only one or a few fragile teeth, a standard bite block may not be sufficiently protective; an individualized approach to dental management with protective gauze padding or a custom bite block may need to be devised.

12.2. Medications Used With ECT

This section covers the medications used for anesthesia and during and immediately after the procedure. Chapter 13 covers the impact of various psychiatric and other medications taken by the patient during the course of ECT.

12.2.1. Anticholinergic Agents

Anticholinergic agents are sometimes given prior to anesthetic induction either to reduce secretions, thereby facilitating airway management, and/or to minimize the possibility of bradyarrhythmias (Anastasian et al. 2014; Shettar et al. 1989) immediately after delivery of the electrical stimulus or during the postictal period.

Electrical stimulation is often associated with a short period of vagally mediated bradycardia (Rasmussen et al. 2007a), sometimes starting with brief asystole (Nagler and Geppert 2011; Robinson and Lighthall 2004). Typically, seizure induction leads to catecholamine release and an associated increase in heart rate. However, if the electrical stimulus is subconvulsive and unopposed by an adrenergic discharge, bradycardia and asystole immediately after the stimulus are more likely (Decina et al. 1984; McCall 1996). Because administration of subconvulsive stimuli is intrinsic to empirical titration for identifying seizure threshold (Sackeim et al. 1987c), many practitioners routinely administer an anticholinergic agent at treatment sessions in which titration is planned to decrease the risk of bradycardia or asystole. Low-dose atropine sulphate has been shown to decrease bradycardia after the ECT electrical stimulus (Anastasian et al. 2014), and there is limited evidence that atropine can decrease ECT associated ventricular arrhythmias (Suzuki et al. 2017). The use of an anticholinergic agent may be especially indicated for patients receiving sympathetic blocking agents (e.g., β-blockers) or in other circumstances in which it is medically important to prevent the occurrence of a vagal bradycardia (Zielinski et al. 1993).

Except as described above, anticholinergic medications are usually unnecessary because they may aggravate preexisting tachycardia in some patients and result in an increase in cardiac workload (Mayur et al. 1998; Rasmussen et al. 1999), ECT-induced hemodynamic changes (Christensen et al. 2019), and autonomic dysfunction (Jadhav et al. 2017). Other potential adverse effects of anticholinergics include urinary retention and constipation or fecal impaction. These adverse effects may be augmented by the muscarinic properties of any other pharmacological agents that the patient is receiving.

Traditionally, anticholinergic agents have been administered either intravenously, 2–3 minutes prior to anesthesia (when used to prevent bradycardia), or intramuscularly or intravenously, 20–60 minutes prior to anesthesia (when used to reduce airway secretions). Intravenous administration has largely replaced intramuscular administration because it obviates the need for an additional injection.

The typical anticholinergic agents used are atropine, 0.4–0.8 mg IV, or glycopyrrolate, 0.2–0.4 mg IV. Glycopyrrolate has the theoretical advantage of being less likely than atropine to cross the blood-brain barrier, whereas atropine may have greater consistency in producing the desired vagal-blocking effect relative to glycopyrrolate. Atropine is also associated with a rebound tachycardia (Kurup and Ostroff 2012). However, controlled comparisons of glycopyrrolate and atropine in ECT have not shown clinically significant differences in effects on cognition, cardiac function, or postictal reports of nausea (Greenan et al. 1983; Kelway et al. 1986; Kramer et al. 1986; Simpson et al. 1987; Sommer et al. 1989; Swartz and Saheba 1989).

12.2.2. Anesthetic Agents

ECT should be performed using only ultrabrief general anesthesia (Bryson et al. 2017; Drop and Welch 1989). The purpose of anesthesia is to produce several minutes of unconsciousness throughout the period of muscle relaxation, including the seizure. Excessive anesthetic dosage may prolong unconsciousness and apnea, raise the seizure threshold, shorten seizure duration, increase the risk of cardiovascular complications, intensify amnesia, and reduce antidepressant efficacy (Boylan et al. 2000; Kronsell et al. 2021; Krueger et al. 1993; Miller et al. 1985). However, if the anesthetic dosage is too low, loss of consciousness may be incomplete, autonomic arousal may occur, and the patient may recall a frightening period of pre- or post-ECT paralysis after the procedure. Thus, the aim is to produce a light level of general anesthesia.

Methohexital is an excellent anesthetic agent for ECT because of its established safety record, effectiveness, and low cost (Vaidya et al. 2012). It has been considered the gold standard for ECT because of its nearly ideal kinetics and because it has only moderate anticonvulsant properties. It is now rarely used outside of ECT and thus may be unfamiliar to many anesthesia providers. The typical starting dose of methohexital is 0.75–1.0 mg/kg given as a single intravenous bolus. Doses at subsequent treatments may be adjusted, up or down, as needed (Bryson et al. 2012a). Another barbiturate, thiopental, is also an effective ECT anesthetic agent (Zahavi and Dannon 2014); however, it is no longer available in the United States, although it is available in other countries. Alternative agents are propofol, etomidate, ketamine, and, less commonly, the ultra-short-acting narcotic agents remifentanil and alfentanil.

Propofol (1.0–2.0 mg/kg IV) is commonly used as an anesthetic agent, and there is accumulating evidence for its efficacy and safety with ECT (Butterfield et al. 2004; Gazdag and Iványi 2007; Gazdag et al. 2004b; Geretsegger et al. 2007; Patel et al. 2006; Rosa et al. 2007). Relative to other anesthetic agents, studies have shown that propofol results in a reduction in seizure duration (Rasmussen 2014) as well as an increase in seizure threshold (Gálvez et al. 2015; Patel et al. 2006). Propofol, like methohexital, frequently causes pain when injected; lidocaine, when used to reduce this injection pain, may have additive anticonvulsant properties. A meta-analysis of 17 trials using etomidate, methohexital, thiopental, and propofol found that propofol significantly reduced seizure duration compared with etomidate and thiopental but had a nonsignificant decrease in seizure duration compared with methohexital (Singh et al. 2015). A retrospective study found that propofol use was associated with a greater likelihood of inadequate seizures than was etomidate use (Graveland et al. 2013). In addition, in individuals with schizophrenia, a randomized crossover study found that seizure duration, as measured by EEG and electromyography, were shorter with propofol than with etomidate, although the seizure quality and number of restimulations were not significantly different (Gazdag et al. 2004a). One strategy to manage decreased seizure duration with propofol has been to decrease the propofol dose and add a short-acting opiate, remifentanil or alfentanil, in order to produce appropriate sedation. Compared with a propofol-only group (0.75 mg/kg), a group of patients who received propofol (0.5 mg/kg) plus a short-acting opiate had longer mean motor seizure durations, required a lower stimulus intensity, and had better recovery parameters (Akcaboy et al. 2005).

Initially, the finding of decreased seizure duration with propofol led some researchers to question the advisability of its routine use for ECT (Swartz 1992). However, it has become increasingly clear that, with the exception of extremely short seizures, seizure duration has limited relevance to the efficacy of ECT when adequate stimulus dosing is used (Loo et al. 2010; Nobler et al. 1993; Sackeim et al. 1991, 1993, 2000). Furthermore, no difference in the therapeutic outcome has been found when propofol is used as the anesthetic agent compared with methohexital (Mårtensson et al. 1994), etomidate (Canbek et al. 2015), or thiopental (Bauer et al. 2009; Canbek et al. 2015). Thus, there is no apparent effect of propofol on the antidepressant efficacy of ECT despite its clear effect in decreasing seizure duration.

Propofol may, in fact, have advantages as compared with other anesthetic agents for ECT. In other medical contexts, propofol is associated with a rapid and "smooth" recovery from anesthesia. Both emergence time (the time from anesthetic administration to eye opening) and recovery time (the time from onset of anesthesia to discharge from the postanesthesia care unit) are shorter with propofol compared with methohexital (Hooten and Rasmussen 2008). Propofol may also reduce the magnitude of hemodynamic changes that accompany ECT (Rasmussen 2014). Furthermore, the available evidence suggests that propofol may reduce immediate post-ECT cognitive effects compared with barbiturate anesthetics (Imashuku et al. 2014).

Use of etomidate (0.15–0.40 mg/kg) or ketamine (1.0–2.0 mg/kg) is typically considered when seizures are brief, missed, or otherwise difficult to elicit (see Chapter 21). Across their respective dosing ranges, seizure duration is longer with etomidate than methohexital or propofol (Avramov et al. 1995; Gazdag et al. 2004b; Saffer and Berk 1998; Trzepacz et al. 1993) and longer with ketamine than thiopental or propofol (Hoyer et al. 2014; Wang et al. 2012).

Etomidate may be particularly useful in patients with heart failure and related conditions because it is less likely to result in hypotensive effects compared with other anesthetic options. Etomidate is associated with less pain on injection than propofol or thiopental (Ye et al. 2017) but has a longer recovery period (Rosa et al. 2008). Myoclonus is common with etomidate shortly after injection. It is not usually problematic during ECT but should not be confused with seizure activity (Lang et al. 2018). Etomidate use is also associated with temporary adrenal suppression, although there is no clear-cut evidence that this effect is clinically relevant in patients receiving ECT (Reveles Jensen et al. 2020). In an acute study of patients given six ECT sessions over 12 days with etomidate as the anesthetic agent (0.3 mg/kg), cortisol levels were initially suppressed within 24 hours of the second and sixth treatment but remained in the normal range and were not significantly different from baseline levels 48 hours after the sixth treatment (Wang et al. 2011). No data are available related to long-term effects of adrenal suppression in patients receiving etomidate for maintenance ECT.

Although ketamine has typically been used with ECT when adequate seizures are difficult to elicit, it has recently become more popular as an ECT anesthetic, either alone or in combination with other agents. This is due to the growing body of evidence suggesting that ketamine has antidepressant properties (Newport et al. 2015; Park et al. 2019); this, in turn, has led to the speculation that ketamine may enhance the antidepressant effect or speed of response in ECT (Ren et al. 2018), particularly when antidepressant response to ECT is delayed or absent. However, clinical trials have shown mixed findings, with some suggesting earlier improvement when ketamine is administered with ECT (Loo et al. 2012; Okamoto et al. 2010; Yoosefi et al. 2014) but others showing no significant overall difference in depressive symptoms after a course of ECT compared with anesthesia with methohexital (Rasmussen et al. 2014), thiopental (Loo et al. 2012; Yoosefi et al. 2014), or propofol (Okamoto et al. 2010). There was also no difference in overall antidepressant response or in depressive symptoms after the first ECT session when anesthesia with thiopental alone was compared with a combination of thiopental and ketamine (Abdallah et al. 2012). Similarly, data on cognition with use of ketamine for ECT has been mixed. Preliminary evidence suggested that ketamine may decrease cognitive effects immediately after ECT compared with methohexital (Krystal et al. 2003), but this was not confirmed in other trials comparing ketamine with methohexital (Rasmussen et al. 2014) or thiopental (Loo et al. 2012). Furthermore, ketamine can cause hypertension and occasionally may produce altered states of consciousness in the postictal period, including hallucinations and dissociation, as well as vestibular side effects (nausea, vertigo, and dizziness) (Rasmussen and Ritter 2014).

The ultra-short-acting narcotic anesthetics remifentanil and alfentanil have sometimes been used for ECT anesthesia, either alone or in combination with other agents (Andersen et al. 2001; Locala et al. 2005; Porter et al. 2008a; Recart et al. 2003; Smith et al. 2003; van den Broek et al. 2004; Vishne et al. 2005b). Most commonly, the dose of methohexital, propofol, or etomidate is decreased and replaced with the narcotic anesthetic for the purpose of increasing seizure length and/or lowering seizure threshold. Most reports of the use of remifentanil or alfentanil in ECT show less prominent changes in heart rate and blood pressure when compared with non-narcotic anesthesia agents (Akcaboy et al. 2005). For example, when used as an adjunctive anesthetic agent, remifentanil can attenuate the ECT-associated increase in heart rate and arterial blood pressure (Nasseri et al. 2009). Short-acting narcotics can also increase the period of apnea following treatment because it takes time for these drugs to be metabolized.

Use of sevoflurane, an inhalational anesthetic gas, is extremely rare with ECT but has been reported to be a satisfactory alternative to intravenous anesthesia (Aoki et al. 2021; Calarge et al. 2003; Hodgson et al. 2004; Toprak et al. 2005; Wajima et al. 2003). Its use has been suggested for patients who are severely needle phobic or those who experience severe pain on injection of intravenous anesthetic agents. If using sevoflurane, all precautions needed with inhalational anesthetics should be observed. In addition, the patient should have intravenous access established after induction and prior to ECT.

Characteristics of anesthetic agents used with ECT are summarized in Table 12–1. Regardless of the anesthetic medication used, the appropriateness of dosage should be determined at each treatment and adjustments made at subsequent treatments.

Table 12–1. *Summary of electroconvulsive therapy (ECT) anesthetic agents*

Anesthetic agent	Usual dose range	Relative anticonvulsant effect	Remarks
Propofol	1.0–2.0 mg/kg	3	Decreased emergence side effects and improved recovery time; pain on injection; decreases seizure length compared with methohexital and etomidate
Thiopental	2.0–3.0 mg/kg	2	No significant advantages over methohexital; no longer available in the United States
Methohexital	0.5–1.2 mg/kg	1	Standard agent for ECT in the United States; pain on injection
Etomidate	0.15–0.4 mg/kg	0	Increases seizure length compared with methohexital and propofol; less cardiovascular depression; myoclonus on injection; potential for adrenal suppression
Ketamine	1.0–2.0 mg/kg	−1 (proconvulsant)	Hypertension, tachycardia; potential for hallucinations, dissociation, nausea, vomiting, and vertigo
Remifentanil or alfentanil	2.5–3.5 mcg/kg remifentanil 10–20 mcg/kg alfentanil	−1	Useful adjunct to increase seizure length with minimal hemodynamic effects

12.2.3. Muscle Relaxants

A skeletal muscle relaxant should be used to modify convulsive motor activity and facilitate airway management. The preferred relaxant agent is succinylcholine (0.5–1.0 mg/kg) administered as an intravenous bolus (Bryson et al. 2012a). Before administering the muscle relaxant, the anesthesia provider should ensure that a patent airway is present and that the patient is unconscious. Otherwise, patients may recall a frightening experience of paralysis while conscious, despite the subsequent elicitation of a generalized seizure.

The purpose of the muscle relaxant is to produce sufficient modification of the convulsive movements to minimize the risk of musculoskeletal injury. Complete paralysis is neither necessary nor desirable. However, for some patients, such as those with osteoporosis or a history of spinal injury, complete relaxation may be indicated, and the muscle relaxant dosage may need to be adjusted upward. Adequacy of muscle relaxation should be determined at each treatment session, and dosage should be modified at successive sessions to achieve the desired effect. One study found that the adequate dose of succinylcholine for muscle relaxation was 0.9 mg/kg, although there was wide variation due to the individualized patient response to succinylcholine (Bryson et al. 2012a). Pretreatment with a small dose of a nondepolarizing muscle relaxant can also be used to reduce the intensity of succinylcholine-induced fasciculations and associated muscle soreness; such soreness often will not recur or can be managed with oral analgesics.

The anesthesia provider should be aware of the medical conditions and medications that may influence the action and choice of muscle relaxant agents (D'Souza et al. 2022). Succinylcholine can trigger excessive potassium release (Martyn and Richtsfeld 2006) and should be avoided in patients with severe burns, muscle rigidity (e.g., neuroleptic malignant syndrome, some patients with catatonia), and neuromuscular disease or injury (e.g., quadriplegia, amyotrophic lateral sclerosis, muscular dystrophy). A nondepolarizing muscle relaxant should be used in these conditions.

A nondepolarizing muscle relaxant may also be indicated in patients with pseudocholinesterase deficiency, cholinesterase inhibition (e.g., exposure to organophosphate pesticides), hypercalcemia, or severe osteoporosis (D'Souza et al. 2022). Pseudocholinesterase deficiency may also be due to an inherited condition. Approximately 4% of the population has a genetic mutation in the gene coding for cholinesterase; the mutations are most common in patients of European descent but uncommon in Asians. A family history of difficulty with anesthesia may be the only indication that a patient is at risk for pseudocholinesterase deficiency. Although pseudocholinesterase deficiency can be confirmed by a laboratory assay, routine determination of pseudocholinesterase levels or dibucaine number is not recommended (Lippi and Plebani 2013). Such determinations should be reserved for patients with a personal or family history of prolonged apnea following exposure to muscle relaxants (Pradhan et al. 2021). If a patient has prolonged paralysis from succinylcholine, a very low dose of succinylcholine or a nondepolarizing muscle relaxant, such as atracurium or rocuronium, may be substituted at subsequent treatments (Hickey et al. 1987; Hicks 1987; Kramer and Afrasiabi 1991; Lui et al. 1993; Pradhan et al. 2021; Stack et al. 1988). An alternative agent should also be used in patients who have a positive test, such as dibucaine number, for pseudocholinesterase deficiency.

Rocuronium is the most commonly used nondepolarizing muscle relaxant (Hoshi et al. 2011; Mirzakhani et al. 2016). Other nondepolarizing muscle relaxants include cisatracurium, atracurium, and vecuronium (Cook and Simons 2021; D'Souza et al. 2022). Relative to succinylcholine, nondepolarizing muscle relaxants generally produce more prolonged paralysis. However, when rocuronium is reversed by sugammadex immediately after the seizure induction, the difference in time to first spontaneous breath or recovery time does not appear to be clinically significant (Hoshi et al. 2011). In comparison with succinylcholine, the combination of rocuronium-sugammadex has also been associated with a decrease in headaches and myalgias (Saricicek et al. 2014), a shortened awakening time (Saricicek et al. 2014), and, in one case report, a decrease in postictal agitation (Postaci et al. 2013). If sugammadex is unavailable to reverse the effects of rocuronium or vecuronium, or when atracurium or cisatracurium have been used, reversal can be achieved by use of neostigmine in combination with glycopyrrolate after seizure induction (Hawkins et al. 2019; Honing et al. 2019).

Before the electrical stimulus is applied, the adequacy of muscle relaxation is ascertained by the diminution or loss of knee, ankle, or plantar withdrawal reflexes, loss of muscle tone, and/or the diminution or failure to respond to a peripheral nerve stimulator. With a depolarizing muscle relaxant such as succinylcholine, it is unlikely that maximal effect has taken place until after muscle fasciculations have disappeared. The last body parts to fasciculate are usually the toes, and the electrical stimulus is usually applied following the disappearance of fasciculations. When a nondepolarizing muscle relaxant is used, the onset and offset of muscle relaxation should be monitored with a peripheral nerve stimulator. A peripheral nerve stimulator is also useful for assessing patients who are at heightened risk for musculoskeletal complications and in whom the extent of relaxation is uncertain. With nondepolarizing muscle relaxants as well as with succinylcholine, older patients often take longer to reach full relaxation than do younger patients (L. A. Lee et al. 2016).

12.2.4. Agents Used to Modify the Cardiovascular Response to ECT

Cardiovascular complications are one of the most common causes of medical morbidity with ECT and tend to occur in patients with cardiac disease (Blumberger et al. 2017; Duma et al. 2019; Nuttall et al. 2004). The ECT seizure is associated with several cardiovascular changes, including an immediate vagal response with bradycardia for a few seconds, followed by sympathetic hyperactivity with tachycardia and hypertension (Kurup and Ostroff 2012; Nagler and Geppert 2011; Rasmussen et al. 2007a; Robinson and Lighthall 2004). These rapid changes in hemodynamics can be accompanied by atrial and ventricular arrhythmias (Kurup and Ostroff 2012). The practice of controlling the hypertension and tachycardia during ECT is driven by the belief that the frequency or severity of cardiac ischemia, arrhythmias, and other cardiovascular adverse events will be reduced (Hermida et al. 2022).

Judgment is warranted when using pharmacological modifications to blunt the cardiovascular effects of ECT and minimize the potential for cardiovascular complications. A strong working relationship with the anesthesia provider is essential in making these decisions; cardiology consultation is of additional benefit in optimizing the management of patients with significant cardiac illness. In patients who are unequivocally at increased risk for vascular complications, such as those with unstable aortic or other vascular aneurysms, it is wise to block the hemodynamic changes in heart rate and blood pressure that accompany seizure induction, and such modifications should be used prophylactically at all treatments (Hermida et al. 2022; Mueller et al. 2009). When patients are tachycardic or hypertensive at baseline before receiving

ECT, there is a concern that further increases in heart rate or blood pressure will not be well tolerated. In patients with unstable hypertension or other cardiac conditions, an attempt should be made to stabilize the patient's medical condition before beginning ECT. However, in most patients, with or without preexisting cardiac illness, many practitioners will forego prophylaxis and monitor cardiovascular changes closely at the initial treatments. The occasional sustained hypertension or significant arrhythmia after seizure induction is then treated acutely, and prophylaxis is considered for subsequent treatments.

When pharmacological modifications are indicated to manage these hemodynamic changes, a number of approaches have been used (Kurup and Ostroff 2012; Saito 2005). In general, most ECT anesthesia providers have relied on β-adrenergic blocking agents and calcium channel blockers to control the cardiovascular effects associated with ECT. The more selective β-adrenergic blocking agents (e.g., esmolol) affect heart rate, but the nonselective agents (e.g., labetalol) also block α-adrenergic receptors and influence both heart rate and blood pressure (Pearce and Wallin 1994; Wiest and Haney 2012). The effect of esmolol is rapid, with a hemodynamic effect within 3 minutes of injection, as compared with 5–10 minutes for labetalol (Boere et al. 2014; Shrestha et al. 2007). Nicardipine has replaced sublingual preparations of nitrates and other calcium channel blockers for control of blood pressure because it can be given intravenously and titrated more precisely than sublingual medications (Zhang et al. 2005). Intravenous nitroglycerin is another agent that can be used to control hypertension but is reserved for situations where tight blood pressure control is deemed critical (Bryson et al. 2012b). Other medications that have been reported to be helpful in modifying the hemodynamic changes with ECT include alfentanil (McCutchen et al. 2023) and dexmedetomidine (Subsoontorn et al. 2021).

12.3. Infection Control Principles in Providing ECT Anesthesia

ECT anesthesia should follow all recommended infection control procedures for the current local environment. The coronavirus disease 2019 (COVID-19) pandemic resulted in the recognition that ECT is an urgent and not an elective procedure for many seriously ill patients. As a result, every effort should be made to keep ECT available for acute and maintenance treatments even during times of resource shortage or infectious disease outbreaks (Espinoza et al. 2020; Maixner et al. 2021; Sienaert et al. 2020).

Modifications to ECT procedures as part of infection control include 1) enhanced patient screening (both for assessment of urgency of need for ECT and infection status), 2) protective equipment for patients and staff, and 3) modifications of the ECT anesthesia technique itself (e.g., to minimize aerosolization of infectious fomites when respiratory infection may be present). Typical bag-mask-valve assisted ventilation used in ECT is associated with spread of airway secretions and should be avoided as much as possible. To this end, ECT anesthesia teams have suggested relying on excellent preinduction oxygenation, with minimal bag-mask-valve ventilation, and only when desaturation occurs. In one study of 106 patients, assisted ventilation was required in only about half. Increased BMI was associated with more frequent need for additional ventilation (Luccarelli et al. 2020a). The lack of hyperventilation during the procedure results in slightly shorter seizures, but this is likely to be of little clinical importance. Viral filters in the breathing circuit are also suggested (Thiruvenkatarajan et al. 2020). Other suggestions include the preferential use of a Jackson Rees circuit instead of an artificial manual breathing unit (AMBU) bag (Limoncelli et al. 2020). Finally, some authors have suggested that supraglottic airway devices (classic laryngeal mask airway, or others) be considered, but there seems to be no consensus on this (Flexman et al. 2020; Thiruvenkatarajan et al. 2020).

Recommendations

12.1. Airway Management

1. Airway management is the responsibility of the anesthesia provider.
2. Prior to each treatment, the anesthesia provider or designee should verify that relevant equipment (e.g., oxygen delivery system, suctioning system, intubation set) is functioning adequately and that necessary supplies for resuscitation are available.

12.1.1. Establishing an Airway

1. For each patient, the ability to provide adequate ventilation should be verified before the muscle relaxant is administered.
2. Patients who may require particular attention with airway management include those who are in the second or third trimester of pregnan-

cy and those with morbid obesity, obstructive sleep apnea, pulmonary disease, or a history of difficult ventilation during prior anesthetics.
3. Intubation should be avoided unless specifically indicated.

12.1.2. Oxygenation

1. Except during stimulus delivery, oxygenation using positive pressure ventilation should be maintained from the onset of anesthetic induction until adequate spontaneous respiration resumes.
2. A respiratory rate of 15–20 breaths per minute using positive pressure is suggested with a concentration of 100% O_2 at a flow rate high enough to maintain effective ventilation with either a bag-mask-valve device or an anesthesia machine.
3. Up to several minutes of preanesthetic oxygenation is helpful for patients at risk of myocardial ischemia or rapid hemoglobin oxygen desaturation after induction of anesthesia.
4. Hyperventilation (40–50 breaths per minute) prior to and during the seizure may be used to improve seizure quality and increase seizure duration.
5. Supplementary oxygen should be available in the recovery area.

12.1.3. Protecting the Teeth and Other Oral Structures

1. The patient's mouth should be checked for the presence of foreign bodies and loose or sharp teeth before initiating anesthesia.
2. Before applying the electrical stimulus, an appropriately sized, flexible, protective foam or rubber bite block should be inserted in the mouth.
3. An individualized approach to dental management with protective gauze padding or a custom bite block may need to be devised when a patient has a structurally different oral cavity.

12.2. Medications Used With ECT

12.2.1. Anticholinergic Agents

1. Anticholinergic premedications need not be given routinely.
2. Atropine or glycopyrrolate may be used to decrease airway secretions or to minimize the risk of vagally mediated bradyarrhythmias or asystole, particularly in patients receiving sympathetic blocking agents or when the electrical stimulation is likely to be subconvulsive, as during a stimulus dose titration procedure.

3. Atropine may be more reliable than glycopyrrolate in preventing bradyarrhythmias, and intravenous administration is preferred for maximum cardiovascular protection from vagally mediated effects.
4. Anticholinergic premedication should be administered intravenously 2–3 minutes before anesthesia when used for prevention of bradycardia or at least 20 minutes prior to anesthesia induction when used for drying of airway secretions.
5. Typical doses are 0.4–0.8 mg IV for atropine and 0.2–0.4 mg IV for glycopyrrolate.

12.2.2. Anesthetic Agents

1. ECT should be carried out using ultrabrief general anesthesia.
2. Regardless of the anesthetic agent being used, doses should be adjusted at successive treatments to provide the desired clinical effect.
3. Methohexital is the most commonly used anesthetic agent, typically at a dose of 0.75–1.0 mg/kg IV given as a single bolus.
4. Propofol (1.0–2.0 mg/kg IV) can also be used for anesthesia with ECT and may be associated with less significant hemodynamic changes, shorter emergence and recovery times, and fewer post-ECT cognitive effects, but it is associated with shorter seizure durations than is methohexital.
5. Etomidate (0.15–0.40 mg/kg IV) has less of an anticonvulsant effect than methohexital or propofol and is less often associated with hypotension.
6. Ketamine (1.0–2.0 mg/kg) is typically used when adequate seizures are difficult to elicit, but its value for potentiating antidepressant effects of ECT is unclear, and side effects include hypertension; tachycardia; and potential for hallucinations, dissociation, nausea, vomiting, and vertigo.
7. Ultra-short-acting narcotic anesthetics (e.g., remifentanil, alfentanil) have sometimes been used for ECT anesthesia, either alone or in combination with other agents, to attenuate heart rate and blood pressure elevations with ECT or when adequate seizures are difficult to elicit.

12.2.3. Muscle Relaxants

1. A skeletal muscle relaxant should be used to minimize convulsive motor activity and to facilitate airway management.
2. Doses of muscle relaxants should be adjusted at successive treatment sessions to achieve the desired effect.

3. The preferred muscle relaxant agent is the depolarizing muscle relaxant succinylcholine (0.5–1.0 mg/kg IV).
4. Muscle relaxation during ECT can also be achieved by using nondepolarizing agents, which should be used in patients who are at increased risk for succinylcholine-induced hyperkalemia (e.g., severe neuromuscular disease, prolonged immobility from catatonia, severe burn injury) or prolonged apnea because of inability to rapidly metabolize succinylcholine.
5. When a nondepolarizing muscle relaxant is indicated, alternative agents are rocuronium, vecuronium, cisatracurium, and atracurium, with reversal achieved using sugammadex (for rocuronium or vecuronium) or neostigmine in combination with glycopyrrolate (with atracurium or cisatracurium).
6. Higher doses may be needed in patients who require complete relaxation to minimize the risk of treatment complications.
7. The anesthesia provider should ensure that the patient is unconscious and that a patent airway is present prior to injection of the muscle relaxant.
8. The adequacy of skeletal muscle relaxation should be ascertained prior to stimulation by identifying
   a. A loss of muscle tone and diminution or disappearance of knee, ankle, or plantar withdrawal reflexes
   b. Failure to respond to electrical stimulation delivered by a peripheral nerve stimulator
   c. Disappearance of muscle fasciculations, when using a depolarizing muscle blocking agent such as succinylcholine
9. A screening assay for pseudocholinesterase deficiency (by determination of the dibucaine number) should be reserved for patients with a personal or family history of prolonged apnea following exposure to muscle relaxants.

12.2.4. Agents Used to Modify the Cardiovascular Response to ECT

1. Anesthesia providers and ECT psychiatrists should be familiar with pharmacological strategies to prevent or treat adverse cardiovascular responses to ECT, including hypertension, hypotension, and arrhythmias.
2. Pharmacological modifications of the cardiovascular response to ECT have risks (e.g., hypotension) as well as benefits; clinical judgment is needed about when to use such strategies.

3. A strong working relationship with the anesthesia provider, a consultation with a physician with expertise in the assessment and treatment of cardiac disease, and an understanding of the cardiovascular effects of ECT are helpful in optimizing the management of patients with cardiovascular conditions or ECT-associated side effects.
4. In patients with unstable hypertension and other cardiac conditions, an attempt should be made to stabilize these conditions before beginning ECT.
5. In patients who are assessed to be at increased cardiovascular risk, consideration should be given to using prophylactic pharmacological modification at all treatments.
6. The most commonly used agents to modify blood pressure increases and tachycardia during ECT are the β-blocking agents esmolol and labetalol, with the calcium channel blocking agent nicardipine used to improve blood pressure control.

12.3. Infection Control Principles in Providing ECT Anesthesia

1. ECT is an urgent and not an elective procedure for many seriously ill patients and should remain available during times of infectious disease outbreaks.
2. The ECT procedure can be modified to minimize aerosolization of infectious fomites by minimizing bag mask ventilation, using preinduction oxygenation, and preferentially using a Jackson Rees circuit instead of an AMBU bag.

CHAPTER 13

Use of Medications During the Course of Electroconvulsive Therapy

13.1. General Considerations

The patient's medications should be carefully reviewed prior to initiating electroconvulsive therapy (ECT) and prior to each treatment to avoid potential adverse effects due to medication-medication and medication-treatment interactions. Many medications can have effects on both the safety and the efficacy of ECT, and the ECT practitioner should assess the risks and benefits of each medication and determine whether concomitant medications may cause adverse side effects or influence the efficacy of a course of ECT.

Understanding the impact of concomitant medication on seizure induction or risks of ECT (e.g., cognitive impairment, cardiovascular effects) is important in balancing the risks and benefits of continuing psychotropic medication during a course of ECT. Some psychotropic medications (e.g., antipsychotics, antidepressants) may decrease the seizure threshold or prolong seizure duration, whereas other psychotropics (e.g., benzodiazepines, anticonvulsants) increase the seizure threshold or impede seizure propagation and duration. The efficacy of ECT is clearly correlated with the quality of the ECT-induced seizure (Sackeim et al. 1987a), and using techniques such as stimulus titration to determine the seizure threshold (see Chapter 14) may mitigate the impact of concomitant medication on achieving an adequate stimulus dose for an individual patient.

When a patient is taking medications that may impede seizure induction or increase the risk of ECT-associated side effects, consideration should be given to decreasing the dosage or discontinuing these agents before beginning the ECT course. Medications prescribed for other medical conditions are usually continued, but the timing of administration and dosage may require adjustment. When medication tapering or discontinuation is indicated, however, it should be done gradually whenever possible. Although ECT may need to be started rapidly and psychotropic medication tapering can be challenging in outpatients, abrupt tapering or discontinuation of many agents (e.g., benzodiazepines, antidepressants) can produce withdrawal effects (e.g., rebound anxiety, nausea, headache) that may be mistaken by the patient or clinician as adverse effects of ECT.

13.1.1. Medications Administered Prior to Each Treatment

Pre-ECT orders for each treatment should specify the medications and dose administered or withheld prior to the treatment. In general, medications thought to exert a protective effect with respect to ECT-induced physiological changes and those necessary to optimize medical status should be given before the treatment and taken with a small sip of water, usually a couple of hours prior to ECT. Examples include antihypertensive and antianginal agents, antiarrhythmics (except lidocaine or its analogues, which may block seizure elicitation) (Devanand and Sackeim 1988; Hood and Mecca 1983), antireflux agents, bronchodilators (except theophylline), glaucoma medications (except long-acting cholinesterase inhibitors), and corticosteroids. If patients are receiving high doses of a diuretic, dose reduction or changes in dose timing may be needed to minimize the risk of hypovolemia and hypotension while taking nothing by mouth (NPO). On the other hand, withholding diuretics may be problematic for patients with heart failure or hypertension.

13.1.2. Medications Withheld Until After Each Treatment

The NPO requirement for ECT may negatively affect patients with diabetes. Hypoglycemic medications, including insulin, are generally withheld until after the treatment (Sundsted et al. 2014). However, some practitioners advocate splitting the morning dose of long-acting insulin and administering half of it before ECT and half after the treatment when indicated (Weiner and Sibert 1996). In either case, a blood glucose level should be obtained for diabetic patients to assess for hyperglycemia or hypoglycemia prior to administering a treatment. Because insulin requirements may fluctuate substantially over the course of ECT (e.g., a patient who has not been eating may start eating again), ongoing monitoring of glucose levels and adjustment of insulin dosing is often necessary (Finestone and Weiner 1984). When glucose control is unstable, a medical or endocrinological consultation may be helpful. In patients without diabetes, ECT does not appear to have a clinically relevant effect on serum blood sugar (Rasmussen and Ryan 2005).

13.2. Medications Often Decreased or Withdrawn Prior to or During an ECT Course

13.2.1. Theophylline

Theophylline has been linked to prolonged seizures and status epilepticus during ECT (Abrams 2002; Devanand et al. 1988a, 1998; Fink and Sackeim 1998; Peters et al. 1984; Rasmussen and Zorumski 1993; Schak et al. 2008), even with blood levels in the therapeutic range for asthma control. Because practice guidelines no longer recommend use of theophylline in the routine treatment of chronic obstructive pulmonary disease (Qaseem et al. 2011), use of other bronchodilators is preferred during the ECT course. If theophylline is used, levels should be kept as low as clinically feasible to minimize the risk of prolonged seizures (Devanand et al. 1988a; Fink and Sackeim 1998; Peters et al. 1984; Rasmussen and Zorumski 1993). Checking levels at the time of treatment can help guide future dose adjustments.

13.2.2. Dopaminergic Medications

Case reports support an association between development of delirium with the administration of ECT (Rudorfer et al. 1992; Zervas and Fink 1992) and the use of levodopa (Sinemet) to treat Parkinson's disease. It is not clear if other dopaminergic medications have the same potential complication; however, levodopa should be held on the morning of ECT and given after the patient has recovered from ECT.

13.2.3. Lithium

There are divergent opinions about the safety of continuing lithium during ECT. Data on the relative risks and benefits of the use of lithium with ECT are limited but indicate that many patients have received lithium during ECT without incident (Dolenc and Rasmussen 2005; Jha et al. 1996; Lippmann and Tao 1993; Mukherjee 1993; Tsujii et al. 2019; Volpe et al. 2003). The one prospective comparative study found no significant adverse outcomes when lithium was given in conjunction with ECT (Thirthalli et al. 2011). Another naturalistic study found that low lithium levels (0.3–0.4 mEq/L) were safe and effective in patients with bipolar disorder receiving ECT (Perugi et al. 2017). However, case reports suggest that some patients receiving lithium during ECT may develop delirium or prolonged seizures (Ahmed and Stein 1987; Ali et al. 2023; el-Mallakh 1988; Naguib and Koorn 2002; Patel et al. 2020; Rudorfer et al. 1987; Sadananda et al. 2013; Sartorius et al. 2005; Small and Milstein 1990; Small et al. 1980; Standish-Barry et al. 1985; Strömgren et al. 1980; Weiner et al. 1980a, 1980b), and such effects may be more likely in individuals with preexisting cerebrovascular disease or head injury. In a large U.S. administrative database study, patients who were treated with ECT and lithium ($N=422$) were 11.7 times more likely to have a diagnosis of delirium than were patients receiving ECT who did not receive lithium ($N=64,148$), with rates of 5.7% and 0.6%, respectively (Patel et al. 2020). However, it was not possible to determine the timing of the delirium diagnosis relative to treatment with ECT or lithium. Nevertheless, the investigators urged caution when using the combination of lithium and ECT. Other investigators have found higher lithium levels to be correlated with longer recovery times post ECT (Thirthalli et al. 2011), and concomitant use of lithium may be associated with a lower seizure threshold on the first ECT treatment (Gálvez et al. 2015).

Consequently, the decision to continue lithium during ECT should be made on an individualized basis, weighing possible risks of concomitant treatment against risks of relapse if lithium is withdrawn. If lithium is being initiated to prevent relapse after ECT, use should be delayed until after the completion of the acute ECT treatment course, if possible. In patients who will be receiving continued treatment with lithium, such as those receiving maintenance ECT, the risk of delirium can be reduced by holding the nighttime lithium dose prior to an ECT treatment. Because the risk of toxicity may be increased at higher serum lithium levels, risk may also be reduced by keeping lithium levels in the low-to-moderate therapeutic range.

13.2.4. Benzodiazepines

Many patients treated with ECT are receiving benzodiazepines for symptoms of insomnia, anxiety, agitation, or catatonia. These medications may also be useful in patients who have difficulty cooperating with ECT treatment preparations because of significant anxiety.

Although seizure duration is not associated with the efficacy of ECT (see Chapter 15), most (Boylan et al. 2000; Gálvez et al. 2015; Krueger et al. 1993; Standish-Barry et al. 1985) but not all (Chiao et al. 2020) studies have shown that benzodiazepines reduce seizure duration in a dose-dependent fashion. Consequently, significant effects of benzodiazepines on seizure threshold or duration could lead to missed seizures (Boylan et al. 2000; Gálvez et al. 2015) (see Chapter 21).

Except in catatonia, for which the combination of benzodiazepines with ECT may increase ECT efficacy (Cronemeyer et al. 2022; Petrides et al. 1997; Unal et al. 2013, 2017), some evidence suggests that concurrent treatment with benzodiazepines diminishes the efficacy of ECT (Greenberg and Pettinati 1993; Nettelbladt 1988; Pettinati et al. 1990; Standish-Barry et al. 1985; Strömgren et al. 1980). For example, in a study by Pettinati et al. (1990), the clinical outcome with right unilateral (RUL) ECT was inferior in depressed patients receiving benzodiazepines compared with patients who were not taking these agents. An additional retrospective study found that patients treated with benzodiazepines who received RUL ECT had a decreased response and longer hospital stays than did patients not taking benzodiazepines (Jha and Stein 1996). This finding contrasts with patients taking benzodiazepines and receiving bitemporal (BT) ECT who had no difference in response as compared with patients not taking a benzodiazepine (Gálvez et al. 2013; Jha and Stein 1996). In addition, 82% (9 of 11) patients taking benzodiazepines who did not respond to RUL ECT had a positive response after the electrode placement was switched to BT ECT (Pettinati et al. 1990). Another retrospective study of patients receiving BT ECT using the dose titration method found that patients taking benzodiazepines had higher remission rates than did patients not taking benzodiazepines (Delamarre et al. 2019), although there were no differences in seizure duration or threshold between the two groups.

Given these contrasting results and the lack of prospective data, the clinician should try to discontinue or lower the dose of benzodiazepines before an ECT course. To limit rebound anxiety and other withdrawal symptoms, attention should be paid to the rate of dose reduction if a benzodiazepine is tapered or stopped. For individuals who are receiving a benzodiazepine for treatment of insomnia, short half-life nonbenzodiazepine medications (e.g., zolpidem, zaleplon, eszopiclone), the melatonin receptor agonist ramelteon, or a low dose of the antidepressant trazodone could be used instead. For patients receiving benzodiazepines to manage ECT-related anxiety, other pharmacological and nonpharmacological management options can be tried (Obbels et al. 2017, 2020a, 2020b). If a benzodiazepine cannot be tapered, and particularly if an adequate seizure cannot be induced in a patient receiving a benzodiazepine, flumazenil (0.5–1.0 mg IV) can be administered at the time of anesthetic induction (Bailine et al. 1994; Berigan et al. 1995; Doering and Ball 1995; Krystal et al. 1998b). Some data also suggest that patients receiving a benzodiazepine may respond preferentially to BT ECT (Delamarre et al. 2019; Gálvez et al. 2013; Jha and Stein 1996; Pettinati et al. 1990).

13.2.5. Anticonvulsant Drugs

Like benzodiazepines, anticonvulsant drugs may increase the seizure threshold and interfere with the expression of ECT-induced seizures (Green et al. 1982; Nobler and Sackeim 1993; Sackeim et al. 1991); however, it may not be possible to discontinue an anticonvulsant medication during ECT. For patients who are receiving an anticonvulsant medication for treatment of bipolar disorder, some practitioners decrease the dosage of anticonvulsant medications before ECT, whereas others prefer to reduce dosage only when it is difficult to produce adequate seizures. For patients receiving maintenance ECT, it is probably sufficient to withhold one or two doses of the medication prior to each treatment. Similarly, for patients receiving anticonvulsants for the treatment of a seizure disorder, the morning dose is usually withheld before ECT. Because of the anticonvulsant properties of ECT (Sackeim 1999), some practitioners maintain patients with seizure disorders at reduced doses of anticonvulsant medications during an acute ECT course. Serum level monitoring may be helpful in maintaining anticonvulsants in the low therapeutic range, thereby minimizing interference with the induction of ECT seizures. In addition, in patients treated with anticonvulsants, use of stimulus titration may help assure that subsequent stimuli are sufficiently suprathreshold to produce therapeutic benefits.

Clearly, the effects of anticonvulsant medication on ECT-induced seizures and therapeutic response are important topics with direct relevance to clinical care, but available research evidence is limited (Rubner et al. 2009; Sienaert and Peuskens 2007; Thirthalli et al. 2010). Several studies have described use of mood-stabilizing anticonvulsant medication in patients with mania who were treated with ECT. In a quasi-randomized controlled trial (RCT) ($N=40$), sodium valproate did not affect cognition or seizure duration with ECT, although it did affect seizure threshold (Haghighi et al. 2013). A second study ($N=42$) that randomly assigned participants to either continue sodium valproate (minimum dose of 750 mg/day) or discontinue sodium valproate found no difference in ECT efficacy between the two groups (Jahangard et al. 2012). In both studies, patients underwent bifrontal ECT for a minimum of six sessions and manic symptoms significantly improved over time, regardless of treatment assignment. Another study randomly assigned 36 patients on valproic acid or carbamazepine to continue full dose of anticonvulsant medication, receive a half-dose of anticonvulsant medication, or discontinue anticonvulsant medication (Rakesh et al. 2017). There were no differences among the three groups on seizure parameters with BT ECT or the primary outcomes of clinical improvement and adverse cognitive side effects, but patients in the full-dose group improved faster than patients in the half-dose group (Rakesh et al. 2017). A retrospective chart review study of patients treated with anticonvulsant medication (67.1% on valproate; 20.2% on carbamazepine, 5.1% on lamotrigine; total $N=79$) during a course of bilateral ECT found no difference in ECT efficacy as compared to patients not receiving anticonvulsant medication ($N=122$). However, patients taking anticonvulsant medication had significantly higher seizure thresholds, shorter motor seizures, greater numbers of missed seizures, and longer hospital stays and needed significantly more treatment sessions to achieve symptomatic improvement (Virupaksha et al. 2010).

Data on concomitant use of lamotrigine with ECT are limited but suggest possible effects on seizure induction or duration. A retrospective chart review of 1,868 ECT treatments (187 patients) found that use of lamotrigine was associated with a greater proportion of sessions with an inadequate seizure duration (100 ECT sessions, lamotrigine dosages of 6.25–200 mg/day; Joo et al. 2017). A retrospective chart review of 19 patients (8 patients taking dosages higher than 200 mg/day) found that the use of lamotrigine was associated with more missed seizures but no clinically significant effect on seizure length or stimulus dose (Sienaert et al. 2011a). A case series of 9 patients receiving combined lamotrigine and ECT found no serious adverse events, significant change in mean seizure duration, or time to reorientation (Penland and Ostroff 2006), although the dosage of lamotrigine was relatively low (approximately 100 mg/day; Freeman 2007). No reports were available on the safety or efficacy of topiramate or gabapentin in combination with ECT.

13.3. Medications Typically Continued During a Course of ECT

13.3.1. Antidepressant Medications

Patients who are referred for ECT have typically not responded fully to medications and have significant rates of relapse (Heijnen et al. 2010; Rasmussen et al. 2009; Sackeim et al. 1990; Shapira et al. 1995), especially in the first few weeks after ECT (Jelovac et al. 2013; Prudic et al. 2013; Sackeim et al. 1993, 2000). Thus, if starting or changing an antidepressant medication, it might be helpful to do so early in the ECT course to avoid a gap in effective treatment in this critical period following an acute ECT course. It is also possible that starting an antidepressant medication early in the ECT course will augment response and help sustain remission (Pluijms et al. 2021). If a decision is made to augment ECT with concomitant antidepressant therapy, it may be wise to review the patient's history of medication treatment before selecting a specific antidepressant, using conservative criteria for the adequacy of trials (e.g., dose, duration, adherence). Although unstudied, it would make sense to administer a different class of antidepressant medication during and after ECT rather than continuing one to which the patient's symptoms had already manifested resistance.

13.3.1.1. Serotonin Reuptake Inhibitors, Serotonin-Norepinephrine Reuptake Inhibitors, and Norepinephrine and Dopamine Releaser and Reuptake Inhibitor

The majority of individuals referred for ECT will already be taking an antidepressant medication. Selective serotonin reuptake inhibitor (SSRI) use is common in patients who have received ECT (Keyloun et al. 2017), although there is limited evidence on concomitant treatment. One small RCT included patients with cardiac issues and suggested that paroxetine can be combined safely with ECT (Lauritzen et al. 1996). In addition, a retrospective review (Baghai et al. 2006) found no significant adverse events and an improved response in patients receiving a concomitant SSRI or mirtazapine with ECT as compared with no concomitant antidepressants. Case reports noted the possibility of increased (Caracci and Decina 1991) or decreased (Gutierrez-Esteinou and Pope 1989) seizure duration with ECT and fluoxetine, but other reports suggested that this combination does not increase the risk for prolonged seizures (Harsch and Haddox 1990; Kellner and Bruno 1989; Zis 1992). Retrospective reviews found that seizure duration was increased by SSRIs but that the increase was not clinically significant (Baghai et al. 2006; Potokar et al. 1997).

Research on the use of a serotonin-norepinephrine reuptake inhibitor (SNRI) in combination with ECT has focused on venlafaxine. In an RCT, venlafaxine (*N*=91) and the tricyclic antidepressant (TCA) nortriptyline (*N*=93) were compared with placebo (*N*=135) in patients receiving BT (*N*=164) or RUL (*N*=155) ECT (Sackeim et al. 2009). In terms of efficacy, the nortriptyline group had a better clinical response and received fewer treatments than did the placebo group, whereas the venlafaxine group did not differ significantly from nortriptyline or placebo. The three groups did not differ in adverse events, although nortriptyline treatment was associated with a better cognitive profile than that of either venlafaxine or placebo. The authors concluded that adding nortriptyline to ECT was associated with a clinically significant improvement in the remission rate and was well tolerated. Venlafaxine was also safe and associated with clinical improvements, although not to the same degree as seen with nortriptyline.

In an open-label study of venlafaxine (Gonzalez-Pinto et al. 2002), four individuals (4 of 110 total sessions) had a brief period of asystole that reverted to normal sinus rhythm after treatment with atropine. Patients who experienced asystole had been receiving a significantly higher average dose of venlafaxine than did individuals who did not experience asystole (337.5 ± 43.30 mg vs. 265.38 ± 78.75 mg); all four had received dosages greater than 300 mg/day. Although the absence of a control group makes it impossible to determine the relationship between the occurrence of asystole and venlafaxine use, the authors recommended using less than 300 mg/day when combining venlafaxine with ECT.

With bupropion, reports of spontaneous seizures with high doses of immediate-release formulations have led to concern that this antidepressant might produce prolonged seizures when combined with ECT (Davidson 1989). Some case reports have described an increase in seizure duration when ECT is given to patients taking bupropion (Conway and Nelson 2001; Dersch et al. 2011), but other reports do not show a change in seizure length (Chiao et al. 2020; Kellner et al. 1994b; Rakesh et al. 2020; Takala et al. 2017) or seizure threshold (Rakesh et al. 2020) with acute bupropion use. Thus, the limited evidence suggests that ECT can be given safely in patients taking bupropion, although caution is recommended for patients receiving high bupropion dosages (Rudorfer et al. 1991).

13.3.1.2. Tricyclic Antidepressants

The TCAs have generally been found to be safe when used in therapeutic doses in combination with ECT (el-Ganzouri et al. 1985; Klapheke 1997; Lauritzen et al. 1996; Nelson and Benjamin 1989; Sackeim et al. 2001a). Although an increase in electroencephalography seizure duration may occur (Chiao et al. 2020), the primary concerns are the potential for cardiac (e.g., bundle branch block, orthostatic hypotension) or anticholinergic (e.g., cognitive) side effects, particularly in geriatric patients or patients with concomitant medical problems.

Early research had methodological weaknesses and inconsistent findings on whether concomitant TCA treatment was associated with faster or greater response to ECT or less likelihood of early relapse (Pritchett et al. 1993). Subsequent studies found evidence that concomitant treatment with a TCA, such as nortriptyline or imipramine, may improve ECT outcome. Lauritzen and colleagues (1996) conducted a double-blind trial in which patients without cardiac disease ($n=52$) were randomly assigned to ECT and imipramine (150 mg/day) or ECT and paroxetine (30 mg/day), whereas those with cardiac disease ($n=35$) received treatment with ECT and paroxetine (30 mg/day) or placebo. ECT was started with BT electrode placement for the first three treatments and was then switched to RUL ECT. The group treated concurrently with imipramine had greater reductions in symptom severity than did the paroxetine comparison group, whereas in cardiac patients the paroxetine and placebo groups did not differ in clinical ratings following ECT or in the number of ECT treatments administered. However, another RCT ($N=47$) found no differences in the rate of response to BL ECT with concomitant receipt of nortriptyline as compared with placebo (Pluijms et al. 2022). In terms of reduction of relapse, patients with major depressive disorder ($N=84$) who had a successful course of ECT were randomly assigned to be maintained on placebo, nortriptyline (75–125 ng/mL), or nortriptyline and lithium (0.5–0.9 mEq/L) (Sackeim et al. 2001a). The 6-month relapse rates were 84%, 60%, and 39%, respectively, demonstrating the superiority of the combination of lithium and nortriptyline in maintaining remission. This study set the gold standard for relapse prevention following ECT. A subsequent RCT comparing venlafaxine ($N=91$), nortriptyline ($N=93$), and placebo ($N=135$) in patients receiving BT ($N=164$) or RUL ($N=155$) ECT found a better clinical response and a need for fewer treatments with nortriptyline as compared with placebo but no difference between nortriptyline and venla-faxine (Sackeim et al. 2009).

In a retrospective study of 84 geriatric patients with unipolar major depression (Nelson and Benjamin 1989), patients were categorized as having received suprathreshold RUL ECT alone, ECT plus low-dose nortriptyline (e.g., serum level 2–49 ng/mL), or ECT plus a therapeutic dose of nortriptyline (e.g., serum level 50–149 ng/mL). Patients who received a combination of ECT and nortriptyline showed no difference in postictal confusion or cardiac side effects but had superior clinical outcome and required significantly fewer treatments than did the group who received ECT alone (8.1 vs. 9.8 treatments). This effect was graded, increasing in magnitude from the low-dose to the therapeutic dose groups, consistent with a benefit of concomitant nortriptyline in enhancing clinical response to ECT.

13.3.1.3. Monoamine Oxidase Inhibitors

There has long been reluctance to administer anesthesia (including that given with ECT) to patients currently or recently receiving nonselective monoamine oxidase inhibitors (MAOIs). In the presence of an MAOI, there has been concern that any pressor agents given to treat a hypotensive episode would not be catabolized and could precipitate a hypertensive crisis. However, available evidence suggests that MAOIs need not be stopped prior to anesthesia (Ebrahim et al. 1993; van Haelst et al. 2012) and that doing so may worsen hemodynamic instability (Sprung et al. 1996) or contribute to worsening of psychiatric symptoms (Abdi et al. 1996).

When MAOIs have been used concomitantly with ECT, few examples of untoward effects have been reported (Bodley et al. 1969; Caudill et al. 2011). Evidence from case reports suggests that MAOIs can be used safely in conjunction with ECT (Beresford et al. 2004; Dolenc et al. 2004b; Freese 1985; Imlah et al. 1965; Kellner et al. 1992b; Monaco and Delaplaine 1964; Muller 1961; Naguib and Koorn 2002; Remick et al. 1987; Wells and Bjorksten 1989). Nonetheless, prudent practice dictates that certain precautions be observed. Hypotension in the presence of MAOIs should not be treated with an indirect-acting vasopressor (e.g., ephedrine). Rather, phenylephrine or a similar agent is recommended. Although meperidine, tramadol, tapentadol, methadone, dextromethorphan, dextropropoxyphene, and pentazocine are contraindicated in combination with an MAOI, these medications would not be expected to be used in the context of ECT; other opioid medications are safe to use in conjunction with an MAOI (Gillman 2005). Evidence on the use of ECT with selective MAOIs (e.g., selegiline, moclobemide) is not available, but theoretically, such medications are likely to have comparable or fewer risks than do nonselective MAOIs.

13.3.2. Antipsychotic Medications

Concomitant use of an antipsychotic medication is common among individuals who are receiving ECT, either to treat symptoms of psychosis or as an adjunctive treatment to antidepressant medications. Dopamine blocking agents, such as metoclopramide and prochlorperazine, have also been used to treat postprocedure nausea and vomiting (see Chapter 19).

With the exception of reserpine, which is no longer used as an antipsychotic agent and is contraindicated with ECT (Bross 1957; Gaitz et al. 1956), antipsychotic medications appear to be safe. In addition, the combination of ECT and antipsychotic medication may be more effective in the treatment of schizophrenia than either form of treatment alone (Ahmed et al. 2017; Ali et al. 2019; American Psychiatric Association 2021; Chanpattana and Sackeim 2010; Chanpattana et al. 1999a; Fink and Sackeim 1996; Grover et al. 2017; Lally et al. 2016; H.T. Lin et al. 2018; Nothdurfter et al. 2006; Pawełczyk et al. 2014; Petrides et al. 2015; Ravanić et al. 2009; Tang et al. 2012; Usta Saglam et al. 2020; Vuksan Ćusa et al. 2018; Wagner et al. 2020; Wang et al. 2018; Zervas et al. 2012); see also Chapter 2.

Initially, there was concern that concomitant use of ECT and clozapine might result in prolonged or spontaneous seizures (Bloch et al. 1996), but this combination also appears to be safe and effective (Benatov et al. 1996; Bhatia et al. 1998; Cardwell and Nakai 1995; Chanpattana 2000; Frankenburg et al. 1993; Grover et al. 2015, 2017; Kupchik et al. 2000; Lally et al. 2016; Safferman and Munne 1992; Sedgwick et al. 1990; Youn et al. 2019). For example, one review of 40 reports including 208 patients receiving combined clozapine and ECT found only 5 patients who developed delirium, 5 with significant tachycardia, and 4 who were described as having prolonged seizures (Grover et al. 2015). The one prospective randomized trial showed that the combination of clozapine plus BT ECT was well tolerated and significantly more effective than clozapine alone, with response rates of 50% versus 0%, respectively (Petrides et al. 2015).

13.3.3. Stimulants

Data on use of stimulants during ECT are limited, and no RCTs are available. A systematic retrospective review did not find an effect of stimulants on seizure threshold or duration (Chiao et al. 2020), although there have been reports of dysrhythmias, hypertension, and decreases in seizure threshold when stimulants are used with ECT (Naguib and Koorn 2002). Thus, a patient who is receiving treatment with a stimulant should be monitored carefully for these side effects. When clinically feasible, stimulants may be held until after the ECT session or discontinued during the acute ECT course.

13.3.4. Cholinesterase Inhibitors

Patients are sometimes referred to ECT while taking cholinesterase inhibitors for dementia. Although published literature on the combination of these agents with ECT is sparse, concerns have been raised about the use of these medications with ECT based on their potential to interact with succinylcholine and contribute to prolonged apnea or bradyarrhythmias (Bhat et al. 2004). Despite these theoretical concerns, case reports, open-label studies, and placebo-controlled trials have not described either of these adverse effects when patients received ECT in conjunction with a cholinesterase inhibitor such as rivastigmine, donepezil, or galantamine (Bhat et al. 2004; Logan and Stewart 2007; Matthews et al. 2008, 2013; Prakash et al. 2006; Rao et al. 2009; Zink et al. 2002). No information is available on ECT in patients using ocular cholinesterase inhibitors to treat glaucoma, but systemic effects are likely to be minimal. Thus, the available evidence does not suggest serious risks associated with the use of cholinesterase inhibitors during treatment with ECT.

13.3.5. Triptans

Some patients referred for ECT may be receiving triptans to prevent post-ECT headache (see Chapter 19), whereas other patients may receive triptans for chronic headaches or migraines (DeBattista and Mueller 1995; Fantz et al. 1998; Markowitz et al. 2001; White et al. 2006). Limited information from case reports suggests that triptans can be used in conjunction with ECT with a low risk of adverse effects.

Recommendations

13.1. General Considerations

1. All medications should be reviewed as part of the pre-ECT evaluation.
2. Medications thought to exert a protective effect with respect to ECT should be given before each treatment.
3. Medications that may interfere with the therapeutic properties of ECT or cause other adverse effects should be decreased or withheld whenever possible.
4. When applicable, medications should be discontinued gradually to reduce withdrawal symptoms.
5. Pre-ECT orders should specify which medications are to be administered and which are to be withheld before each treatment.
6. Classes of agents generally given before an ECT treatment include (but are not limited to) antihypertensives, antianginals, antiarrhythmics (with the exception of lidocaine), antireflux agents, bronchodilators (except theophylline), glaucoma medications (except long-acting cholinesterase inhibitors), and corticosteroids.
7. Hypoglycemic agents are generally withheld until after each treatment, although administration and dosing of insulin, particularly long-acting insulin, typically needs to be adjusted for each individual patient.

13.2. Medications Often Decreased or Withdrawn Prior to or During an ECT Course

1. Theophylline should be discontinued or decreased because of the risk of prolonged seizures or status epilepticus.
2. To reduce the risk of delirium, levodopa should be held the morning of ECT and given in the recovery area.
3. To reduce the risk of delirium, lithium is typically discontinued or kept at low serum levels during an acute ECT course and held the evening before ECT in patients receiving maintenance ECT.
4. When clinically feasible, benzodiazepines should be tapered prior to an ECT course, or flumazenil should be given before each ECT to minimize the effects of benzodiazepines on seizure activity.
5. Decisions about continuation of anticonvulsant medications depend on the indication for treatment and a risk-benefit analysis for the individual patient.

6. When used for treatment of a seizure disorder, the morning anticonvulsant dose is often held, and the anticonvulsant blood levels are kept as low as clinically feasible.
7. When an anticonvulsant is used for treatment of a mood disorder, the dosage may be decreased during an acute ECT course, particularly if it is difficult to elicit a seizure with ECT, whereas with maintenance ECT, one or two doses of the anticonvulsant are typically withheld prior to each treatment.

13.3. Medications Typically Continued During a Course of ECT

1. The SSRIs and SNRIs are safe when used with patients receiving ECT.
2. Bupropion appears to be safe in patients receiving ECT, although patients taking high dosages of bupropion may have a longer duration of ECT-induced seizures.
3. TCAs have been shown to be safe when used in combination with ECT, and the TCA nortriptyline may increase ECT efficacy and decrease relapse rates.
4. MAOIs do not need to be routinely discontinued prior to a course of ECT, although treating clinicians should be aware of medications that are contraindicated for use with MAOIs such as indirect-acting vasopressors and some opioid medications.
5. Antipsychotic medications are safe for use with ECT.
6. When clinically feasible, stimulants should be discontinued or held until after the ECT session because of possible side effects, including decreases in the seizure threshold, dysrhythmias, and hypertension.
7. Decisions about continuing cholinesterase inhibitors should consider the potential cognitive benefits of treatment for the patient as well as the theoretical but not yet substantiated possibility of associated asystole, bradycardia, or prolongation of the muscle-relaxing effects of succinylcholine.
8. Triptans can be continued during treatment with ECT.

CHAPTER 14

The Electrical Stimulus and Placement of Stimulus Electrodes

14.1. Waveform Characteristics

According to standard nomenclature proposed for transcranial electrical stimulation, the electrical stimulus delivered by electroconvulsive therapy (ECT) devices involves high-intensity transcranial electrical stimulation with a pulsed waveform given at an intensity sufficient to induce a seizure (Bikson et al. 2019). Furthermore, ECT devices generate trains of rectangular pulses that alternate in direction (i.e., polarity) (Figure 14–1).

Waveforms differ markedly in their efficiency in eliciting seizures (Peterchev et al. 2010; Sackeim et al. 1994). Generally speaking, as compared with a sine wave stimulus, a brief pulse stimulus can produce a seizure with a lower stimulus intensity, expressed in either units of charge (millicoulombs [mC] or milliampere-seconds [mA-sec]) or energy (joules [J] or watt-seconds) (Weiner 1980). It is believed that the leading edge of each phase of the waveform is responsible for neuronal depolarization and seizure induction. Through the process of accommodation, the firing threshold of neurons can be increased by applying a slow-rising current, as occurs with a sine wave stimulus. In contrast, the fast-rising current with a rectangular brief pulse stimulus will result in cell firing at lower current intensity (Koester 1985).

As shown in Figure 14–1, the traditional sine wave stimulus is slow to reach maximum intensity and has a long phase duration. Therefore, at the beginning of each phase, stimulation intensity is too low to produce effective depolarization, and the neuronal threshold will increase. After peak intensity is reached with the sine wave, the long-phase duration results in more stimulation than necessary to induce the seizure, which is thought to contribute to the inefficiency of stimulation and the

A

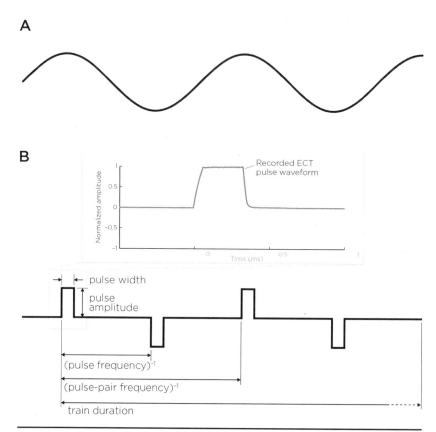

B

Figure 14–1. *(A) Sine wave. (B) Brief pulse waveform as recorded and with stimulus parameters labeled.*

To obtain the recorded ECT pulse waveform, the ECT device was discharged onto a resistive load (e.g., 300 Ω). The voltage across the load was recorded using an oscilloscope, and the current was calculated using Ohm's law. In the lower part of the figure, the amplitude or height of each pulse reflects the current administered, as measured in milliamps (mA). The peak currents of ECT devices range from 500 to 900 mA; however, with constant current stimulation, this amplitude will be consistent across all pulses. The duration of each pulse is the pulse width and typically varies between 0.25 and 2.0 ms. The number of pulse pairs (bidirectional pulses) per second determines the frequency of the stimulus. A total of 80 pulses or 40 pulse pairs per second is equivalent to a frequency of 40 Hz. Depending on the device, the frequency may vary from 10 to 120 Hz. The total duration of the pulse train determines the stimulus duration. Depending on the device, this may vary from 0.5 to 8.0 seconds.

MST = magnetic seizure therapy.

Source.   Zhi-De Deng. Used with permission.

greater extent of cognitive side effects when ECT is administered with a sine wave stimulus as compared with a rectangular pulse stimulus. In contrast, the rectangular pulsed waveform reaches peak intensity virtually instantaneously. The duration of each pulse is relatively short, with a rapid return to baseline. Therefore, brief pulse stimulation is more electrically efficient than sine wave stimulation in eliciting seizures.

Comparative studies have generally found sine wave and brief pulse stimulation to be equivalent in efficacy, but brief pulse is superior in tolerability (Andrade et al. 1988a; Carney et al. 1976; Scott et al. 1992; Valentine et al. 1968; Weiner et al. 1986a). More specifically, short-term cognitive side effects (Carney et al. 1976; Valentine et al. 1968; Weiner et al. 1986a) and interictal electroencephalogram (EEG) slowing (Weiner et al. 1986b) are considerably more severe with sine wave stimulation. Consequently, sine wave stimulation in ECT is not justified and should not be used.

14.2. Stimulus Parameters

The maximal output of ECT devices depends on local regulations. ECT devices available in the United States are limited by the U.S. Food and Drug Administration to a maximal output of 576 mC or approximately 100 J at a 220-ohm (Ω) impedance (Krystal et al. 2000a). Devices available in other parts of the world have double this maximal output, up to 1,200 mC.

Although the relative efficiency of manipulating pulse amplitude (current) is beginning to be explored (see Chapter 24), available ECT devices generate a constant current stimulus, in which the peak current is either fixed or set by the user. Use of a constant current mode of delivery also guarantees the delivery of a predetermined charge. By Ohm's law (voltage=current×impedance), voltage varies as a function of the impedance (or resistance in the case of direct current) to the passage of the current. Thus, depending on the impedance, the device adjusts the voltage administered during the stimulation to keep the current at the desired level. A very high impedance, due to a poor quality of contact at the interface between the electrodes and the skin, will result in an excessive output voltage, which can theoretically produce skin burns. For this reason, available ECT devices are equipped with voltage limiters that prevent delivery of excessive voltage under abnormally high impedance conditions. Devices that deliver either a constant voltage or a constant energy were available in the past, but there is no conceptual justification for such designs.

With constant current brief pulse devices, several other features of the stimulus may be varied. More specifically, in addition to altering the peak current amplitude, the clinician may adjust some or all of the following parameters: the width of pulses, the frequency of pulses, and the duration of the pulse train (see Figure 14–1). Stimulus intensity controls on ECT devices should allow sufficient flexibility in one or more of these parameters to treat patients with a broad range of seizure thresholds. It should also be noted that radically different configurations of stimulus parameters may be associated with identical summary measures of overall stimulus intensity, such as charge or energy. For example, the charge of a bidirectional brief pulse stimulus delivered with a pulse frequency of 40 Hz, a pulse width of 1.4 ms, a pulse amplitude of 800 mA, and a train duration of 2 seconds will be 179.2 mC. An identical charge would be delivered by doubling the frequency to 80 Hz, decreasing the pulse width to 1.0 ms, and shortening the train duration to 1.4 seconds.

A considerable body of research has addressed the effects of modifying pulse width on the efficiency of stimulation. In general, it appears that extending the pulse width of the ECT stimulus beyond 1.0 ms is the least efficient method of increasing the stimulus intensity. In contrast, pulse widths of 0.5–0.75 ms are more efficient in seizure elicitation than are pulse widths of longer duration (Ithal et al. 2020; Rasmussen et al. 1994; Swartz and Larson 1989; Swartz and Manly 2000).

Ultrabrief pulse widths (e.g., 0.25–0.3 ms) may be particularly efficient at seizure elicitation (Lisanby et al. 1997). Studies in animals (Hovorka et al. 1960; Hyrman et al. 1985; Liberson 1945, 1947) and humans (Cronholm and Ottosson 1963; Goldman 1949; Liberson 1948; Pisvejc et al. 1998; Robin and de Tissera 1982) have established that ultrabrief pulse configurations can reliably elicit generalized seizures at a substantially lower absolute electrical dosage than standard brief pulse stimulation can. In fact, the chronaxie, which is the optimal current duration to produce central neuronal depolarization, may be of the order of only 0.1–0.2 ms (Peterchev et al. 2010; Sackeim et al. 1994). Ultrabrief pulse widths that are closer to the chronaxie are, thus, more efficient than are longer pulse widths that deliver more charge to depolarize a neuron than necessary (Peterchev et al. 2010). For this reason, use of ultrabrief pulse width right unilateral (RUL) ECT is an effective way of lowering the threshold for seizure induction and permits most patients to be treated at sufficient stimulus intensities with existing U.S. devices (Kellner et al. 2016b).

Research has examined whether suprathreshold stimulation with ultrabrief pulses can preserve the efficacy of ECT while further reducing cognitive side effects. In a systematic review and meta-analysis of studies that compared brief and ultrabrief pulse RUL ECT, brief pulse RUL ECT was more efficacious but had greater effects on global cognition, retrograde memory, and anterograde learning and recall than did ultrabrief pulse RUL ECT (Tor et al. 2015). Individual randomized controlled trials (RCTs) included two that found comparable efficacy of ultrabrief pulse RUL (0.3 ms at 6–8 times seizure threshold) and brief pulse RUL (1.0–1.5 ms at 5–6 times seizure threshold) with a superior cognitive side effect profile for ultrabrief pulse RUL (Loo et al. 2014; Sackeim et al. 2008). However, another medium-size RCT found greater efficacy and a more rapid response with brief pulse as compared with ultrabrief pulse when RUL ECT was given twice weekly at 8 times seizure threshold using brief pulse (1.0 ms) or ultrabrief pulse (0.3–0.4 ms) waveforms (Spaans et al. 2013). Of the other studies in the meta-analysis, many were underpowered, used limited cognitive assessments, had short periods of follow-up, or varied in the extent to which the stimulus intensity was above the seizure threshold (Tor et al. 2015; Verwijk et al. 2012). Data from observational studies also provide a mixed picture. A pooled retrospective analysis of brief pulse RUL ECT (at 5 times seizure threshold) compared with ultrabrief pulse RUL ECT (at 6 times seizure threshold) found comparable response rates for the two groups but a trend for faster improvement and higher remission rates in patients who received brief pulse as compared with ultrabrief pulse RUL ECT (Loo et al. 2013). In addition, data on RUL ECT from the Swedish National Quality Register showed no differences at 6-month follow-up in remission rate or subjective memory impairment among the groups that had a stimulus pulse width of <0.5, 0.5, or >0.5 ms (Tornhamre et al. 2020). However, another retrospective study (Ramalingam et al. 2016) found a greater need for switching electrode placements or pulse widths in the midst of the ECT course when ultrabrief pulse RUL ECT was used as compared with other brief pulse RUL or bilateral (BL) ECT. Taken together, the available evidence with RUL ECT suggests potential advantages for ultrabrief pulse widths (0.3 ms) in terms of cognitive side effects as compared with brief pulse widths of 1.0–1.5 ms, but brief pulse RUL ECT offered some advantages in efficacy in some but not all studies. Comparisons of RUL ultrabrief stimuli and brief pulse widths of 0.5 ms require additional study, as does the impact of stimulus intensity above the seizure threshold on the efficacy and side effects of ultrabrief stimuli.

Fewer studies have been done using ultrabrief BL ECT. An initial report suggested that response with ultrabrief BL ECT (2.5 times seizure threshold) may be less robust than that with ultrabrief RUL ECT or brief pulse BL or RUL ECT (Sackeim et al. 2008). In contrast, several small RCTs found no differences in efficacy or neuropsychological effects of ultrabrief pulse (0.3 ms) ECT using bifrontal (BF) (at 1.5 times seizure threshold) or RUL (at 6 times seizure threshold) electrode placement (Sienaert et al. 2009, 2010). A small RCT of bitemporal (BT) ECT that compared ultrabrief (0.3 ms at 3 times seizure threshold) and brief pulse treatment (1.0 ms at 1.5 times seizure threshold) found that efficacy and cognitive outcomes did not differ at the end of the ECT course (Martin et al. 2020b). A small retrospective study of BL ECT found no differences in response or remission rates with stimulus pulse widths of 0.25 ms versus 0.5 ms (Niemantsverdriet et al. 2011). Additional studies of ultrabrief BL ECT are needed, but it seems possible that stimuli will need to be at least 3 times seizure threshold for optimal efficacy.

The effects of changing stimulus parameters other than pulse width are less well studied. Preliminary evidence indicates that increasing the train duration of a brief pulse constant current stimulus is somewhat more efficient in seizure elicitation than increasing pulse frequency (Devanand et al. 1998; Isenberg et al. 2016; Swartz and Larson 1989), and lower pulse frequencies are more efficient than higher frequencies in seizure elicitation (Peterchev et al. 2010).

14.3. Electrode Placement

14.3.1. Choice of Electrode Placement

The most commonly used electrode placements include BT, BF, and RUL electrode placements. RCT evidence indicates that these three common electrode placements have significant and comparable degrees of antidepressant efficacy when the stimulus intensity is adequately dosed relative to the patient's seizure threshold (Kellner et al. 2010; Sienaert et al. 2009, 2010). Because these electrode placements differ in the location where electrodes are positioned on the head, they differ in the parts of the brain that are stimulated (see Figure 14–2).

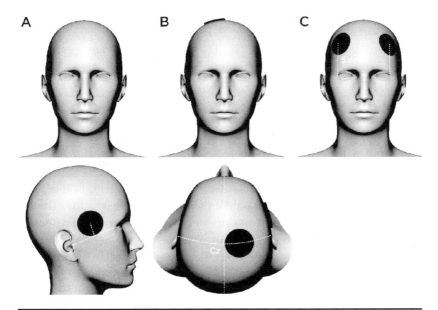

Figure 14–2. *Location of stimulus electrodes with (A) bitemporal (BT), (B) right unilateral (RUL), and (C) bifrontal (BF) electrode placement.*
See Plate 1 to view this figure in color.
(A) With BT ECT, stimulus electrodes are placed on both sides of the head, with midpoints approximately 1 inch above the center of a line connecting the tragus and external canthus. When using 2-inch-diameter electrodes, the bottom of the electrode will be tangential to the line, as illustrated above. **(B)** With RUL ECT, one electrode is placed on the right temple as done with BT, and the other is located at the intersection of the midpoints of the lines going from left to right tragus and from inion to nasion. The midpoint of these lines defines the vertex, and with 2-inch electrodes, the top of the electrode is adjacent to the vertex. **(C)** With BF ECT, each electrode is placed 5 cm above the outer edge of each orbit, along a line parallel to the sagittal plane.
Source. Zhi-De Deng. Used with permission.

Electrode placement may affect the severity and duration of cognitive side effects. Generally speaking, BT ECT produces more short- and long-term adverse cognitive effects than does RUL ECT (d'Elia 1970; Dominiak et al. 2021a; Fromholt et al. 1973; Janicak et al. 1991; McElhiney et al. 1995; Sackeim et al. 1986, 1993, 2007, 2008; Squire 1986; Weiner et al. 1986a). In addition, BT as compared with unilateral ECT is associated with a greater likelihood of developing a transient delirium, at times requiring interruption or premature discontinuation of the ECT course (Daniel and Crovitz 1982, 1986; Miller et al. 1986; Sackeim et al. 1993). Months after the treatment course, the extent of amnesia for autobiographical events may be greater in patients who received BT compared with RUL ECT (Lisanby et al. 2000; McElhiney et al. 1995; Sackeim et al. 2000, 2007; Sobin et al. 1995; Weiner et al. 1986a). These cognitive advantages of RUL as compared with BT ECT are thought to be maintained across psychiatric diagnoses (Sackeim 1992), although evidence from clinical trials is limited. In terms of BF ECT, an initial study (Bailine et al. 2000) and subsequent meta-analysis (Dunne and McLoughlin 2012) showed less decline in Mini-Mental State Examination (MMSE) scores with BF as compared with BT ECT. However, an additional multicenter randomized double-blind controlled trial compared BF (at 1.5 times seizure threshold), BT (at 1.5 times seizure threshold), and RUL ECT (at 6 times seizure threshold) in patients with a major depressive episode. The investigators found no significant differences in antidepressant response or changes in MMSE score or measures of executive function, although response to BT ECT was more rapid than with RUL ECT (Kellner et al. 2010). Furthermore, RUL ECT was not statistically different from BT or BF ECT on measures of anterograde memory or retrograde amnesia, although it did show an advantage on reorientation score at 20 minutes after ECT (Kellner et al. 2010). In this study, BT ECT was superior to BF ECT on two measures of anterograde amnesia (Kellner et al. 2010).

In diagnostic groups other than major depressive disorder, less information is available on the effects of electrode placement on the efficacy of ECT. It has been suggested that BT electrode placement is particularly indicated for patients with acute mania (Milstein et al. 1987), although evidence on this point is contradictory (Black et al. 1986, 1989a; Mukherjee et al. 1988). In schizophrenia, comparative trials of RUL and BT ECT have not detected a difference in efficacy (Bagadia et al. 1988; Doongaji et al. 1973; el-Islam et al. 1970; Wessels 1972). However, this issue is still unresolved because these studies had small samples and other methodological problems (Krueger and Sackeim 1995). More recently, in an RCT, BF ECT was found to be superior in speed of response and efficacy compared with BT ECT in schizophrenia (Phutane et al. 2013). More research is needed to definitively establish the relative efficacies of RUL, BT, and BF ECT in psychiatric conditions other than major depressive disorder.

Even in major depressive disorder, a small subgroup of patients may respond only to BT ECT (Price and McAllister 1986; Sackeim et al. 1993). Although controversy exists in this regard (Strömgren 1984), some practitioners recommend an adequate course of moderately su-

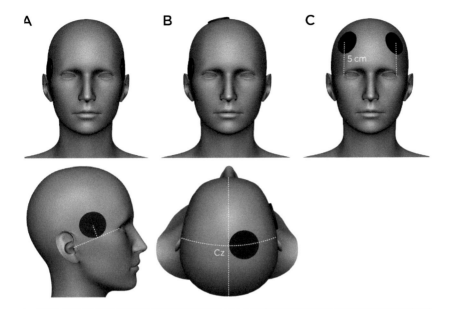

Plate 1. *(Figure 14–2) Location of stimulus electrodes with (A) bitemporal (BT), (B) right unilateral (RUL), and (C) bifrontal (BF) electrode placement.*

(A) With BT ECT, stimulus electrodes are placed on both sides of the head, with midpoints approximately 1 inch above the center of a line connecting the tragus and external canthus. When using 2-inch-diameter electrodes, the bottom of the electrode will be tangential to the line, as illustrated above. **(B)** With RUL ECT, one electrode is placed on the right temple as done with BT, and the other is located at the intersection of the midpoints of the lines going from left to right tragus and from inion to nasion. The midpoint of these lines defines the vertex, and with 2-inch electrodes, the top of the electrode is adjacent to the vertex. **(C)** With BF ECT, each electrode is placed 5 cm above the outer edge of each orbit, along a line parallel to the sagittal plane.

Source.   Zhi-De Deng. Used with permission.

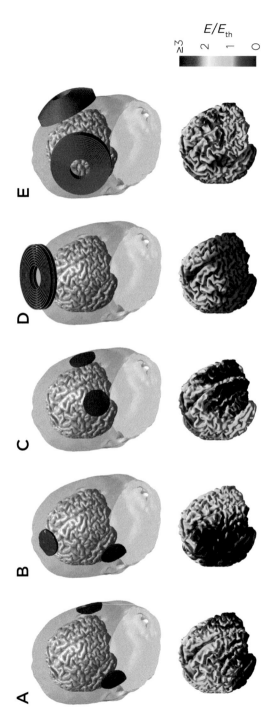

Plate 2. (*Figure 24–1*) *Simulation models of (A) bitemporal ECT, (B) right unilateral ECT, (C) bifrontal ECT, (D) MST with circular coil placed over vertex, and (E) MST with twin coil placed over midline prefrontal cortex. Stimulation strength (E-field magnitude relative to neural activation threshold, E/E_{th}; see Deng et al. 2011) on the cortical surface at current of 800 mA for ECT and 100% of maximum stimulator output for MST.*

ECT = electroconvulsive therapy; MST = magnetic seizure therapy.
Source. Zhi-De Deng. Used with permission.

E/E_{th}

≥3

2

1

0

prathreshold BT treatment before concluding that a patient's symptoms are resistant to ECT (Abrams 1986, 1997; Crismon et al. 1999; Sackeim et al. 1993, 2000).

The extent to which practitioners use RUL, BF, or BT ECT varies considerably (Farah and McCall 1993). Some practitioners use RUL, BF, or BT ECT exclusively. Others start patients with RUL ECT and switch to BT or BF ECT if patients do not respond or if response is excessively slow (Abrams and Fink 1984; Kellner and Farber 2016). For example, patients are often switched to BT or BF ECT if they have not shown sufficient improvement after six RUL treatments. In the face of inadequate response, another option is to increase the stimulus intensity with RUL ECT before switching to BT or BF ECT. Given restrictions on the maximal electrical output of ECT devices in the United States, patients with very high seizure thresholds may also need to be treated with BT or BF ECT if it is not possible to administer substantially suprathreshold stimulation with RUL ECT (see section 14.7). Rather than beginning with RUL ECT, an alternative approach is to start all patients with BT or BF ECT, switching to RUL ECT if cognitive side effects become severe. Another option is to use BT or BF ECT selectively in patients whose psychiatric or medical status requires a greater assurance of rapid clinical response. For patients with a skull defect, such as a skull fracture or metal plate embedded in the skull, the electrode placement should be chosen to avoid stimulating over or adjacent to the skull defect because doing so might alter the current flow, with unclear clinical implications (Amanullah et al. 2012).

Practitioners should be skilled in administering both unilateral and BL ECT (either BF or BT or both). Given the intricacies involved in choosing among electrode placements, practitioners should have a clear understanding of the variations in therapeutic and adverse effects with each electrode placement. In addition, they should appreciate that electrode placement interacts with other factors (e.g., waveform, pulse width, dosage above seizure threshold) and influences clinical or adverse effects. Thus, decisions about electrode placement should be made in concert with decisions about stimulus intensity and other stimulus parameters. Furthermore, because electrode placement affects therapeutic and adverse effects, decisions about electrode placement should be discussed with the patient's attending physician, if different from the ECT psychiatrist, and with the consenter as part of the informed consent process (see Chapter 10).

14.3.2. Electrode Positioning

The BT electrode positioning involves estimating, on each side of the head, the midpoint of the line connecting the external canthus and the tragus. The midpoint of the stimulus electrode is then placed approximately 1 inch above this point (see Figure 14–2). Therefore, with a 2-inch electrode, the bottom of the electrode is tangential to the line connecting the external canthus and the tragus.

The BF electrode positioning has evolved over the years. After an early study with closely spaced BF stimulus electrodes demonstrated decreased memory effects but limited efficacy compared with traditional BT placement (Abrams and Taylor 1973), later investigations used a wider placement for BF ECT, achieved by placing an electrode 5 cm above the outer angle of each orbit on a line parallel to the sagittal plane (Lawson et al. 1990; Letemendia et al. 1993). Given the closer spacing of the BF electrodes compared with the BT or RUL placements, it is important to avoid the risk of electrical shunting that can result from having excessive gel or liquid on the forehead creating a current path between the two electrodes. An asymmetrical electrode placement has also been described that uses a frontal position on the left side and the standard frontotemporal position on the right side (Swartz 1994), but there is limited evidence regarding its safety and efficacy relative to other more common electrode placements.

Although various placements have been used for RUL ECT, a configuration that maximizes interelectrode distance may be optimal with regard to efficacy and seizure elicitation (Pettinati et al. 1986). Among the unilateral placements, the d'Elia (1970) location is recommended. This placement involves determining the intersection of the lines connecting the two auditory tragi and the nasion and inion. The midpoint of the parietal electrode is then placed approximately 1 inch lateral to this point (see Figure 14–2). The frontotemporal electrode is in the same position as in traditional BT BL ECT. A prefrontal unilateral placement should be avoided because of difficulties in seizure elicitation (Erman et al. 1979).

In right-handed patients, RUL ECT produces less disruption of verbal functions than does left unilateral ECT or BL ECT (Daniel and Crovitz 1983). However, in left-handed patients, the optimal stimulus electrode placement is uncertain. It is estimated that approximately 70% of left-handed patients are lateralized for language functions in a manner similar to that of right-handed patients, 15% have bilateral representation of language, and 15% have reversal of the typical pattern, with right hemisphere superiority for language functions (Bryden 1982; Bryden and Steenhuis 1991; Peters 1995; Rasmussen and Milner 1977). In this light, most practitioners prefer to administer RUL ECT independent of handedness, although a recent review of the literature provides information on the safety and efficacy of left unilateral ECT (Kellner et al. 2017). Although its use has been uncommon, it has been suggested that the laterality of unilateral electrode placement could be alternated over the first few treatments to determine which placement is associated with less severe acute confusion and verbal amnesia (Pratt et al. 1971).

If handedness is considered in determining electrode placement, it is important to recognize that the hand used in writing and the patient's report of handedness are fallible indicators (Peters 1995). Many strongly left-handed individuals write with the right hand. Individuals who are basically right-handed may report being ambidextrous or left-handed (or vice versa) because of inconsistencies in hand usage for different activities. Inquiries should be made concerning a set of specific activities, such as throwing a ball, use of a knife and fork, use of scissors, and so on. Standardized sets of items are readily available (e.g., Oldfield 1971; Porac and Coren 1981; Rackowski et al. 1976). Predominant hand usage should determine assignment of handedness. Assessment of asymmetry in other domains (e.g., eyedness or footedness) is not germane.

14.4. Stimulus Electrode Types

Generally speaking, a larger electrode surface area will result in lower impedance to the passage of the current. In general, firm pressure of the electrode against the scalp helps minimize impedance. The metal electrodes may be applied to the scalp using a snugly fitting band or handheld electrodes. Handheld electrodes must be insulated so that the user is not in contact with the electrode or with exposed wiring connecting the stimulus cable to the electrode. Instead of using metal electrodes and conductant gel, another approach is the use of disposable ECT stimulating pads that have an adhesive and conducting gel already included. Disposable adhesive pad electrodes, like the snugly fitting band, have the advantage of not requiring an operator to hold them in place when BL ECT is performed. Nevertheless, adhesive electrodes can be difficult to apply if there is extensive hair at the BT electrode placement sites, and a handheld electrode is still typically needed at the rostral (vertex) site with unilateral ECT. In the past, saline-soaked pads were used as the conductant on electrodes, but this is no longer recommended.

14.5. Stimulus Electrode Site Preparation

Careful attention should be paid to the preparation of the scalp stimulus electrode sites and to the contact between the electrodes and the scalp. An increase in impedance will occur if there is inadequate preparation or poor contact, and with constant current devices, an overly high impedance will prevent the stimulus from being delivered.

A standard procedure for electrode site preparation should be developed by each facility. One method involves cleansing the skin with a solvent such as rubbing alcohol. After the site has dried, an abrasive conductant is rubbed into the scalp to lower site impedance. These gels are often referred to as *electrode gel* or *electrolyte gel* and are sold by medical supply companies. Conductant gel is then applied to the electrodes to ensure an adequate interface. If the electrode site is covered by a significant amount of hair, as is likely to be the case for the rostral (upper) electrode with unilateral placement, it is often sufficient to simply part the hair prior to rigorous application of the solvent and abrasive conductant; however, for individuals with coarse, curly hair textures it may be necessary to style hair in widely spaced cornrows to permit effective electrode contact. Routine shaving of the hair is unnecessary. Care should be taken to prevent smearing of any conducting medium across the scalp between the electrodes because this will produce an alternate path for the stimulus current. Because the smeared conducting medium has a low impedance, a greater proportion of current will pass across the scalp instead of entering the brain. This shunting of current results in a lessened ability to elicit a seizure.

14.6. Impedance Testing

Modern ECT devices have built-in capacity to assess the integrity of the ECT circuit prior to the administration of the stimulus. During this procedure, which is an important part of safe ECT practice, an imperceptible current is passed, and the impedance in the total circuit is determined. The normal range for this static impedance is from 100 to 3,000 Ω. An abnormally low static impedance is most often due to smearing of conductive medium between the electrodes, but it may also occur if the patient has heavy perspiration or has administered a cream, gel, or spray to the hair. Excessively high impedance may be due to poor contact between an electrode and the scalp, incomplete or improper preparation of the electrode sites, poor contact between the electrodes and the stimulus cable, a break in the stimulus cable, or a poor connection or disconnection of the stimulus cable from the device.

If an abnormally high or low value of static impedance is observed, the cause should be ascertained and remedied before proceeding with the treatment. The presence of a value of static impedance in the normal range should be verified by administration of another testing procedure or via a continuous readout of impedance values from devices so equipped. Even if static impedance values are in a generally acceptable range (e.g., less than 3,000–5,000 Ω depending on the device), a marked increase in static impedance prior to stimulation should alert the practitioner to the fact that electrode contact at the sites may not be optimal. However, regardless of static impedance levels, when dynamic impedance is extremely high, all present U.S. ECT devices have built-in voltage-limiting features (typically at 400–450 volts), which prevent the delivery of the stimulus.

14.7. Stimulus Dosing

Several considerations influence the dosage of the ECT stimulus. Patients have marked variability (as much as fiftyfold) in the electrical threshold for eliciting an adequate seizure (Boylan et al. 2000; Coffey et al. 1995a; Colenda and McCall 1996; Enns and Karvelas 1995; Lisanby et al. 1996; Sackeim et al. 1987c; Shapira et al. 1996). Factors such as electrode placement, stimulation parameters, sex, anesthetic dosage, and concomitant medications are known to affect the seizure threshold (Beale et al. 1994b; Boylan et al. 2000; Chiao et al. 2020; Francis-Taylor et al. 2020; Gálvez et al. 2015; Gangadhar et al. 1998; Kronsell et al. 2021; Krueger et al. 1993; Luccarelli et al. 2021b; Peterchev et al. 2010; Sackeim et al. 1987c, 1991; Unal et al. 2021). Seizure threshold also increases with age, and very low thresholds for seizure elicitation are particularly likely in children and adolescents (Ghaziuddin et al. 2020; Petrides et al. 2009).

The minimum electrical dosage with respect to seizure threshold is a function of both stimulus electrode placement and waveform, with both RUL and ultrabrief stimuli being associated with a need for higher stimulus intensity to assure clinical response (Sackeim et al. 1993, 2000, 2008). Regardless of electrode placement, the speed of clinical response may be slower with barely suprathreshold stimuli than with higher-intensity stimuli (Nobler et al. 1997; Robin and de Tissera 1982; Sackeim et al. 1993, 2000). With RUL electrode placement, stimuli barely above threshold have been found to be therapeutically weak (Krystal et al. 1995; Letemendia et al. 1993; Sackeim et al. 1987b, 1993, 2000). The efficacy of RUL ECT notably improves when stimulus intensity is moderately suprathreshold (e.g., 150% above or 2.5 times the initial threshold), but this form of RUL ECT may still be inferior in clinical outcome to BT ECT (Sackeim et al. 1993, 2000). However, studies demonstrate that when RUL ECT stimulation is markedly suprathreshold (e.g., 500% above or 6 times the threshold), its efficacy is equivalent to BT ECT (Kellner et al. 2010; McCall et al. 2000; Sackeim et al. 2000, 2008). This finding coincides with evidence that RUL ECT is particularly efficacious when a high fixed electrical dosage is used (Abrams et al. 1991; d'Elia 1992; McCall et al. 1995, 2000). Consequently, for treating major depressive disorder, RUL ECT should be used with a minimum electrical dosage exceeding initial threshold by more than 150% (2.5 times) initial seizure threshold, particularly with ultrabrief stimulus waveform, for which 500% (6 times) initial seizure threshold is required (Sackeim et al. 2008). An even higher intensity relative to threshold (up to 500% above or 6 times threshold) may exert greater efficacy with relatively little difference in cognitive side effects (Kellner et al. 2010; Sackeim et al. 2000). With BL (including BT and BF) ECT, the maximal dosage administered with brief pulse stimuli should be, at most, moderately suprathreshold (i.e., 1.5–2.5 times threshold) for most patients (Kellner et al. 2010). Increasing the stimulus dosage above this value with brief pulse BL ECT only rarely enhances efficacy and is likely to accentuate cognitive side effects (Ottosson 1960; Sackeim et al. 1993). Fewer data are available regarding stimulus dosing with ultrabrief BL ECT (Sackeim et al. 2008), but intermediate doses, between those required for brief pulse BL and ultrabrief pulse RUL, are likely necessary to maximize the likelihood of an adequate therapeutic response. Regardless of electrode placement and stimulus waveform, further increases in stimulus intensity are often needed over an acute ECT series because of the fact that seizure threshold rises to a variable and unpredictable extent (Sackeim et al. 1987c).

As a consequence of the significant variability in seizure threshold based on electrode placement, stimulus characteristics, and patient-specific factors, an approach to individualizing stimulus dosing is needed. For this reason, many practitioners use an empirical titration procedure (Sackeim et al. 1987a) because they prefer to be cognizant of the degree to which stimulus dosage exceeds seizure threshold. Other practitioners use a formula to specify electrical dosage that accounts for one or more of the factors that predict seizure threshold (Petrides and Fink 1996b; Petrides et al. 2009). Delivery of a fixed electrical dose for all patients is not recommended.

14.7.1. Empirical Stimulus Titration

Empirical stimulus titration provides the most precise method for estimating seizure threshold, and a number of studies argue that stimulus titration is the preferred method of dosing to optimize outcomes (Ittasakul et al. 2019). Particularly with RUL ECT, which is highly dose-dependent, stimulus titration is a more accurate way to ensure safe and effective treatment (Tiller and Ingram 2006).

With this approach, a titration procedure is usually conducted at the first treatment, and possibly later in the course if clinical improvement has stalled and an increase in seizure threshold is suspected. At each treatment, the parameters of administered stimuli and the number of stimulations should be documented. At the initial treatment, a stimulus dosage is selected that is expected to result in an adequate seizure in only a minority of patients. (The manufacturer's manual can be consulted for sample seizure threshold titration schedules and associated suprathreshold dosing parameters.)

Because subconvulsive stimuli result in vagal stimulation and parasympathetic-mediated bradycardia (Decina et al. 1984; McCall et al. 1994), some practitioners elect to premedicate with an anticholinergic agent (atropine or glycopyrrolate) when empirical titration is used (Zielinski et al. 1993). Use of an anticholinergic agent may be particularly important if patients are also pretreated with a β-blocking agent (Decina et al. 1984; McCall 1996).

Once it is established that the stimulus was subconvulsive and did not elicit sustained motoric or EEG manifestations of a seizure, the stimulus intensity is increased and the patient is restimulated. The interval between restimulations should be approximately 20 seconds to observe for delayed seizures that may occur with barely suprathreshold stimuli and to reduce residual effects of the previous subconvulsive stimulus (see Chapter 21). With most stimulus dose titration protocols, the distribution of seizure threshold values is such that most patients have an adequate seizure by the second or third stimulation; however, each facility should adopt a policy on the maximal number of restimulations permitted during a session; four or five stimulations is a common cutoff. In addition, a larger dose increment should be used for the final restimulation in a dose titration procedure. Limited evidence suggests that cognitive side effects are not intensified by the administration of subconvulsive stimuli followed by convulsive stimuli as compared with convulsive stimuli alone (Prudic et al. 1994).

With empirical titration, the subconvulsive stimulus prolongs unconsciousness and, unless there are prolonged delays between stimuli, it is uncommon to need additional anesthetic medications. Nevertheless, a half-dose of muscle relaxant should be administered if behavioral observations (e.g., spontaneous movements or respiration) suggest that muscle relaxant effects are wearing off. Some anesthesia providers believe that the patient should be pretreated with an anticholinergic agent if a second dose of a muscle relaxant is administered.

14.7.2. Formula-Based Stimulus Dosing

To limit the possibility or number of subconvulsive administrations, some practitioners prefer to use a formula-based approach to determine stimulus intensity. The simplest formulas adjust stimulus intensity to the patient's age (Abrams and Swartz 1989) or to half the patient's age (Petrides and Fink 1996b; Petrides et al. 2009). More complex formulas can also be used that account for additional predictive factors such as electrode placement and sex, but such formulas account for only 40% or less of the variability in initial seizure threshold (Boylan et al. 2000; Coffey et al. 1995a; Colenda and McCall 1996; Enns and Karvelas 1995; Krueger et al. 1993; Sackeim et al. 1991; Shapira et al. 1996). Error in the formula-based estimate may result in administration of either markedly suprathreshold threshold stimulation, which aggravates short-term cognitive side effects, or barely suprathreshold stimulation, which may be ineffective with RUL ECT, particularly with younger individuals (Enns and Karvelas 1995; Shapira et al. 1996). The risk of an excessive stimulus dose is higher in older adults, particularly older women (Landry et al. 2020). In addition, when the value obtained from a formula grossly underestimates seizure threshold, a subconvulsive stimulus will be administered, and the practitioner will engage in a form of empirical titration. Although some manufacturers still recommend using full-age dosing for RUL ECT, empirical stimulus titration is preferred. If a formula-based dosing is to be used for BT and BF dosing, it is recommended to use half-age rather than full-age dosing to avoid excessive cognitive side effects, particularly for older individuals.

14.7.3. Fixed-Dose Stimulus Dosing

Routine use of a high fixed-dose stimulus intensity is not recommended. Instead, this strategy should be reserved exclusively for patients with sufficiently serious concomitant medical conditions in which avoidance of subconvulsive stimulation is a priority. Although high fixed-dosage stimulation maximizes the probability of response to RUL ECT (Abrams 2002; Abrams et al. 1991; McCall et al. 1995, 2000), the problems in the use of formula-based dosing apply even more so to the use of a high fixed dose. Given the marked individual differences in seizure threshold, some patients treated with a high fixed dose may receive an electrical stimulus intensity that exceeds seizure threshold by tenfold, twentyfold, or more. Such a dosing strategy is likely to aggravate cognitive side effects without gains in efficacy relative to more moderate dosing. Furthermore, in rare patients with an exceptionally high initial seizure threshold, use of a fixed dosing strategy can result in barely suprathreshold stimulation. Consequently, approaches that adjust stimulus dosing on the basis of patient- or treatment-related factors are generally recommended in preference to fixed-dose stimulus dosing.

14.7.4. Stimulus Dosing Adjustments During the Treatment Course

The determination of stimulus dosage should also consider that seizure threshold changes over the treatment course, with many patients manifesting large increases—for example, 25%–200% (Coffey et al. 1995b; Sackeim 1999; Sackeim et al. 1987c). Because of this phenomenon, dosage may need to be adjusted upward to maintain a consistent suprathreshold level. Signs that a midcourse dosage adjustment may be necessary include progressive lack of clinical response or worsening seizure quality. A midcourse retitration may be performed to confirm that the threshold has increased, and the stimulus dosage can be adjusted accordingly. In patients who show slow or inadequate clinical response and no more than mild cognitive side effects, an even further dosage increase may be considered. In patients for whom a level of stimulation has consistently produced adequate seizures but who experience severe cognitive side effects, a switch to a RUL placement, spacing of treatments over longer intervals, or a decrease in stimulus intensity may be considered.

Recommendations

14.1. Waveform Characteristics

1. A sine wave stimulus should not be used because of the greater severity of cognitive side effects and the lack of evidence of any therapeutic advantage relative to brief pulse or ultrabrief pulse stimuli.
2. Ultrabrief pulse width, coupled with unilateral electrode placement and adequate dosage relative to seizure threshold, is an appropriate method to minimize cognitive side effects.

14.2. Stimulus Parameters

1. Maximal output of ECT devices depends on local regulations.
2. A constant current stimulus is recommended.
3. Constant voltage or constant energy devices should not be used.
4. Stimulus intensity controls on ECT devices should allow sufficient flexibility in one or more parameters (e.g., pulse width, pulse frequency, pulse train duration) to treat patients with a broad range of seizure thresholds.
5. Manipulations of train duration and pulse width appear to be the most efficient methods of altering stimulus intensity.
6. Use of ultrabrief pulse width RUL ECT is associated with a low threshold for seizure induction and permits most patients to be treated at sufficient stimulus intensities with existing U.S. devices.

14.3. Electrode Placement

14.3.1. Choice of Electrode Placement

1. ECT psychiatrists should be skilled in administering ECT using different electrode placements.
2. Practitioners should understand the ways in which differing electrode placements influence therapeutic and adverse effects.

3. The choice of electrode placement should be based on an ongoing analysis of applicable risks and benefits for the individual patient.
4. The choice of electrode placement should be decided by the ECT psychiatrist in consultation with the consenter and the attending physician (if different from the ECT psychiatrist).
5. Decisions about electrode placement should be made in concert with decisions about stimulus intensity and should include consideration of efficacy and cognitive effects.

14.3.2. Electrode Positioning

1. With BT ECT, electrodes should be placed on both sides of the head, with the midpoint of each electrode approximately 1 inch above the midpoint of a line extending from the tragus of the ear to the external canthus of the eye.
2. With BF ECT, electrodes should be placed 5 cm above the outer edge of the orbit on a line parallel to the sagittal plane.
3. With unilateral ECT, the preferred (d'Elia) configuration places one electrode in the standard position used with BT ECT and places the midpoint of the second electrode 1 inch lateral to the vertex of the scalp; virtually all unilateral ECT is administered on the right side to minimize verbal memory impairment.
4. Stimulus electrodes should be placed far enough apart so that the amount of current shunted across the scalp is minimized.
5. Care should be taken to avoid stimulating over or adjacent to a skull defect.

14.4. Stimulus Electrode Types

1. Metal electrodes may be applied to the scalp using a snugly fitting band or handheld electrodes, using firm pressure to minimize impedance and ensure good contact during stimulus delivery.
2. Handheld electrodes must be insulated so that the user is not in contact with the electrode or with exposed wiring connecting the stimulus cable to the electrode.
3. Instead of metal electrodes and conductant gel, disposable ECT stimulating pads that include adhesive and conducting gel can be used.
4. When disposable ECT stimulating pads are used with unilateral ECT, a handheld electrode is still typically needed at the rostral (vertex) site.

14.5. Stimulus Electrode Site Preparation

1. Scalp areas in contact with stimulus electrodes should be cleansed and gently abraded or properly prepared following manufacturer guidance for self-adhesive electrodes.
2. Before each use, the contact area of the stimulus electrodes should be coated with a conducting gel, paste, or solution (except in the case of self-adhesive electrodes).
3. Conducting gel should be confined to the area under the stimulus electrodes and should never spread across the hair or scalp between stimulus electrodes.
4. When stimulus electrodes are placed over an area covered by hair, a conducting abrasive medium should be rubbed into the scalp, and the hair beneath the electrodes should be parted. For individuals with coarse, curly hair textures it may be necessary to style hair in widely spaced cornrows to permit effective electrode contact. Clipping the underlying hair is unnecessary.

14.6. Impedance Testing

1. A means of ensuring the electrical continuity of the stimulus path, such as a static impedance test, is recommended.
2. The cause of abnormally low or high static impedance should be ascertained and remedied before proceeding with the treatment.

14.7. Stimulus Dosing

1. Restimulation at a higher stimulus intensity should be considered whenever seizure monitoring indicates that an adequate ictal response has not occurred.
2. Dosage relative to seizure threshold should take into account electrode placement:
   a. For brief pulse RUL ECT, dosing should be between 150% and 500% above (i.e., 2.5–6 times) initial seizure threshold, whereas for ultrabrief pulse RUL, a 500% increase (i.e., 6 times initial threshold) is indicated.
   b. For brief pulse BT and BF ECT, dosing should be between 50% and 150% above initial seizure threshold (i.e., 1.5–2.5 times initial threshold), whereas for ultrabrief pulse BT and BF ECT, dosing

should be between 150% and 500% above (i.e., between 2.5–6 times initial threshold).

3. Dosage should be individualized for each patient:

   a. Empirical titration is the most precise method for identifying seizure threshold. At subsequent treatments, dosing is adjusted relative to this empirically determined estimate of seizure threshold.

   b. Formula-based procedures adjust electrical intensity for factors such as electrode placement, sex, age, anesthesia dosage, and concomitant medications.

   c. Among the formula-based approaches to stimulus dosing for BT and BF ECT, it is recommended to use half-age rather than full-age formulas for older individuals to avoid excessive cognitive side effects, whereas full-age formulas may be needed in younger individuals to avoid understimulation.

   d. A high fixed-dose strategy should not be used routinely and should be reserved for rare situations in which serious concomitant medical conditions preclude the safe use of subconvulsive stimulation.

CHAPTER 15

Seizure Monitoring During ECT

15.1. General Considerations

Given the central role of seizure induction with electroconvulsive therapy (ECT), seizure monitoring is essential. The management of missed, abortive, inadequate, or prolonged seizures is predicated on proper seizure monitoring; these topics will be discussed in Chapter 21.

The available research suggests that seizure duration, whether measured at an individual treatment or cumulatively across the treatment course, is of relatively limited clinical utility as an indicator of treatment efficacy (Kales et al. 1997; Lalla and Milroy 1996; Nobler et al. 1993; Sackeim 1999; Sackeim et al. 1987c, 1991). This may, at least in part, reflect that seizure duration appears to have a complex association with stimulus intensity. When stimulus intensity is extremely close to the seizure threshold, the patient may manifest a brief or abortive seizure (see Chapter 21). Motor manifestations of these seizures are typically 15 seconds or less. With a small increment in stimulus intensity to a barely suprathreshold level, the patient often manifests a long seizure with low-amplitude electroencephalogram (EEG) expression and an absence of postictal EEG suppression (Krystal et al. 1993, 1995; Nobler et al. 1993). When stimulus intensity is substantially above threshold, seizure duration decreases, but EEG seizure expression is more robust (higher amplitude), and the probability of postictal EEG suppression is greater (Krystal et al. 1993, 1995; Luber et al. 2000; Nobler et al. 1993; Riddle et al. 1993; Sackeim et al. 1991; Zis et al. 1993).

Given this information, it is unlikely that knowledge of seizure duration alone is sufficient to determine whether a patient has had an adequate treatment. However, when measured from the end of the stimulus, a seizure duration that is less than 15 seconds in both motor (convulsive) and EEG manifestations is likely to be insufficient for full therapeutic benefit. Some seizures of long duration may also be therapeutically ineffective if the stimulus intensity is barely suprathreshold. Some practitioners calculate total seizure time from multiple stimulations to determine treatment adequacy, but no empirical justification exists for this practice. For example, a patient who has had two abortive seizures in a session, each of 11 seconds, should not be considered to have had an adequate treatment simply because the total seizure time exceeded a 15-second criterion.

Although seizure duration typically decreases over the treatment course, practitioners should also be alert to marked changes in seizure duration. For example, if seizure duration decreases from 100 to 40 seconds with successive treatments, the later treatment may have been problematic because of marginally suprathreshold stimulation or other limiting factors. In contrast, a stimulus that is moderately or markedly suprathreshold may be fully effective but result in motor or EEG manifestations between 15 and 30 seconds and occasionally less, particularly in geriatric patients, who usually have shorter seizure durations than do younger individuals (Boylan et al. 2000; Krueger et al. 1993; Sackeim et al. 1991; Strömgren and Juul-Jensen 1975). Further increments in stimulus intensity with these patients may result in decreased seizure duration and accentuation of cognitive side effects.

15.2. Ictal Motor Activity

The duration of the seizure and the method of measurement should be documented at each treatment. The simplest and most reliable method for assessing seizure duration is timing the duration of motor (convulsive) movements. However, these movements are much attenuated or absent with the use of muscle relaxants (e.g., succinylcholine). Therefore, regardless of muscle relaxant dosage, it is recommended that distribution of such an agent to the hand or foot be blocked to allow for timing of unmodified convulsive movements without risk to the patient. Before the muscle relaxant is administered, a blood pressure cuff should be inflated to a pressure above the expected peak systolic pressure during the seizure (e.g., 250 mm Hg). This cuff should not be the same one used to monitor blood pressure.

Another reason for use of the cuff technique is that on rare occasions the anesthetic dose will be insufficient, and patients may retain consciousness while paralyzed. Movement in the cuffed limb will alert the treatment team to this occurrence and should be promptly followed by administration of additional anesthetic agent.

All present U.S. ECT devices have the capability for physiological monitoring of the motor response (electromyography and/or motion detection). Although such techniques provide documentation of the motor response, they detect movement in only one body part and have not been shown to be more reliable than visual observation. In fact, even with use of the cuff procedure, convulsive movements may be visible for a longer duration in other body regions, particularly in the neck and face. Thus, in determining the full duration of motor activity caused by the seizure, the disappearance of all such movements should be taken as the motor seizure endpoint. In contrast, patients may sometimes have an adequate seizure without motor manifestations being apparent (Mayur et al. 1999; Scott and Riddle 1989). This circumstance may occur because the cuff is inflated too late, because the ictal blood pressure increase exceeds the inflated pressure of the cuff, or for other reasons.

Immediately after the seizure, the cuff should be deflated to minimize the duration of diminished blood flow to the extremity. Furthermore, particular care is necessary in use of this technique in patients at risk for skin or musculoskeletal complications or who have severe peripheral vascular disease, deep vein thrombosis, lymphedema in the lower extremities, or sickle cell disease (Mankad et al. 2010). In such patients, the cuff technique should be omitted. Optimal placement is on the distal portion of a limb (ankle is generally preferable to wrist) because it has been documented that full limb convulsive movements in patients with severe osteoporosis can lead to fracture (Levy 1988).

15.3. Ictal Electroencephalography

Seizures should always be monitored with EEG in addition to observations of motor activity. EEG seizure activity is commonly of significantly longer duration than motor convulsive movements (Warmflash et al. 1987). Also, patients may occasionally have prolonged cerebral seizures (see Chapter 21, section 21.1) or return of seizure activity (tardive seizures as detailed in Chapter 19) that do not manifest in motor movements.

At minimum, one channel of EEG activity should be monitored with a digital display and paper record. Recording a paper copy of two channels of EEG data is preferred over recording from a single channel. With two channels of EEG data, it is less likely that artifacts will cause problems in reading the EEG than when recording over a single channel. Having two channels of EEG data can also help in determining whether a seizure was elicited and in identifying its endpoint.

15.3.1. Electroencephalographic Recording Site Determination and Preparation

It is good practice to maintain a consistent protocol for EEG site determination and preparation. The most common sites for recording EEG during ECT involve either a frontal-frontal montage or a frontal-mastoid montage. The frontal-frontal montage is likely to show diminished EEG activity because an EEG channel records the voltage difference between two electrodes, and synchronous voltage changes at both electrodes will cancel. In contrast, a reference point on the mastoid, the bony prominence behind the ear, is more likely to approximate a relatively inactive site, maximizing the recorded EEG seizure expression. For this reason, a frontal-mastoid montage is preferred (Krystal and Weiner 1993; Weiner et al. 1991). In addition, use of a left-sided montage assists in determining seizure generalization with right unilateral (RUL) ECT. Thus, if only one EEG channel is used, common practice is to record from the left frontal and left mastoid regions. With this montage, the frontal electrode(s) should be situated at least 1 inch above the midpoint of the eyebrow. Placing this electrode higher on the forehead (i.e., 1–3 inches) can increase the amplitude of EEG seizure expression, whereas a high placement of the mastoid electrode will reduce contamination of the EEG with pulse artifact.

Careful attention should be paid to the preparation of the EEG sites. Poor contact and other causes of excessive impedance at EEG sites are by far the most common reason for poor EEG recordings. Such artifact interferes with determining seizure occurrence, the quality of seizure expression, and the time point and extent of suppression at seizure termination. The steps involved in preparing EEG sites are similar to those used in preparing sites for ECT electrodes (see Chapter 14).

Both the frontal and mastoid sites should be cleaned with a solvent such as rubbing alcohol and then patted dry. An abrasive conductant should be rubbed into the skin with a cotton swab or other applicator in the area of the electrode. Restricting the area of the abrasive conductant helps ensure that the electrode adheres well to the skin. Alternatively, a wider area may be vigorously abraded and the abrasive conductant wiped dry from the skin. The electrodes are then placed in the proper positions. A disposable EEG electrode consisting of silver-silver chloride and a conductive gel is commonly used to record EEG in ECT. If metal electrodes are used (gold cup, silver-silver chloride), the same preparation steps should be employed. However, the electrode should be filled with a conductant and taped to the skin.

15.3.2. Electroencephalographic Monitoring

After the EEG leads are connected to the EEG electrodes, the adequacy of the EEG lead placement and recording ability should be ascertained before administering anesthetic and muscle-relaxing agents. The amplification of the EEG should be adjusted so that low-voltage fast-frequency activity is clearly discernible and that high-amplitude EEG activity such as may occur with anesthesia or during ECT seizures does not exceed the range of the signal display and does not overlap other channels if recorded. If the EEG amplification setting is too high, postictal EEG suppression may appear as seizure activity, leading to erroneous diagnosis of a prolonged seizure. On the other hand, if the EEG amplification setting is too low, it may lead to a false diagnosis of a missed seizure. Once an appropriate amplification level is identified, it generally should not be changed. When two channels of EEG are recorded, it is important to determine which channel reflects left-sided and which reflects right-sided activity, and it is useful to record this information on the hard copy output. The configuration is easily discerned by tapping the frontal EEG electrodes and observing which channel manifests high-amplitude artifact (Parker et al. 2001).

EEG monitoring should continue until the clinician is certain that seizure activity has terminated. Termination is most often indicated by a period of markedly attenuated activity (suppression), which occurs after the high-amplitude sharp and slow wave activity that occurs during the seizure. Unfortunately, the determination of EEG seizure endpoint can be challenging because of factors such as poor seizure expression and/or postictal suppression or with seizures that terminate slowly or in an erratic manner. Consequently, the clinician should be familiar with the different manifestations of seizure termination and expression as well as the range of artifacts that may result in apparent EEG seizure activity when none is present (e.g., anesthetic effects, movement, electrocardiogram [ECG] artifact). An automated EEG and/or motor seizure endpoint detection feature is sometimes used but may not be as accurate as visual endpoint determination (Krystal and Weiner 1995).

15.3.3. Electroencephalographic Seizure Adequacy Measures

Some ECT devices have included measures that convey information about EEG changes during and after the seizure. Similar EEG measures are also obtained qualitatively or quantitatively by some ECT practitioners. Various factors are likely to influence ictal and postictal EEG expression, including patient age, treatment number, initial seizure threshold, the anesthetic used, and medication status (Azuma et al. 2007; Francis-Taylor et al. 2020; Krystal et al. 1993, 1995, 1996, 2003; McCall et al. 1996a, 1996b; Nobler et al. 1993). Nevertheless, better clinical outcome is associated with seizures that are accompanied by higher-amplitude spike-and-wave activity and followed by greater postictal EEG suppression, as well as other indices derived from the EEG data recorded during and immediately after seizures (Azuma et al. 2007, 2011; Edwards et al. 2003; Folkerts 1996; Francis-Taylor et al. 2020; Jagadisha et al. 2003; Krystal et al. 1995; Luber et al. 2000; Minelli et al. 2016; Nobler et al. 1993; Perera et al. 2004; Suppes et al. 1996; Ten Doesschate et al. 2019). A meta-analysis incorporating 44 studies suggested a modest relationship between these EEG indices and therapeutic outcome (Francis-Taylor et al. 2020), although some patients will still show a strong therapeutic response when seizures do not display these characteristics. Results of the meta-analysis support the utility of monitoring ictal EEG indices in detecting when a decrement in seizure expression or postictal suppression occurs in an individual over the treatment course. Such changes may indicate that a rise in seizure threshold has occurred, and this information could be incorporated into treatment decision-making, where appropriate (Francis-Taylor et al. 2020; Krystal et al. 2000b, 2000c). Ictal EEG indices can also be considered in concert with clinical outcome data when deciding on a change in treatment to boost therapeutic potency.

Recommendations

15.1. General Considerations

1. Seizure monitoring consists of observing the presence and duration of both ictal motor activity and ictal EEG activity.
2. Seizure duration should be monitored to ensure an adequate ictal response and to detect prolonged seizure activity.
3. When measured from the end of the stimulus, a seizure duration that is less than 15 seconds in both motor (convulsive) and EEG manifestations is likely to be insufficient for therapeutic benefit, although longer seizures may also be ineffective if the stimulus intensity is barely suprathreshold.

15.2. Ictal Motor Activity

1. Seizure duration should be documented at each treatment and should be monitored by timing the longest duration of convulsive movements in any body region.
2. Visual observation is the simplest and most reliable means of monitoring the ictal motor response.

3. Determination of the length of the ictal motor response can be facilitated by placing a blood pressure cuff at the wrist or ankle prior to muscle relaxant infusion and inflating it substantially above the anticipated systolic pressure during the seizure.
4. The duration of cuff inflation should be minimized.
5. The cuff technique should be omitted in patients at risk for skin or musculoskeletal complications or who have severe peripheral vascular disease, deep vein thrombosis, lymphedema in the lower extremities, or sickle cell disease.

15.3. Ictal Electroencephalography

Scalp EEG monitoring should be carried out on at least a one-channel basis and visualized using a digital display and paper record; monitoring of two EEG channels is preferred.

15.3.1. Electroencephalographic Recording Site Determination and Preparation

1. EEG recording electrodes should be positioned to maximize the detection of ictal EEG activity, with the use of a frontal-mastoid montage being preferred.
2. Because excessive impedance at EEG sites is the most common cause of poor EEG recordings, careful attention should be paid to EEG site preparation and the adequacy of electrode contact with the scalp.

15.3.2. Electroencephalographic Monitoring

1. The adequacy of the EEG lead placement and recording ability should be ascertained before administering anesthetic and muscle-relaxing agents.
2. EEG monitoring should continue until the clinician is certain that seizure activity has terminated.
3. The ECT psychiatrist should be aware of the different manifestations of EEG seizure onset and termination as well as artifacts likely to occur during monitoring, such as ECG, pulse, electromyography activity, and anesthesia effects.

15.3.3. Electroencephalographic Seizure Adequacy Measures

1. Better clinical outcome may be associated with indices derived from EEG data, such as seizures that are accompanied by higher-amplitude

spike-and-wave activity and followed by greater postictal EEG suppression.

2. Ictal and postictal seizure indices can be considered in concert with clinical outcome data when making decisions about needed changes in stimulus parameters to optimize therapeutic response.

CHAPTER 16

Postictal Recovery Period

16.1. Management in the Treatment Area

Physiological monitoring should continue until it is safe for the patient to be transferred from the treatment area to the recovery area. The patient should not be transferred from the treatment area until spontaneous respiration has resumed, with adequate tidal volume and return of pharyngeal reflexes. Vital signs and electrocardiogram (ECG) should be sufficiently stable so that the patient can return to a lower level of observation. Complications that may occur in the treatment area are cardiovascular complications, prolonged apnea, and prolonged seizures (see Chapter 19, section 19.2, and Chapter 21, section 21.1).

16.2. Management in the Recovery Area

The recovery area should be a low-stimulus environment to promote smooth recovery. Management of the patient in the recovery area should be supervised by the anesthesia provider, who should be readily available in case of emergency. The recovery nurse should provide continuous observation and supportive care. Vital signs should be assessed at a minimum of 15-minute intervals, starting with arrival in the recovery area. The patient should be gently reoriented to their pretreatment baseline, and time to reorientation should be measured. Recovery care should include assessing for common electroconvulsive therapy (ECT) side effects such as headache, nausea, and myalgia (see Chapter 19, section 19.3).

The patient is safe to leave the recovery area when awake with stable vital signs and otherwise prepared to return to ward care (for inpatients) or to the care of responsible significant others (for outpatients). To ensure that general instructions and any specific aftercare recommendations are communicated effectively, the recovery nurse should provide a handoff to the individual accompanying the patient home or back to the inpatient service. If safe to do so, the patient should be encouraged to drink and/or eat before leaving the recovery area.

16.3. Postrecovery Care

Once recovery is complete, the patient should continue to receive the supportive care established on discharge from the recovery area. This postrecovery care focuses on returning to a pretreatment diet, ambulating safely (if the patient was ambulatory before the treatment), and assessing the effectiveness of interventions to manage side effects. Postrecovery care generally lasts for at least 1 hour from the time of discharge from the recovery area, depending on the patient's age and level of frailty.

For inpatients, postrecovery care may take place on the inpatient unit. For outpatients, postrecovery care begins in the treatment facility, continues until outpatient discharge criteria are met, and concludes at the patient's home, where loved ones or other responsible adults are able to monitor the patient. The specific location within the treatment facility may vary, including an area adjacent to the recovery area, part of the recovery area itself, or a discharge lounge. Although it is preferable to have separate pretreatment and posttreatment areas, small facilities may find it necessary to commence postrecovery care in the pretreatment area.

Criteria should be established for the discharge of outpatients from the facility. Such criteria typically include ambulatory status, cognitive status, and removal of the intravenous catheter. The level of functioning should be compatible with a safe journey home. Because ECT may affect cognitive and motor function, patients should be accompanied home by a responsible adult. Patients who are receiving an acute course of ECT should not drive or operate heavy equipment at least until the acute course is complete (see Chapter 8, section 8.3.3). Patients in a maintenance course of ECT should not drive for at least 24 hours after the ECT treatment. Recommendations regarding driving should be individualized by considering factors specific to each patient such as age, functional status, the severity of side effects from ECT, and the prescribing of concomitant medications that may also influence driving safety.

Recommendations

16.1. Management in the Treatment Area

1. Physiological monitoring should continue until it is safe for the patient to be transferred from the treatment area to the recovery area.
2. Key criteria for transferring the patient from the treatment area include return of spontaneous respiration (with adequate tidal vol-

ume and return of pharyngeal reflexes), stabilization of vital signs, and absence of adverse effects requiring immediate medical evaluation or intervention.

16.2. Management in the Recovery Area

1. Recovery care should be delivered primarily by the recovery nurse and overseen by the anesthesia provider, who should be readily available.
2. Recovery care should include continuous observation and supportive care, monitoring vital signs at a minimum of every 15 minutes until stable, reorienting the patient to their pretreatment baseline, assessing for common ECT side effects, and notifying the anesthesia provider of any situation potentially requiring medical intervention.
3. It is safe for the patient to leave the recovery area when they are awake with stable vital signs and prepared to return to ward care (for inpatients) or to the care of responsible significant others (for outpatients).
4. Before the patient leaves the recovery area, a handoff communication between the recovery nurse and the receiving party should have occurred.

16.3. Postrecovery Care

1. Postrecovery care focuses on observing the patient's general functioning and orientation, returning to a pretreatment diet, ambulating safely (if the patient was ambulatory before the treatment), and assessing the effectiveness of interventions to manage ECT side effects.
2. For inpatients, postrecovery care may take place on the inpatient unit. For outpatients, postrecovery care begins in the treatment facility, continues until outpatient discharge criteria are met, and concludes at the patient's home.
3. Discharge of the patient should follow criteria established at the facility.
4. Patients in an acute course of ECT should not drive or operate heavy equipment at least until the course is complete. Patients in a maintenance course of ECT should not drive for at least 24 hours after the ECT treatment.

CHAPTER 17

Evaluation of Outcome

17.1. Measurement-Based Care

Measurement-based care involves the use of psychometrically sound rating scales to document changes in symptoms or domains of interest with treatment as well as to determine whether symptoms or adverse effects of treatment are present or absent (Fortney et al. 2017). Multiple lines of evidence suggest that measurement-based care is feasible and that it has multiple benefits relative to standard care (Guo et al. 2015). Such benefits include systematic documentation of psychiatric symptoms, assistance in treatment-related decision-making, increases in patient awareness and insight, and improvements in therapeutic response, rates of remission, and overall outcomes (Guo et al. 2015; Trivedi et al. 2006). In patients who are receiving electroconvulsive therapy (ECT), changes in rating scale scores over time are particularly helpful to identify whether the degree of improvement has accelerated, decelerated, or reached a plateau as well as to document the extent of residual symptoms at the completion of the ECT course. Thus, measurement-based care is increasingly viewed as a best practice for documenting therapeutic outcomes, including changes in quality of life (QOL), with ECT as well as assessing for adverse effects, including effects on cognition (Gill and Kellner 2019). In addition, before beginning an ECT course, it is recommended that each patient have a documented treatment plan that indicates the illness to be treated as well as specific criteria for therapeutic response and remission.

There are multiple rating scales that can be employed in measurement-based care, each with strengths and weaknesses (Möller 2009). Thus, it is important that each ECT facility determine which rating scales will be feasible and useful for patients in their respective practice. Factors to consider when choosing specific rating instruments include 1) who will complete the rating instrument (e.g., clinician-rated, self-rated), 2) length of rating scale assessment (e.g., amount of time required, burden for patients and clinicians), 3) patient variables (e.g., age, language, race/ethnicity, culture, reading level, education, health literacy), 4) rating scale psychometrics, 5) availability of appropriate scale norms, 6) mode of administration (paper and pencil, computer or other electronic device), and 7) cost. Depending on predictive values, sensitivity, and specificity, some rating scales may be better suited to brief screening, whereas other rating scales may be better suited for detailed assessments of symptoms and for outcome monitoring. Scales that ask the patient to rate symptoms over several weeks may not be sufficiently sensitive to change, which can be problematic during an acute course of ECT (American Psychiatric Association 2016).

Implementing measurement-based care into ECT practice requires consideration of additional factors, including 1) designating team member(s) who will oversee measurement-based care; 2) determining how measurement-based care will be integrated into ECT sessions; 3) identifying where rating scale information will be documented in the medical record; and 4) determining how changes in ratings will be tracked over the ECT course, which can include use of a database registry. Clinical therapeutic effects, cognitive effects (see Chapter 20), and QOL exemplify the domains to be assessed in ECT practice that are typically incorporated into measurement-based care.

Although available information suggests that ambulatory patients are generally cooperative with completion of rating instruments (Duffy et al. 2008; Narrow et al. 2013; Zimmerman and McGlinchey 2008), some patients may be unwilling to do so. More commonly, individuals may not be able to collaborate in completion of either a patient- or clinician-rated scale because of significant depression, catatonia, psychosis, or cognitive difficulties (American Psychiatric Association 2016).

Rating scales should always be used as a supplement and not a replacement for clinical assessment (American Psychiatric Association 2016). Overreliance on quantitative measures may lead to missing other key elements of the patient's symptoms and life circumstances. In addition, a focus on summative scores can result in answers to crucial questions (e.g., extent of suicidal ideation) being overlooked.

17.2. Evaluation of Clinical Therapeutic Effects

17.2.1. Global Impression Rating Scales

The Clinical Global Impression (CGI) scale is a publicly available scale that is commonly used for assessing clinical effects associated with treatment (Forkmann et al. 2011; Guy 1976). The CGI is completed by the clinician and includes three items that assess severity of illness; global improvement; and efficacy, which is the ratio of treatment associated therapeutic effect and side effects. The complement to the CGI is the Patient Global Impression (PGI) scale (Guy 1976), which is completed by the patient and documents change in clinical status, disease severity, and disease improvement. The CGI and PGI can be useful for assessing a patient's current overall clinical state and change in global clinical status, but it may also be useful to include rating instruments that are specific and sensitive to assessing psychiatric symptoms.

17.2.2. Depression Symptom Rating Scales

A plethora of clinician-rated and self-report depression symptom severity measures have been used in research studies of ECT in adults with major depressive disorder (MDD) (Husain et al. 2004; Kellner et al. 2006, 2016b; Lisanby 2007; Wade et al. 2020). These scales can also be used in clinical practice to document the presence and magnitude of depressive symptoms at baseline as well as to monitor the change in depressive symptoms and severity during the ECT course (Brus et al. 2017; Fried et al. 2016b; Kellner et al. 2015; McClintock et al. 2011b). Among the collection of more than 250 depression rating scales (Santor et al. 2006), there is significant variation in psychometric properties, including reliability, validity, sensitivity to change over time, and dimensionality (McClintock et al. 2011b). In addition, many of these scales require training for reliable and valid administration, scoring, and interpretation. Content of scales also differs. Although individual items, available factor subscores, and total scores from depression scales provide useful information, not all scales assess the elements of the DSM-5 (American Psychiatric Association 2013) MDD criteria, for example (Fried et al. 2016a). Furthermore, many of the depression symptom severity rating scales instruct the rater to assess symptoms over the past week or more. Because symptomatic change with ECT is often rapid and may require more frequent assessment, it can be useful to reduce the interval being examined to a few days, as has been done in research studies of ECT (Kellner et al. 2006, 2016b).

Of the many depression symptom severity rating scales used in clinical trials, the most commonly used clinician-rated scales are the Hamilton Rating Scale for Depression (HRSD; Hamilton 1960) and the Montgomery-Åsberg Depression Rating Scale (MADRS; Montgomery and Åsberg 1979) (Fried et al. 2016b; Zimmerman et al. 2015). The clinician-rated and self-report versions of the Inventory of Depressive Symptomatology (IDS-C, IDS-SR; Rush et al. 1996) and Quick Inventory of Depressive

Symptomatology (QIDS-C, QIDS-SR; Rush et al. 2003) have also been used in multiple clinical investigations, including Sequenced Treatment Alternatives to Relieve Depression (STAR*D; Rush et al. 2006).

There are multiple versions of the HRSD, based on the total number of items, which ranges from 6 to 31. In ECT research, out of 100 studies identified in a relatively recent review, approximately half used the 17-item HRSD to assess depression severity (Kellner et al. 2015), whereas other studies used the 24-item HRSD (e.g., Kellner et al. 2016b, 2016a). The HRSD has strengths, including sound psychometric properties and long-standing global use in clinical and research practice, but it does not address all of the DSM-5 MDD symptom criteria and asks about symptoms of anxiety as well as depression (McClintock et al. 2011c; Zimmerman et al. 2005). Another issue with the HRSD is the inconsistency in differential rating of symptoms, with some items rated on a 3-point Likert scale and others on a 5-point scale (McClintock et al. 2011b; Zimmerman et al. 2005). In addition, some versions of the HRSD do not have a primary reference that describes them (McClintock et al. 2011b; Zimmerman et al. 2005). Training is important to assuring good interrater reliability among clinicians administering the HRSD, and this is particularly true for early versions of the HRSD, which did not provide well-structured instructions (Carrozzino et al. 2020).

The MADRS comprises 10 items rated on a 7-point Likert scale and was designed to be sensitive to change with antidepressant treatment (Montgomery and Åsberg 1979). If needed, methods are available to convert total scores between the MADRS and the 17-item HRSD (Leucht et al. 2018). As with the HRSD, the MADRS captures some, but not all, symptoms of the DSM MDD criterion. Moreover, the MADRS has been found to be multidimensional, with potential for unreliability in measurement of some items (Craighead and Evans 1996). Also, without training, there could be poor interrater reliability among clinicians administering the MADRS.

Self-ratings of depression symptom severity are used increasingly in clinical practice (Brown et al. 2018; Soda et al. 2020) and have also been used in ECT research in adults (Brus et al. 2017; Ghasemi et al. 2014; Tornhamre et al. 2020). Similar to clinician-rated scales, patient self-report scales can give helpful information on the presence, severity, and change of depressive symptoms with treatment (Zimmerman et al. 2018).

The self-report versions of the IDS (Rush et al. 1996) and the QIDS (Rush et al. 2003), with 30 and 16 items, respectively, are publicly available and psychometrically sound measures of the DSM-IV-TR (American Psychiatric Association 2000) MDD domain criteria. Each IDS and QIDS item is rated on a 4-point Likert rating scale, and scoring generates a severity score for each MDD domain as well as a total score of overall depressive symptom severity. Whereas the IDS is multidimensional in measuring both anxiety and depressive symptoms, the QIDS is unidimensional and assesses only depressive symptoms (Rush et al. 2003).

The nine-item version of the Patient Health Questionnaire (PHQ-9; Kroenke et al. 2001) is a reliable and valid self-report rating instrument available in the public domain that is based on the nine items in the DSM-IV-TR criteria for MDD. The PHQ-9 assesses depression severity for each criterion on a 4-point Likert scale on the basis of the relative number of days in the past 2 weeks that the symptom was present. As such, it may be less sensitive to change in the severity of individual symptoms. The PHQ-9 also provides an item that assesses the impact of depressive symptoms on activities of daily living.

The Beck Depression Inventory II (BDI-II; Beck et al. 1996) is a licensed self-report instrument comprising 21 items that are rated on a 4-point Likert scale on the basis of symptoms during the past 2 weeks. The BDI-II does not assess all DSM-5 MDD criterion items, although it has strong psychometric properties.

More recently, the Symptoms of Major Depressive Disorder Scale (SMDDS) was created as a new self-report of depression symptom severity that can be completed using a web-based format (Bushnell et al. 2019). It was developed following U.S. Food and Drug Administration (FDA) recommendations and is qualified by the FDA for exploratory use in antidepressant clinical trials (Bushnell et al. 2019). The SMDDS contained 36 items at its initial development, but through research, it was found that 16 items rated on a 5-point Likert scale provided valuable information regarding DSM-5 depression criteria, with strong psychometric properties. Although this measure was reported to be publicly available (Bushnell et al. 2019), there may be a fee to use it in practice.

For patients with MDD with psychotic features, one review (Østergaard et al. 2015) recommends the use of the Psychotic Depression Assessment Scale (PDAS) (Østergaard et al. 2014). The PDAS was empirically designed to specifically assess depressive and psychotic symptoms in adult patients with MDD and psychotic features. The scale comprises 11 items (6 items from the 17-item HRSD and 5 items from the Brief Psychiatric Rating Scale [BPRS]) that are rated on a 5-

point Likert scale that ranges from 0 to 4. The overall total score provides an indicator of depression and psychotic symptom severity level. A semistructured interview for the PDAS was created to assist in administration and scoring (Østergaard et al. 2015).

Selexted depression rating scales are outlined in Table 17–1. These scales have a number of advantages and disadvantages, and ECT practitioners should determine which scales are most appropriate for use in their practice settings.

17.2.3. Anxiety Symptom Rating Scales

Anxiety symptoms are often present with other neuropsychiatric illnesses. Generalized anxiety disorder is particularly comorbid with MDD (Olariu et al. 2015), and ECT can be modestly beneficial for comorbid anxiety and depressive symptoms (Huang et al. 2019). Many patients experience anxiety related to treatment with ECT (Obbels et al. 2017, 2020a, 2020b). Thus, it may be prudent to employ an anxiety symptom severity rating scale to assess for such symptoms. Multiple clinician-rated and self-report rating scales have been developed to assess for the presence and magnitude of anxiety symptoms (Balon 2007; Julian 2011; Therrien and Hunsley 2012).

Clinician-rated scales include the Hamilton Anxiety Rating Scale (HARS; Hamilton 1959) and the $HRSD_{17}$ and IDS-C anxiety ($HRSD_{17ANX}$, IDS-C_{ANX}) subscales (McClintock et al. 2011b). The HARS consists of 14 items rated on a 5-point Likert scale via a semistructured interview based on responses to behavioral questions. Although widely used, the HARS has been questioned with regard to its validity (Porter et al. 2017). The $HRSD_{17ANX}$ and IDS-C_{ANX} each contain 5 items from their respective larger scales (McClintock et al. 2011b). The $HRSD_{17ANX}$ items are rated on a 3-point or 5-point Likert scale, and the IDS-C_{ANX} items are rated on a 4-point Likert scale; both instruments provide information on the absence or presence of significant anxiety symptoms. Because both the $HRSD_{17}$ and IDS-C are multidimensional, depressive and anxiety symptoms can be measured by either rating scale.

Self-report scales include the Anxiety Symptoms Questionnaire (ASQ; Baker et al. 2019), the Beck Anxiety Inventory (BAI; Beck et al. 1988), the ECT-Related Anxiety Questionnaire (ERAQ; Obbels et al. 2020a), the seven-item Generalized Anxiety Disorder scale (GAD-7; Spitzer et al. 2006), the Screen for Adult Anxiety Related Disorders

Table 17–1. *Selected depression symptom rating scales*

Scale	Format	Number of items	Approximate time to complete	Language	Cost	Remission
Beck Depression Inventory II (BDI-II)	Self-report	21	10 minutes	Multiple languages	Licensed with associated fee	Total score ≤13
Hamilton Rating Scale for Depression (HRSD)	Clinician rated	Varies depending on version. The 17-item version was the first to be published. Since that time, multiple versions have been created (e.g., 6-, 21-, 24-, and 28-item versions).	Varies depending on version. The 17- and 21-item versions have been reported to take 15–20 minutes.	Multiple languages	Available in public domain	Varies depending on version. For the 17-item HRSD, total score ≤7
Inventory of Depressive Symptomatology (IDS)	Clinician rated and self-report	30	10–15 minutes	Multiple languages	May have associated fee depending on use (e.g., clinical, research)	Total score ≤13
Montgomery-Åsberg Depression Rating Scale (MADRS)	Clinician rated and self-report	10	15–20 minutes	Multiple languages	Available in public domain	Total score ≤5

Table 17–1. *Selected depression symptom rating scales (continued)*

Scale	Format	Number of items	Approximate time to complete	Language	Cost	Remission
Patient Health Questionnaire-9 (PHQ-9)	Self-report	9	1–5 minutes	Multiple languages	Available in public domain	Total score ≤4
Quick Inventory of Depressive Symptomatology (QIDS)	Clinician rated and self-report	16	5–7 minutes	Multiple languages	May have associated fee depending on use (e.g., clinical, research)	Total score ≤5

(SCAARED; Angulo et al. 2017), and the State Trait Anxiety Inventory (STAI; Spielberger et al. 1970, 1983).

The ASQ is a psychometrically sound self-report anxiety symptom severity rating instrument for use in adults (Baker et al. 2019). It comprises 17 items that document the frequency and intensity of each item as rated on a 10-point scale (Baker et al. 2019). Research supports the use of the BAI, which comprises 21 items rated on a 4-point Likert scale that assess anxiety symptom severity. However, the BAI has been critiqued for being unable to discriminate between the severity of anxiety and depressive symptoms when studied in adult primary care populations (Muntingh et al. 2011). The ERAQ is a 17-item self-report scale with sound psychometric properties designed specifically for adult patients treated with ECT to inform the presence and severity of anxiety symptoms associated with ECT (Obbels et al. 2020a). The rating scale was initially created in the Dutch language and has been translated into English. The GAD-7 is a psychometrically sound measure rated on a 4-point Likert scale predicated on DSM-IV diagnostic criteria (American Psychiatric Association 1994) that detects the presence and severity of generalized anxiety disorder (Spitzer et al. 2006). The 44-item self-report SCAARED was developed specifically to assess for DSM-5 anxiety disorders in young adults (ages 18–27) and has sound psychometric properties (Angulo et al. 2017). Because it assesses anxiety symptoms over the previous 3 months, it may be useful for baseline assessment but would require an adapted time frame to measure treatment-related effects on anxiety (e.g., from the past 3 months to the past few days). The STAI consists of 40 items rated on a 4-point Likert scale that assess both state and trait features of anxiety (Spielberger et al. 1970, 1983). Although research shows the STAI to have strong psychometric properties, the scale is multidimensional, which limits its specificity in measuring pure anxiety (Balsamo et al. 2013).

Selected anxiety rating scales are outlined in Table 17–2.

17.2.4. Hypomanic and Manic Symptom Rating Scales

ECT is an established treatment for bipolar disorder in depressive, hypomanic, or manic episodes, including episodes with mixed features (Abbott et al. 2019; Perugi et al. 2020). Moreover, some patients with MDD could potentially develop hypomanic or manic symptoms during the ECT course, as is the case with other antidepressant therapies. As such, it can be helpful to use rating scales to assess for any such symptoms. Research on ECT in bipolar disorder has most often used a clinician-rated instrument such as the Young Mania Rating Scale (YMRS;

Table 17–2. *Selected anxiety rating scales*

Scale	Format	Number of items	Approximate time to complete	Language	Cost	Remission
Beck Anxiety Inventory (BAI)	Self-report	21	10 minutes	Multiple languages	Licensed with associated fee	Total score ≤7
ECT-Related Anxiety Questionnaire (ERAQ)	Self-report	17	15 minutes	Dutch, English	Available in public domain	Unspecified remission criteria
Generalized Anxiety Disorder Scale-7 (GAD-7)	Self-report	7	3 minutes	Multiple languages	Available in public domain	Total score <5
Hamilton Anxiety Rating Scale (HAM-A)	Clinician rated	14	10–15 minutes	Multiple languages	Available in public domain	Total score <17
Screen for Adult Anxiety Related Disorders (SCAARED)	Self-report	44	Not reported	Multiple languages	Available in public domain	Not reported
State Trait Anxiety Inventory (STAI)	Self-report	40	10 minutes	Multiple languages	Licensed with associated fee	Unspecified remission criteria

Young et al. 1978) or the Clinician-Administered Rating Scale for Mania (CARS-M; Altman et al. 1994).

Multiple clinician-rated and self-report rating scales exist for assessing hypomanic and manic symptoms (Picardi 2009). One comprehensive symptom content analysis identified seven such scales that are in common use on the basis of their frequency count in the published literature (Chrobak et al. 2018). Of those, clinician-rated scales included the Bech-Rafaelsen Mania Rating Scale (BRMRS; Bech et al. 1978), the CARS-M (Altman et al. 1994), and the YMRS (Young et al. 1978), whereas the self-report rating scales included the Bipolar Spectrum Disorder Scale (BSDS; Ghaemi et al. 2005), the Hypomania Checklist 32 (HCL-32; Angst et al. 2005), the Mood Disorder Questionnaire (MDQ; Hirschfeld et al. 2000), and the Mood Swings Questionnaire (MSQ; Parker et al. 2006).

Collectively, the rating scales assessed 64 hypomanic and manic symptoms, with limited overlap in symptom assessment among the scales (Chrobak et al. 2018). As such, the scales were determined to be noninterchangeable, with each having specific benefits and limitations. For example, with regard to assessment of DSM-5 hypomanic and manic symptoms, the BSDS assessed the least number of hypomanic and manic symptoms (five), whereas the MDQ and the HCL-32 assessed the most (nine).

Three additional self-rating scales for hypomanic and manic symptoms have been found to be psychometrically sound (Altman 1998): the Internal State Scale (ISS; Bauer et al. 1991), the Self-Report Manic Inventory (SRMI; Shugar et al. 1992), and the Altman Self-Rating Mania Scale (ASRM; Altman et al. 1997). The ISS contains 17 items rated on a visual analogue scale that assess the presence and magnitude of both depressive and manic symptoms. The SRMI consists of 47 items that assess the presence and magnitude of manic symptoms that are rated either true or false. The ASRM comprises 5 items rated on a 5-point Likert scale that document the presence and severity of manic symptoms, including elevated mood, inflated self-esteem, decreased need for sleep, pressured speech, and psychomotor agitation.

Selected mania rating scales are outlined in Table 17–3.

17.2.5. Psychosis Symptom Rating Scales

Consistent evidence has demonstrated the utility of ECT to treat psychotic symptoms, including hallucinations and delusions across an array of neuropsychiatric illnesses (e.g., MDD with psychotic features, postpartum depression, schizophrenia) (Ali et al. 2019; Rosenquist et al. 2014; Rundgren et al. 2018; Sanghani et al. 2018) in adults across the

Table 17–3. *Selected hypomanic and manic symptom rating scales*

Scale	Format	Number of items	Approximate time to complete	Language	Cost	Remission
Altman Self-Rating Mania Scale (ASRM)	Self-report	5	5 minutes	Multiple languages	Available in public domain	Total score <6
Bech-Rafaelsen Mania Rating Scale (MAS)	Clinician rated	11	15–30 minutes	Multiple languages	Available in public domain	Total score <15
Clinician-Administered Rating Scale for Mania (CARS-M)	Clinician rated	15	15–30 minutes	Multiple languages	Available in public domain	Unspecified remission criteria
Young Mania Rating Scale (YMRS)	Clinician rated	11	15–30 minutes	Multiple languages	Available in public domain	Total score <12

lifespan (Heijnen et al. 2019). Interestingly, in patients with MDD, psychotic features are predictive of clinical response and remission with ECT (Avery and Lubrano 1979; Buchan et al. 1992; Clinical Research Centre 1984; Heijnen et al. 2019; Hobson 1953; Lykouras et al. 1986; Mandel et al. 1977; Pande et al. 1990; Petrides et al. 2001; Sobin et al. 1996; Spashett et al. 2014; van Diermen et al. 2020).

For patients with psychotic features, particularly those with schizophrenia, there are many rating scales (Kane 2013) that can be used to document the presence (or absence) and magnitude of such features before, during, and after the ECT course. Of the many scales, two are used primarily in clinical and research practice: the BPRS (Overall and Gorham 1962) and the Positive and Negative Syndrome Scale (PANSS; Kay et al. 1987). Both scales are administered by clinicians, assess an array of psychotic features, have sound psychometric properties, and have been found to be useful in clinical and research practice (Schooler 2017). However, neither scale includes items that assess cognitive symptoms of schizophrenia (Howes et al. 2017).

The original BPRS consisted of 16 items (Overall and Gorham 1962), with each item rated on a 7-point Likert scale on the basis of behavioral observation and direct responses to questions. In 1974, the BPRS was modified with the addition of 2 new items (for a total of 18 items) that measure excitement and disorientation. Since its publication, the 18-item BPRS is more commonly used than the 16-item scale in practice (Schooler 2017). Later, the BPRS-Expanded (BPRS-E; Lukoff et al. 1986) was created. This scale consists of 24 items inclusive of the 18-item BPRS (Overall 1974) plus an additional 6 items that assess bizarre behavior, neglect, suicidal ideation, elevated mood, distractibility, and psychomotor hyperactivity (Lukoff et al. 1986). A meta-analysis suggested that the BPRS-E is multidimensional and assesses four primary factors: positive symptoms, negative symptoms, affect, and activation (Dazzi et al. 2016). On the basis of the meta-analysis findings, the authors recommended that the BPRS-E consist of 26 items, with the inclusion of specific items of bizarre behavior, conceptual disorganization, impoverished thinking, poor attention, and inappropriate affect (Dazzi et al. 2016). Because the BPRS may be lengthy to give in its entirety, it may be possible to use select items based on meta- and factor-analyses that highlight key items to administer for clinical outcomes (Shafer 2005). Overall, the different versions of the BPRS are useful, providing multiple units of information, including a total score of overall psychotic symptom severity, subscale scores to examine psychotic and neuropsychiatric symptom domains, and individual item scores to examine specific symptom features.

The PANSS (Kay et al. 1987) consists of 30 items, 18 of which are from the original BPRS (Overall and Gorham 1962) and the other 12 of which are from the Psychopathology Rating Schedule (Singh and Kay 1975). The items on the PANSS are rated on a 7-point Likert scale and divided into three subscales, including positive symptoms, negative symptoms, and general psychopathology. Multiple studies have found that the PANSS is multidimensional, and most studies converge on a five-factor structure, though the factors have been found to vary by study (Shafer and Dazzi 2019). A 2019 meta-analysis, which was consistent with prior meta-analyses, identified the five factors of the PANSS as positive symptoms, negative symptoms, affect, resistance, and disorganization (Shafer and Dazzi 2019). Moreover, the study found that the item of lack of judgment and insight was unrelated to a single dimensional factor and actually had a negative association with the positive symptoms and disorganization factors.

For patients with MDD with psychotic features, the PDAS can be used as described in section 17.2.2.

Selected psychosis rating scales are outlined in Table 17–4.

17.2.6. Catatonia Symptom Rating Scale

ECT is highly efficacious for the treatment of catatonia (Fink 2019; Luchini et al. 2015; Pelzer et al. 2018; Rosenquist et al. 2018). Multiple rating scales have been developed to assess catatonic symptoms (Sienaert et al. 2011b). One of the first catatonia rating scales, the Bush-Francis Catatonia Rating Scale (BFCRS; Bush et al. 1996a), comprises 23 items that were predicated on multiple diagnostic classification systems available at the time, including DSM-IV and the *International Classification of Diseases,* 10th Edition (ICD-10). The authors also created a brief version of the measure that consisted of 14 items that could be used as a screening instrument for catatonia (Bush et al. 1996a). Both the full and the brief BFCRS document the absence or presence and severity of catatonia symptoms (e.g., immobility, mutism, staring) and were found to be psychometrically sound (Bush et al. 1996a). For these reasons, as well as for its ease of use in practice, the BFCRS is most often recommended for the assessment of catatonia (Sienaert et al. 2011b). Of other catatonia rating scales (Sienaert et al. 2011b), the Northoff Catatonia Rating Scale (NCRS; Northoff et al. 1999) and the Braunig Catatonia Rating Scale (BCRS; Bräunig et al. 2000) also have sound reliability.

Table 17–4. *Selected psychosis symptom rating scales*

Scale	Format	Number of items	Approximate time to complete	Language	Cost
Brief Psychiatric Rating Scale (BPRS)	Clinician rated	16, 18, or 24 items, depending on version	20–30 minutes	Multiple languages	Available in public domain
Positive and Negative Syndrome Scale (PANSS)	Clinician rated	30	40–50 minutes	Multiple languages	Available in public domain

Selected catatonia rating scales are outlined in Table 17–5.

17.2.7. Quality-of-Life and Functioning Scales

Definitions for QOL and health-related QOL (HRQOL) vary, but in general, QOL incorporates objective and subjective accounts of overall health and general well-being, whereas HRQOL has commonly been conceptualized as self-perceived health status or the impacts of health on QOL (Karimi and Brazier 2016). In addition to beneficial effects on psychiatric symptoms, acute and maintenance ECT have been associated with improvements in QOL and HRQOL with various neuropsychiatric illnesses (e.g., MDD, schizophrenia) in adult and geriatric populations (Garg et al. 2011; Giacobbe et al. 2018; Güney et al. 2020; McCall et al. 2013, 2017, 2018).

The majority of ECT research has used the Medical Outcomes Study Short Form Survey (SF-36; Ware and Gandek 1994; Ware and Sherbourne 1992) to assess QOL, and one study (Garg et al. 2011) used the World Health Organization (WHO) Quality of Life BREF (WHOQOL-BREF; World Health Organization 1998a). Additional QOL rating scales include the full WHOQOL (World Health Organization 1998b), and the National Institutes of Health (NIH) Neuro-QOL (Gershon et al. 2012).

The SF-36 is a widely used self-report measure of QOL that consists of 36 items that produce three primary scores for overall QOL, physical QOL, and mental QOL, as well as subscales titled Physical Functioning, Physical Role, Bodily Pain, General Health, Vitality, Social Functioning, Emotional Role, and Mental Health (Ware and Gandek 1994; Ware and Sherbourne 1992). The SF-36 has a differential scoring system, with some items rated as yes or no and others rated on multiple Likert item scales that range between 3 and 6. Although the scoring system can be complex because of the need to transform certain items, the SF-36 has been found to have strong psychometric properties and has normative demographic data available (McHorney et al. 1993).

The WHO Disability Assessment Schedule 2.0 (WHODAS 2.0) also provides ratings of functioning, with domain-specific scores for cognition, mobility, self-care, getting along, life activities (household and work), and participation (World Health Organization 2010). It is available in a 36-item version, which is part of the "emerging measures" described in DSM-5-TR (American Psychiatric Association 2022) and requires about 20 minutes to complete. A 12-item version, which requires about 5 minutes to complete, is also available. The WHODAS 2.0

Table 17–5. *Selected catatonia symptom rating scales*

Scale	Format	Number of items	Approximate time to complete	Language	Cost
Braunig Catatonia Rating Scale (BCRS)	Clinician rated	21	45 minutes	Multiple languages	Available in public domain
Bush-Francis Catatonia Rating Scale (BFCRS)	Clinician rated	23	5 minutes	Multiple languages	Available in public domain
Northoff Catatonia Rating Scale (NCRS)	Clinician rated	40	Unspecified	Multiple languages	Available in public domain

can be completed by the patient, a proxy, or an interviewer (either in person or by phone). It has been studied internationally in reliability and validity testing (World Health Organization 2010). Although the WHODAS 2.0 may be multidimensional (Saltychev et al. 2021), it appears to be applicable across cultures, in general population samples, and in clinical samples, including individuals with mental illness (Federici et al. 2017; Holmberg et al. 2021; Sjonnesen et al. 2016).

The WHOQOL and WHOQOL-BREF were developed by the WHO to be culturally sensitive instruments for use in multiple countries to assess QOL. The WHOQOL and WHOQOL-BREF comprise 100 items and 26 items, respectively, that are rated on a 5-point Likert scale. Both measures are completed by self-report, have been found to have strong psychometric properties, and produce an overall index of QOL as well as multiple QOL subindices (Grassi et al. 2020; World Health Organization 1998a, 1998b).

The Neuro-QOL is a relatively newer computerized adaptive QOL measure completed by self-report. The rating scale was developed by the National Institute of Neurological Disorders and Stroke specifically for use in patients with neurological illnesses. The Neuro-QOL has been found to be psychometrically sound, has available demographic normative data, and provides an overall score and multiple subscales of QOL (Gershon et al. 2012; Hanmer et al. 2020).

Selected QOL and functioning scales are outlined in Table 17–6.

Recommendations

17.1. Measurement-Based Care

1. Before beginning an ECT course, it is recommended that each patient have a documented treatment plan that indicates the illness to be treated and specific criteria for therapeutic response and remission.
2. Use of measurement-based care facilitates assessment and documentation of therapeutic outcomes, changes in QOL, and adverse effects, including effects on cognition.
3. Implementing measurement-based care into ECT practice requires the following:
   a. Designating team member(s) who will oversee measurement-based care

Table 17–6. *Selected quality-of-life and functioning rating scales*

Scale	Format	Number of items	Approximate time to complete	Language	Cost
Medical Outcomes Study Short Form Survey (SF-36)	Self-report	36	10–20 minutes	Multiple languages	Licensed with associated fee
National Institutes of Health Neuro-QOL	Self-report	Computer adaptive test, so number of items may vary	Time varies depending on number of items	Multiple languages	Licensed with associated fee
World Health Organization Disability Assessment Schedule 2.0 (WHODAS 2.0)	Self-report, proxy, or interviewer	12- and 36-item formats	5–20 minutes depending on number of items	Multiple languages	Available in public domain
World Health Organization Quality of Life (WHOQOL)	Self-report	100	30 minutes	Multiple languages	Available in public domain
WHOQOL-BREF	Self-report	26	15 minutes	Multiple languages	Available in public domain

   b. Determining how measurement-based care will be integrated into ECT sessions
   c. Identifying where rating scale information will be documented in the medical record
   d. Determining how changes in rating scale results will be tracked over the ECT course
4. Choice of specific rating scales for use in measurement-based care should include consideration of the following:
   a. Who will complete the rating instrument (clinician-rated or self-rated)
   b. Length of rating scale assessment (e.g., amount of time required, burden for patients and clinicians)
   c. Patient variables (e.g., age, language, race/ethnicity, culture, reading level, education, health literacy)
   d. Rating scale psychometrics and sensitivity to change
   e. Availability of appropriate scale norms
   f. Mode of administration (paper and pencil, computer, telephone)
   g. Rating scale cost
5. Rating scales should always be used as a supplement and not a replacement for clinical assessment.

17.2. Evaluation of Clinical Therapeutic Effects

1. Scales assessing clinical global improvement and QOL can be useful in assessing the overall efficacy of ECT.
2. Selection of symptom-based rating scales to assess therapeutic benefits of ECT should be tailored to the primary goals of treatment (e.g., resolution of depression, anxiety, mania, catatonia, or psychosis).

CHAPTER 18

Frequency and Number of Treatments

18.1. Frequency of Treatments

During the acute phase of treatment, electroconvulsive therapy (ECT) is administered two or three times per week on alternating days. In the United States, ECT is typically performed three times per week on a Monday/Wednesday/Friday schedule. If delirium or other severe cognitive dysfunction develops during a course of three times weekly ECT, a reduction in the frequency of treatment should be considered. Relative to a schedule of three times per week, twice-weekly treatment results in the same degree of final clinical improvement, but short-term cognitive effects may be less severe, and the rate of response may be slower (Gangadhar et al. 1993; Lerer et al. 1995; McAllister et al. 1987; Shapira et al. 1998). In some circumstances, interrupting the ECT course or reducing the schedule to once per week may be necessary, although treating once per week throughout the ECT course may limit efficacy (Janakiramaiah et al. 1998; Kellner et al. 1992a).

In the past, treatments were sometimes delivered more often than thrice weekly; however, routine use of daily treatments is not indicated because it increases the risk of cognitive dysfunction without clear evidence of therapeutic benefit. Some practitioners argue that daily ECT, regardless of electrode placement, may be useful early in the treatment course when a particularly rapid response is necessary, as in individuals with severe mania or malignant catatonia (Fink et al. 2016), high suicidal risk, or severe inanition. Although restimulation may be needed following a missed or inadequate seizure, producing more than one adequate seizure in the same session is rarely justified. If essential in urgent clinical circumstances, such as in the treatment of patients with neuroleptic malignant syndrome (McKinney and Kellner 1997) or intractable seizure disorder (Griesemer et al. 1997), the number of adequate seizures elicited in a treatment session should be limited to two (Roemer et al. 1990). Multiple monitored ECT, a form of treatment in which more than one adequate seizure is produced in the same treatment session under continuous anesthesia (Maletzky 1981), is no longer acceptable.

The frequency of maintenance ECT treatment is discussed in Chapter 23.

18.2. Number of Treatments

The goal of the acute phase of treatment with ECT is full remission with complete resolution of symptom burden and return to the premorbid level of functioning. However, the total number of ECT treatments in an acute course is a function of clinical improvement as well as the tolerability of treatment. Evaluation of response should focus on measurable changes in target symptoms (see Chapter 17) and side effects of treatment (see Chapters 19 and 20), with assessment performed at regular intervals. Such measurement-based care can enable the treatment team to identify side effects, if they occur, and to define full remission, partial response, and nonresponse in quantitative terms.

Patients vary in the number of acute phase treatments necessary to achieve a full clinical response. Thus, it is not possible to prespecify a fixed number of treatments that a patient will need. Typically, in patients with a mood disorder, the acute course of ECT will be between 6 and 12 treatments. However, some patients manifest full remission after only a few treatments (Husain et al. 2004). Other patients may not begin to show substantial improvement until they have received 10 or more treatments (Nobler et al. 1997; Sackeim et al. 1993; Segman et al. 1995). Clinical observations suggest that this may be particularly true when an initially inadequate response led to a modification in the ECT technique (e.g., a change from right unilateral [RUL] to bilateral electrode placement). A higher number of treatments may also be needed in individuals with schizophrenia (Chanpattana and Andrade 2006; Petrides et al. 2015).

For those patients whose illness fully remits, the acute treatment course should be tapered rather than stopped abruptly in order to decrease the likelihood of relapse (Gill and Kellner 2019; Kellner et al. 2016a). Such a taper may be considered the beginning of the maintenance phase of treatment. Maintenance treatment may consist of ECT, pharmacotherapy, psychotherapy, or some combination thereof (see Chapter 23).

For those patients who show improvement but have persistent symptoms or functional impairment, adjusting the ECT technique can be considered. For example, a change in electrode placement from RUL or bifrontal to bitemporal (BT) can further optimize ECT efficacy and speed of response (Finnegan et al. 2016; Lapidus and Kellner 2011; Sackeim et al. 2020). Other specific modifications can include delivering additional ECT treatments, increasing the pulse width from ultrabrief to brief (Sackeim et al. 2020; Tor et al. 2015), reducing doses of medications that may be interfering with seizure elicitation (e.g., anticonvulsants, anesthetic induction agents; Kronsell et al. 2021), and using medications to augment efficacy (e.g., addition of an antidepressant in patients with depression, addition of clozapine or another antipsychotic medication in patients with schizophrenia, use of pre-ECT flumazenil in a patient taking a benzodiazepine). Increasing the delivered charge can enhance response, and repeating stimulus titration can ensure that stimulation dosages are adequate and sufficiently above seizure threshold (Kellner et al. 2016b; Sackeim et al. 2000).

If it is decided that the treatment technique has been optimal (e.g., use of bilateral electrode placement at an increased stimulus intensity), termination of ECT should be considered in patients who have shown substantial but incomplete clinical improvement yet remain unchanged after two to three additional treatment sessions. Continuing with additional high-intensity BT ECT has been reported to be successful in a research setting in some patients whose conditions did not respond to ECT otherwise (Sackeim et al. 1993, 2020). Nonetheless, the risks of such an extended series should be weighed against those of a persisting episode.

Each facility should have a policy, in accordance with regulatory and accreditation requirements, regarding the number of treatments that may be given in an acute course before reassessing and documenting the need to continue ECT treatment. This number is typically between 12 and 20 treatments (Sackeim et al. 2020), but if a patient shows minimal or no response after 6–10 treatments, the indication for continued ECT should be reassessed. The recommendation to administer additional ECT treatments should be discussed with the patient as part of a new informed consent process (Chapter 10). When a course of treatment extends beyond this range, consultation with another psychiatrist with privileges in ECT may be helpful. Management of situations where there has been an overall lack of response to an acute series of ECT is discussed in Chapter 22.

The goal of the maintenance phase of treatment with ECT is to maintain the improvement achieved during the acute phase. When a patient's illness has responded to ECT, the transition from the acute phase to the maintenance phase is important. If the course is abruptly terminated, a patient may experience symptom relapse within 1 or 2 weeks of ECT and need to return for another course of treatment (Kellner et al. 2006). Provision of ECT on a weekly basis during the first few weeks of maintenance pharmacotherapy was tested empirically in the Prolonging Remission in Depressed Elderly (PRIDE) study and was shown to provide protection from relapse during the period when pharmacological effects are building (Kellner et al. 2016a). Strategies for using maintenance ECT to prevent relapse and recurrence are discussed in Chapter 23.

In some patients, additional acute courses of ECT may be helpful or necessary because of the natural history of relapse or recurrence of the psychiatric condition being treated. The decision to commence an additional acute course of ECT involves assessing the quality of the previous response to the treatment, including occurrence of adverse effects. In particular, the presence and severity of persistent cognitive deficits should be considered, especially if bilateral electrode placement was used previously or is planned in the upcoming course (McElhiney et al. 1995; Sackeim et al. 2000; Weiner et al. 1986a).

There is no evidence that repeated courses of ECT lead to permanent structural brain damage (Devanand et al. 1994; Weiner 1984) or that a limit on the maximum lifetime number of treatments with ECT is appropriate (Devanand et al. 1991; Lippman et al. 1985). However, frequent relapses despite maintenance treatment suggest that those strategies be reconsidered and modified (Sackeim 1994; Sackeim et al. 1990). For patients whose illness requires repeated treatment of acute episodes with ECT, attention should be given to the adequacy of post-ECT pharmacotherapy in terms of the type, dosage, and duration of medication. If, after a tapered course of ECT, adequate pharmacotherapy is ineffective in preventing relapse or cannot be tolerated because of side effects, or if the patient prefers it, additional ECT should be considered as a maintenance treatment (see Chapter 23).

Recommendations

18.1. Frequency of Treatments

1. During the acute phase of treatment, ECT is delivered two or three times per week.
2. A reduction in treatment frequency should be considered if delirium or other severe cognitive dysfunction occurs.

18.2. Number of Treatments

1. The total number of treatments in an acute course of ECT should be a function of clinical improvement and side effect tolerability.
2. In major depression, an acute ECT course generally consists of 6–12 treatments, although response and remission may occur either earlier or later.
3. For those patients whose illness fully remits, the acute treatment course should be tapered rather than stopped abruptly in order to decrease the likelihood of relapse, with the taper considered as the beginning of the maintenance phase of treatment.
4. In the absence of significant clinical improvement after 6–10 treatments, the indication for continued ECT should be reassessed, with consideration given to modification of ECT technique (e.g., change from unilateral to bilateral electrode placement, increase in stimulus dosage, use of medications to potentiate the clinical response).
5. A larger number of ECT treatments may be required in some individuals with schizophrenia or when a change in ECT technique has taken place because of lack of response.
6. Each facility should develop a policy regarding the number of treatments after which a formal assessment of the need for continued ECT should be evaluated and discussed with the consenter.
7. Additional acute courses of ECT are sometimes necessary because of relapse or recurrence of the psychiatric condition, but the previous response to the treatment, including any occurrence of adverse effects, should be considered before beginning an additional acute course of ECT.

CHAPTER 19

General Adverse Events

19.1. Mortality

Precise rates of the mortality attributable to electroconvulsive therapy (ECT) are difficult to determine because of intrinsic methodological issues, such as uncertainty about cause of death, the time frame for linking death to ECT, and variability in reporting requirements. Published estimates from large and diverse patient series over several decades report up to 4 deaths per 100,000 ECT treatments (Abrams 1997; Babigian and Guttmacher 1984; Blumberger et al. 2017; Crowe 1984; Fink 1979; Heshe and Roeder 1976; Kramer 1985; Nuttall et al. 2004; Reid et al. 1998; Shiwach et al. 2001; Tørring et al. 2017; Watts et al. 2011; Weiner 1979).

Despite the frequent use of ECT in geriatric patients and patients with significant medical conditions (Sackeim 1998; Weiner et al. 2000), the mortality rate appears to have decreased in recent years because of advances in the medical practice of ECT. For example, a pooled analysis, based on data from 15 studies in 32 countries and 766,180 treatments, found an ECT-related mortality rate of 2.1 deaths per 100,000 treatments (Tørring et al. 2017). No ECT-related deaths were found In the Veterans Affairs (VA) National Center for Patient Safety database that contained information from all VA hospitals between 1999 and 2010 (Watts et al. 2011). These rates compare favorably with reported rates of mortality related to anesthesia, which have been estimated at 8.5 per 100,000 in developed countries (Bainbridge et al. 2012) and 10.85 per 100,000 in elective surgical procedures in individuals age 60 or older (Braghiroli et al. 2021).

Longitudinal studies of depressed patients have also shown that hospitalized patients who received ECT had similar or lower mortality rates at 1-year follow-up than patients who received other treatment modalities or no treatment (Kaster et al. 2022; Munk-Olsen et al. 2007; Rhee et al. 2021; Watts et al. 2021). Furthermore, evidence from large administrative database and registry studies shows longer-term rates of suicide after ECT to be comparable or less than suicide rates in individuals who did not receive ECT (Kaster et al. 2022; Kucuker et al. 2021; Rhee et al. 2021; Rönnqvist et al. 2021; Watts et al. 2022). Thus, taken together, the available evidence supports the relative safety of ECT as well as benefits in reducing suicide mortality and all-cause mortality among hospitalized patients with depression.

19.2. Cardiovascular, Cerebrovascular, and Pulmonary Complications

Cardiovascular and pulmonary complications are the leading causes of significant medical adverse events and death from ECT (Blumberger et al. 2017; Burke et al. 1987; Nuttall et al. 2004; Osler et al. 2022; Pitts 1982; Rice et al. 1994; Welch and Drop 1989; Zielinski et al. 1993; see Chapter 9, sections 9.2.1 and 9.2.2). Consequently, in the immediate postictal period, the treatment team should be ready to manage cardiovascular complications, including cardiac arrest, arrhythmias, ischemia, hypertension, and hypotension.

Although most cardiac arrhythmias in the immediate postictal period are benign and resolve spontaneously, given their high rate of occurrence, an electrocardiogram (ECG) should be monitored during and immediately after the procedure. Vital signs (e.g., pulse, systolic and diastolic blood pressure) should also be monitored during treatment and recovery periods and should be stable before the patient leaves the recovery area.

The type, likelihood, and severity of post-ECT cardiac complications are correlated with the presence of preexisting cardiac illness (Bryson et al. 2013; Cristancho et al. 2008; Huuhka et al. 2003; Prudic et al. 1987; Rice et al. 1994; Zielinski et al. 1993) (see Chapter 9, section 9.2.1). With the development of modern anesthetic techniques, ECT can be administered safely in patients with a number of cardiac conditions (Christopher 2003). Nevertheless, patients at increased risk include those with uncontrolled hypertension, recent myocardial infarction (<60 days), unstable angina, decompensated heart failure, severe aortic stenosis, uncontrolled atrial fibrillation, unrepaired abdominal aortic aneurysms >5.0 cm, and tachyarrhythmias or bradyarrhythmias associated with hypotension or requiring urgent medical attention (Sundsted et al. 2014; Tess and Smetana 2009).

With the advent of highly sensitive assays for cardiac troponins, several studies have examined whether cardiac troponin levels are increased in association with ECT. Several small pilot studies have yielded mixed findings and are far from definitive (Briggs et al. 2011). Two studies showed an increase in cardiac troponin levels in 8% of 100 patients (Duma et al. 2017) and 11.5% of 70 patients (Martinez et al. 2011). Another study of 20 patients found increased cardiac troponin levels in 15% of the sample but no evidence of a significant change in cardiac function or clinical complications (Matz et al. 2019). An additional study of 44 patients found no significant ECG changes or changes in cardiac troponin levels 1 hour and 6 hours, respectively, after the ECT procedure (Próchnicki et al. 2019). These findings are comparable to the results of a large prospective international cohort study of more than 15,000 patients ages 45 years and older who underwent inpatient noncardiac surgery. That sample also showed increases in cardiac troponin levels in 8%, but only 35% of those patients had ECG evidence of ischemia, and only 15.8% experienced an ischemic symptom (Botto et al. 2014). The implications of this finding of increased cardiac troponin levels with ECT is unclear in terms of cardiovascular outcomes (Briggs et al. 2011; Duma et al. 2017), particularly because the rate of myocardial infarction with ECT is very low, at less than 1 per 1,000 ECT treatments (Duma et al. 2019).

Overall rates of cardiovascular events are also low in patients who have received ECT. In fact, in a large Swedish registry study (Nordenskjöld et al. 2022), patients who had received ECT (N=5,476) were less likely to have experienced a major adverse cardiovascular event during 1 year of follow-up than were propensity-matched patients with moderate to severe major depression who did not receive ECT (1.4% vs. 2.3%, respectively; hazard ratio, 0.65; 95% CI 0.49–0.85).

Cerebrovascular complications are notably rare despite the temporary increases in cerebral blood flow and intracranial pressure with the induction of an ECT seizure (Hsiao et al. 1987). With the use of modern anesthesia, the hemodynamic response to ECT can be better controlled to reduce the risk of cerebrovascular complications (Saito 2005; Viguera et al. 1998). However, patients at higher risk include those with signs or symptoms of an intracranial lesion (e.g., papilledema, focal neurological deficits, mass effect or brain edema on MRI) and those with an acute hemorrhagic stroke in the preceding 30 days, particularly if blood pressure remains poorly controlled (Sundsted et al. 2014).

Pulmonary complications can also occur in the recovery period after ECT. Patients with asthma and chronic obstructive pulmonary disease (COPD) are at higher risk for postictal pulmonary complications, and their oxygenation should be monitored during and after the procedure. Such patients may also benefit from use of bronchodilators or other inhalers on the morning of ECT prior to treatment.

The primary differential diagnoses for patients who develop respiratory distress while recovering from ECT include improper airway management with upper airway obstruction, pulmonary embolism (PE), and aspiration pneumonia. Airway management can be addressed by mask ventilation and ensuring that the patient maintains an adequate oxygen saturation. Patients may demonstrate wheezing or decreased breath sounds, stridor, tachycardia, use of accessory muscles, and difficulty speaking if their airway is not patent. Once the upper airway is clear of obstruction, other causes for respiratory distress should be addressed.

Aspiration is another cause of respiratory distress and can lead to pneumonitis. Risk factors for aspiration include failing to maintain a nothing by mouth (NPO) status prior to treatment; use of enteral tube feeding; and presence of obesity, late-stage pregnancy (Rose et al. 2020), hiatal hernia, bowel obstruction, and neuropathy including that due to diabetes (Kurnutala et al. 2013). When risk is significant, the anesthesia team should consider intubation, and conditions such as a bowel obstruction should be addressed before proceeding with ECT, if possible. Aspiration risk is also increased in patients taking antipsychotic medications (Cicala et al. 2019; Herzig et al. 2017; Manjunatha et al. 2011) and may be greater in patients receiving clozapine, presumably because of hypersalivation (Cicala et al. 2019; Estime et al. 2019). If aspiration occurs, it can be identified by decreased breath sounds on pulmonary examination and findings on a subsequent chest X-ray. Aspiration pneumonitis has high morbidity and mortality and should be managed in an acute medical setting.

A PE is another potential etiology of oxygen desaturation post-ECT and is most commonly caused by a deep vein thrombosis (DVT). ECT patients may be at risk for PE because of extended immobility due to depression or catatonia. Other risk factors for PE include obesity, smoking, supplemental estrogen use, pregnancy, inherited clotting disorders, cardiovascular disease, and, more recently, coronavirus disease 2019 (COVID-19). Patients who are immobile for long periods of time should be given prophylactic care, which can include anticoagulant medication, compression stockings, leg elevation, and prescribed physical activity. In a patient at high risk for DVT or PE, putting a cuff or tourniquet on an ankle to observe the motor seizure should be avoided because it can cause pooling of blood in the extremity and further increase risk. Acute onset of pulmonary edema has also been reported in patients receiving ECT (Cochran et al. 1999; Fryml et al. 2018; Hatta et al. 2007; Manne et al. 2012; Mansoor et al. 2016; Myers et al. 2007; Nykamp et al. 2021; Oliva et al. 2022; Price et al. 2005; Sargent and Reeves 2008; Sekimoto et al. 2022; Takahashi et al. 2012).

Prolonged postictal apnea is defined as the absence of any respirations and is a rare event. In virtually all patients, it resolves spontaneously. Regardless of duration, however, maintaining adequate oxygenation is critical until respiration resumes. During the recovery period, clinically significant apnea is uncommon, but when it occurs, it is most often related to obstructive sleep apnea or obstruction due to positioning (McCall et al. 2009; Trakada et al. 2017). More rarely, contributors can include central sleep apnea or reduced respiratory drive from respiratory alkalosis in a patient with severe COPD.

Prolonged paralysis and postictal apnea can occur if a higher than needed dose of succinylcholine is used. Subsequent treatments can use either a lower dose of succinylcholine or a nondepolarizing muscle relaxant, such as atracurium or rocuronium (Hickey et al. 1987; Hicks 1987; Kramer and Afrasiabi 1991; Lui et al. 1993; Stack et al. 1988). Less commonly, a patient with prolonged apnea may have a full or partial pseudocholinesterase deficiency that slows the metabolism of choline ester drugs (Packman et al. 1978; Pantuck 1993; Robertson 1966; Watts et al. 2011). In these individuals, an alternative nondepolarizing muscle relaxant agent should be used. Although tests for pseudocholinesterase deficiency are available, routine determination of these values is not recommended (Lippi and Plebani 2013), unless required by local regulations. Instead, determinations of pseudocholinesterase levels or dibucaine number should be reserved for patients with a personal or family history of prolonged apnea following exposure to muscle relaxants (Lippi and Plebani 2013). Other causes of cholinesterase deficiency include liver disease, chronic anemias, malignancy, tuberculosis, and medications including phenothiazines and glucocorticoids (Jensen and Mogensen 1996; Robertson 1966). Medications such as cholinesterase inhibitors (e.g., donepezil, galantamine) used in patients with Alzheimer's disease can interact with succinylcholine and prolong the duration of paralysis or apnea (Crowe and Collins 2003; D'Souza et al. 2022). Although one randomized trial showed no differences in rates of prolonged paralysis or bradycardia in patients who received placebo as compared with those receiving cholinesterase inhibitors (Matthews et al. 2013), caution is warranted in patients who are receiving these medications. If a nondepolarizing neuromuscular blocking agent is used instead, care should be taken to assure that full neuromuscular blockade is achieved; a higher dose of medication may be needed to achieve an appropriate level of neuromuscular blockade in patients taking cholinesterase inhibitors.

19.3. Headache, Muscle Soreness, and Nausea

Headache is a common side effect of ECT (Devanand et al. 1995; Freeman and Kendell 1980; Gomez 1975; Mulder and Grootens 2020; Sackeim et al. 1987d; Tubi et al. 1993; Weiner et al. 1994) and may be particularly frequent in younger patients, especially children and adolescents (Devanand et al. 1995; Rey and Walter 1997; Walter and Rey 1997). Although estimates of post-ECT headache frequency vary from 5% to 45%, the precise incidence is difficult to determine because of methodological issues, including the high rates of headache in patients with depression, the potential effects of concurrent medication or medication withdrawal, and differences in headache assessment across studies.

In most patients, post-ECT headache is mild (Freeman and Kendell 1980; Sackeim et al. 1987d), although some patients report severe pain associated with nausea and vomiting. Typically, the headache is frontal in location with a throbbing character. Although the etiology of post-ECT headache is unknown, its typical throbbing nature suggests a similarity to vascular headache (Weiner et al. 1994; Weinstein 1993). Suggested mechanisms include the acute increase in blood pressure and cerebral blood flow with ECT, electrically induced spasm of the temporalis muscle (Abrams 2002; Weiner et al. 1994), and changes in serotonin receptor sensitivity (Weiner et al. 1994). However, the occurrence of post-ECT headache does not appear to be related to bitemporal as compared with right unilateral electrode placement (Devanand et al. 1995; Fleminger et al. 1970; Sackeim et al. 1987d; Tubi et al. 1993), stimulus dosage (Devanand et al. 1995), or therapeutic response to ECT (Devanand et al. 1995; Sackeim et al. 1987d). It is not known whether preexisting headache syndromes (e.g., migraine) increase the risk of post-ECT headache, but ECT may exacerbate a previous headache condition (Weiner et al. 1994).

Treatment of post-ECT headache is symptomatic. Patients who experience frequent post-ECT headaches may benefit from prophylactic treatment such as aspirin, acetaminophen, or nonsteroidal anti-inflammatory drugs (NSAIDs) given as soon as possible after ECT or even immediately before the ECT treatment. Most patients also benefit from bed rest in a quiet, darkened environment.

Typically, aspirin, acetaminophen, and NSAIDs are highly effective, particularly if given promptly after the onset of pain (Leung et al. 2003). Because it can be given intravenously, the NSAID ketorolac is often used as a symptomatic or prophylactic treatment. Nevertheless, potential side effects of NSAIDs should be considered, including gastrointestinal bleeding, risk of renal failure, compromised hemostasis, and increased levels of lithium. In addition, intravenous ketorolac should not be used late in pregnancy; while breastfeeding; with renal impairment; or in patients with hypersensitivity to NSAIDs or acetylsalicylic acid, including aspirin-sensitive asthma.

Triptans have also been used as a symptomatic treatment for post-ECT headache (DeBattista and Mueller 1995; Fantz et al. 1998; Markowitz et al. 2001; White et al. 2006). In a patient with severe refractory post-ECT headache, subcutaneous or intranasal sumatriptan given several minutes before ECT was also found to provide effective prophylaxis (DeBattista and Mueller 1995; White et al. 2006). However, caution is warranted before using a triptan in a patient with cardiovascular issues (Diener 2020; Dodick et al. 2020; Ghanshani et al. 2020). Other medications that have been effective in treating ECT-associated headaches include topiramate (Ye et al. 2013) and propranolol (Hawken et al. 2001). Status migrainosus after ECT that was refractory to triptan therapy has been treated with dihydroergotamine (Stead and Josephs 2005).

Following ECT, some patients report generalized muscle soreness, which can be treated symptomatically with analgesic agents such as aspirin, acetaminophen, or an NSAID. These side effects are most common after the first treatment and in younger patients but may not be reported subsequently (Dinwiddie et al. 2010). Muscle soreness due to intense fasciculations following administration of a depolarizing muscle relaxant (e.g., succinylcholine) can be alleviated at subsequent treatments by changing to a nondepolarizing agent, such as rocuronium (Saricicek et al. 2014). Alternatively, muscle soreness due to excessively vigorous convulsive movements can be managed with an increase in the dose of muscle relaxant. Although the degree of muscle soreness has often been attributed to either the magnitude of fasciculations or motor activity, two studies did not find a correlation between these variables and the severity of myalgias (Dinwiddie et al. 2010; Rasmussen et al. 2008).

Jaw pain sometimes occurs because of direct electrical stimulation of the pterygoid, masseter, and temporalis muscles with resulting muscle contraction, which is not attenuated by the muscle relaxant (Minneman 1995). Such pain can be reduced by ensuring closure of the teeth around the bite block and exerting firm, upward pressure under the chin to minimize the resultant abrupt clamping of the jaw. If jaw pain does occur, it can be treated with aspirin, acetaminophen, or an NSAID.

Estimates of the prevalence of nausea after ECT vary from 1% to 23% of patients (Gomez 1975; Sackeim et al. 1987d), but as with headache, methodological issues make the incidence difficult to quantify. Nausea may occur because of headache or its treatment with narcotics, particularly in patients with vascular-type headache. Nausea may also occur independently as a side effect of anesthesia, because of the withdrawal or institution of psychotropic medications, or by other unknown mechanisms.

When nausea accompanies the headache, the primary treatment should focus on the relief of the headache as outlined earlier. Otherwise, post-ECT nausea is typically well controlled with the serotonin 5-HT$_3$ receptor antagonists ondansetron and dolasetron, which can be given intravenously several minutes before or after ECT. Dopamine-blocking agents such as phenothiazine derivatives (e.g., prochlorperazine), trimethobenzamide, or metoclopramide can also be used but have the potential to cause hypotension and extrapyramidal symptoms. Intravenous promethazine is not recommended because of problems with severe tissue injury in the event of extravasation (Le and Patel 2014). If nausea is severe or accompanied by vomiting, these agents should be administered parenterally or by suppository. Another consideration in recurrent nausea is changing the anesthetic agent to propofol, which may be less likely to contribute to post-ECT nausea (Bailine et al. 2003). Transdermal scopolamine has also been used for treating postprocedural nausea (Pergolizzi et al. 2012).

19.4. Postictal Agitation

At one or more treatments, a minority of patients (7%–10%) may develop postictal agitation characterized by motor agitation, disorientation, and poor response to commands (Augoustides et al. 2002; Auriacombe et al. 2000; Devanand et al. 1989). For some patients, postictal agitation may occur at one or two treatments and never recur; however, postictal agitation often recurs in subsequent treatments (Devanand et al. 1989; Kikuchi et al. 2009).

Care should be taken to distinguish among delirium with postictal agitation, agitation due to prolonged apnea, and status epilepticus, including nonconvulsive status epilepticus. Often, however, the precipitating cause of the agitation is unknown. For example, one retrospective case control study of 24 patients with postictal agitation and 24 controls with no postictal agitation found no difference in the two groups in degree of pretreatment agitation, anesthetic or succinylcholine dose, number of ECT treatments received, mean seizure duration, number of titrated treatments with subconvulsive stimulation, type of EEG endpoint, or ultimate clinical outcome (Devanand et al. 1989).

Recovery from postictal agitation may take from 5 to 45 minutes, and patients are usually amnestic for the episode. Importantly, postictal agitation may result in physical injury either to a patient who thrashes against hard objects or to staff members who attempt to protect the patient. In addition, patients may dislodge the intravenous line, complicating management. Depending on severity, postictal agitation may be managed supportively or pharmacologically.

Supportive management of postictal agitation includes one-to-one nursing and ensuring that the recovery area is free of bright lights and that noise is minimized. Pharmacological strategies, such as administering an intravenous bolus of propofol (Augoustides et al. 2002; O'Reardon et al. 2006), methohexital (Cristancho et al. 2008), midazolam, or other short-acting benzodiazepine (Labbate and Miller 1995), are particularly effective when the patient becomes agitated while emerging from anesthesia. Intravenous haloperidol has also been used to treat postictal agitation, although its use may be associated with ventricular ectopy (Greene et al. 2000). In severe postictal agitation, dexmedetomidine can be used (Bryson et al. 2013; Feenstra et al. 2023; Qiu et al. 2020; Sterina et al. 2023). Alternatively, the patient can be sedated with an induction dose of propofol and allowed to emerge slowly from anesthesia. If intravenous access is lost, benzodiazepines and antipsychotic medications can be given intramuscularly.

Strategies to prevent the recurrence of postictal agitation at subsequent ECT treatments include reviewing the patient's medications and limiting medications (e.g., lithium, dopaminergic agents) that have been associated with postictal agitation (el-Mallakh 1988; Nymeyer and Grossberg 1997; Rudorfer et al. 1992; Sadananda et al. 2013). Another prophylactic strategy includes premedication with low-dose dissolvable olanzapine (Hermida et al. 2016), an oral sedating antihistamine such as promethazine (Vishne et al. 2005a), or intravenous midazolam or dexmedetomidine (Mizrak et al. 2009). Other suggestions include increasing the dose of the induction anesthetic agent (Devanand and Sackeim 1992), changing the induction agent to propofol (Butterfield et al. 2004; Eranti et al. 2009), or administering an intravenous bolus of propofol after the ECT seizure (Tzabazis et al. 2013).

19.5. Treatment-Emergent Mania

As with antidepressant medications, a small minority of patients with depression may switch into a hypomanic or manic episode during the ECT course (Andrade et al. 1988b, 1990; Angst et al. 1992; Devanand et al. 1988b, 1992). Although such a shift is rare, patients with bipolar disorder may be the most likely to exhibit it. Interestingly, manic patients with mixed features have also been observed to switch into a depressive episode. The practitioner should be alert to such changes in mood states (Valentí et al. 2008; Vieta 2005).

Treatment-emergent manic symptoms and delirium with euphoria have a number of phenomenological similarities (Devanand et al. 1988b), and it is important to distinguish between the two syndromes. With the latter, patients are typically confused, with pronounced memory disturbance that is evident immediately following the treatment and persists for hours to days. Furthermore, states of delirium with euphoria are often characterized by giddiness or a carefree disposition, but other classical features of hypomania such as racing thoughts, hypersexuality, and irritability may be absent. In contrast, treatment-emergent hypomanic or manic syndromes include the full range of classical hypomanic or manic features but generally occur in the context of a clear sensorium. Thus, evaluating cognitive status may be particularly helpful in distinguishing delirium with euphoria from treatment-emergent manic symptoms.

Several approaches exist for managing hypomanic or manic symptoms that emerge during the ECT course (Cloutier et al. 2021). Some practitioners continue the ECT, whereas others increase the time between treatments, decrease the stimulus intensity, or change from bilateral to unilateral electrode placement. Another option is to postpone further ECT and observe the patient's course to determine whether the manic symptoms remit spontaneously or whether ECT should be resumed for persistent mania or return of depressive symptoms. The ECT course can also be terminated, and manic or residual depressive symptoms can be addressed with pharmacotherapy, such as lithium carbonate, anticonvulsants (e.g., valproic acid), or an antipsychotic medication.

Recommendations

19.1. Mortality

1. Precise rates of the mortality attributable to ECT are difficult to determine, but best estimates suggest a rate of fewer than 4 deaths per 100,000 treatments, with apparent decreases in mortality rates in recent years despite the frequent use of ECT in geriatric patients and patients with significant medical conditions.
2. Evidence from longitudinal studies has shown that mortality rates following hospitalization are lower among depressed patients who received ECT than among patients who received other treatment modalities or no treatment.

19.2. Cardiovascular, Cerebrovascular, and Pulmonary Complications

1. Although most cardiac arrhythmias in the immediate postictal period are benign and resolve spontaneously, an ECG should be monitored during and immediately after the procedure.
2. Vital signs (e.g., pulse, systolic and diastolic blood pressure) should be monitored during treatment and recovery periods and should be stable before the patient leaves the recovery area.
3. The type, likelihood, and severity of post-ECT cardiac complications are correlated with the presence of preexisting cardiac illness; patients at increased risk include those with uncontrolled hypertension, recent myocardial infarction (<60 days), unstable angina, decompensated heart failure, severe aortic stenosis, uncontrolled atrial fibrillation, and unrepaired abdominal aortic aneurysms >5.0 cm, or tachyarrhythmias or bradyarrhythmias associated with hypotension or requiring urgent medical attention.

4. Patients at higher risk of cerebrovascular complications include those with signs or symptoms of an intracranial lesion (e.g., papilledema, focal neurological deficits, mass effect or brain edema on MRI) and those with an acute hemorrhagic stroke in the preceding 30 days, particularly if blood pressure remains poorly controlled.

5. Postictal pulmonary complications are more frequent in patients with asthma and COPD; such patients may benefit from use of bronchodilators or other inhalers on the morning of ECT prior to treatment.

6. Patients who are catatonic or immobile should receive prophylactic treatment to prevent venous thromboembolism.

7. Prolonged postictal apnea is rare but requires that adequate oxygenation be maintained until it resolves.

8. When prolonged apnea occurs, treatment is guided by the underlying cause, which is most often issues with airway management, a higher than needed dose of succinylcholine, or slowed metabolism of succinylcholine.

19.3. Headache, Muscle Soreness, and Nausea

1. Post-ECT headache can be treated with aspirin or acetaminophen along with bed rest in a quiet, darkened environment.

2. Patients who experience frequent post-ECT headaches may benefit from prophylactic treatment such as aspirin or acetaminophen given as soon as possible after ECT or even immediately before the ECT treatment.

3. An NSAID (e.g., intravenous ketorolac) can also be given for acute or prophylactic treatment of post-ECT headache, but potential side effects of NSAIDs include gastrointestinal bleeding, risk of renal failure, compromised hemostasis, and increased levels of lithium. In addition, intravenous ketorolac should not be used late in pregnancy, while breastfeeding, with renal impairment, or in patients with hypersensitivity to NSAIDs or acetylsalicylic acid, including aspirin-sensitive asthma.

4. Muscle soreness or jaw pain can be treated with analgesic agents such as aspirin, acetaminophen, or an NSAID.

5. Muscle soreness that appears to be related to intense fasciculations after administration of a depolarizing muscle relaxant (e.g., succinylcholine) can be reduced in subsequent treatments by switching to

a nondepolarizing agent, whereas muscle soreness related to vigorous convulsive movements can be managed with an increase in the muscle relaxant dose.

6. Jaw pain can be reduced by ensuring closure of the teeth around the bite block and exerting firm, upward pressure under the chin to minimize the clamping of the jaw due to direct electrical stimulation of the pterygoid, masseter, and temporalis muscles.

7. Nausea and vomiting can be addressed by treating any associated headache, by administering a serotonin 5-HT$_3$ receptor antagonist (e.g., ondansetron, dolasetron) or dopamine-blocking agent (e.g., prochlorperazine, trimethobenzamide, metoclopramide), or by changing to propofol as an anesthetic agent at subsequent ECT treatments.

19.4. Postictal Agitation

1. It is important to distinguish between postictal agitation and other possible causes of confusion or agitation such as status epilepticus or apnea.

2. The patient's pharmacotherapy regimen should be examined to identify medications (e.g., lithium, carbidopa) that may be associated with postictal agitation.

3. Pharmacological management of postictal agitation can include administering an intravenous bolus of propofol, methohexital, midazolam, or other short-acting benzodiazepine.

4. Prophylactic strategies include increasing the dose of the induction anesthetic agent in subsequent ECT treatments; changing the induction agent to propofol; giving a bolus of propofol after the ECT seizure; or premedicating with low-dose dissolvable olanzapine, an oral sedating antihistamine (e.g., promethazine), or intravenous midazolam or dexmedetomidine.

19.5. Treatment-Emergent Mania

1. Although a small minority of patients with depression may switch into a hypomanic or manic episode during the ECT course, it is important to distinguish treatment-emergent manic symptoms from delirium with euphoria.

2. When hypomanic or manic symptoms emerge during an ECT course, management options include

   a. Continuing ECT
   b. Increasing the time between treatments
   c. Decreasing the stimulus intensity
   d. Changing from bilateral to unilateral electrode placement
   e. Postponing additional ECT until it is clear whether manic symptoms persist or depression recurs
   f. Terminating the ECT course and instituting pharmacotherapy

CHAPTER 20

Cognitive Side Effects of Electroconvulsive Therapy

20.1. Objective Cognitive Side Effects

20.1.1. Characteristics of Objective Cognitive Side Effects

Cognitive side effects associated with electroconvulsive therapy (ECT) have been studied for decades (Ingram et al. 2008; McClintock et al. 2014; Sackeim 1992; Semkovska and McLoughlin 2010; Squire 1986) and are often of significant concern to patients and their families. Accordingly, clinicians who administer or refer patients for ECT should be familiar with the characteristics and magnitude of cognitive side effects, and this information should be conveyed during the consent process (see Chapter 10).

Table 20–1 lists ECT treatment factors that have been associated with variations in the type and magnitude of cognitive side effects during and following treatment with ECT (Anderson et al. 2017; Butterfield et al. 2004; Geretsegger et al. 2007; Lisanby 2007; Lisanby et al. 2000; Loo et al. 2008; Sackeim et al. 1993, 2000, 2007, 2008; Sienaert et al. 2009; Tor et al. 2015; Weiner et al. 1986b).

A number of other aspects of cognitive changes with ECT are notable. First, confounding factors can make it difficult to interpret cognitive changes with ECT. Psychiatric illnesses such as major depressive disorder (MDD) (Butters et al. 2000; Martin et al. 2020b; McClintock et al. 2010; Zakzanis et al. 1998), bipolar disorder (Mann-Wrobel et al. 2011), and psychosis (Bowie et al. 2018) can have adverse impacts on neurocognitive functions, including processing speed, attention, verbal fluency, learning and memory, working memory, and executive function (Lisanby et al. 2020; McClintock et al. 2014; Semkovska and McLoughlin 2010; Semkovska et al. 2011; Zakzanis et al. 1998). Consequently, many patients will have cognitive difficulties before receiving ECT.

Table 20–1. *Treatment factors that may increase or decrease the severity of cognitive adverse effects*

Treatment factor[a]	Treatment feature associated with increased cognitive side effects	Steps to be taken to reduce cognitive side effects
Stimulus waveform[b]	Brief pulse	Change to ultrabrief pulse
Electrode placement	Bitemporal	Change to right unilateral
	Bifrontal	Change to right unilateral
Stimulus intensity	Grossly suprathreshold	Reduce electrical dose to a level that is not excessive yet is still sufficiently suprathreshold to maintain efficacy
Spacing of treatments	ECT administered three times per week	Decrease treatment frequency to once or twice a week
Concomitant psychotropic medications	Lithium or agents with independent adverse cognitive effects	Reduce dose or stop implicated psychotropics
Anesthetic medications	High dose may contribute to amnesia	Reduce dose as appropriate for light level of anesthesia

[a]See Chapters 12, 13, 14, and 18 for additional information about treatment-related factors and their effects on cognition.
[b]A sine wave stimulus waveform is also associated with increased cognitive side effects, but use of this waveform is not recommended.

These cognitive difficulties may be particularly likely in young patients in their first psychotic episode (Wyatt 1991, 1995). Furthermore, presence of neurological disease may also predispose patients to greater cognitive impairment with ECT. This can occur in older patients, in whom depression may presage a neurodegenerative process (Chen et al. 1999; Devanand et al. 1996), as well as in individuals with preexisting dementia who may be receiving ECT to treat mood disorders or improve behavioral disturbances (Acharya et al. 2015; Hermida et al. 2020b; Isserles et al. 2017). In addition, changes in psychiatric symptoms with treatment may mediate performance on some cognitive measures. Indeed, global cognitive status typically improves as symptoms respond, at least in part because of improvements in attention (Bayless et al. 2010; Semkovska and McLoughlin 2010). Furthermore, patients whose depression has remitted after the ECT course tend to show better performance on cognitive measures as compared with those whose depression has not remitted (Butters et al. 2000; Grützner et al. 2019; Hasselbalch et al. 2011, 2012; Riddle et al. 2017), despite the fact that depression symptom severity is unrelated to neurocognitive performance (Keilp et al. 2018; McClintock et al. 2010).

Second, the type and severity of cognitive alterations change rapidly with time following each treatment. The most prominent cognitive side effects are observed in the immediate postictal period, when patients experience a period of disorientation, which is usually brief and may be associated with postictal agitation (see Chapter 19, section 19.4). During this period of disorientation, processing speed, attention, verbal fluency, executive function, and memory exhibit transient impairments, which recede at variable rates (Calev et al. 1991a; McClintock et al. 2014; Sackeim 1986; Semkovska and McLoughlin 2010). The magnitude of other ECT-induced cognitive effects also tends to diminish over time, a fact that should be considered when scheduling and interpreting follow-up cognitive tests.

Third, patients vary considerably in the extent and severity of cognitive side effects that they develop following ECT. Information about factors that contribute to these individual differences is limited. Although ECT is generally tolerable in older adults and in individuals with mild cognitive impairment or dementia (Acharya et al. 2015; Hermida et al. 2020b), the extent of global cognitive impairment before the ECT course may predict a greater magnitude of retrograde amnesia for autobiographical information after the ECT course and at later follow-up assessments (Sobin et al. 1995). Similarly, some (Martin et al. 2018; Sobin et al. 1995) but not all (Sienaert et al. 2010) research suggests that the magnitude and persistence of inconsistencies in autobiographical memory may be predicted by the duration of disorientation immediately after ECT treatment. Patients who have a preexisting neurological disease (e.g., Alzheimer's disease, Parkinson's disease) or insult (e.g., stroke) may also be more likely to exhibit memory impairment and delirium with ECT (Figiel et al. 1991; Mulsant et al. 1991). ECT-induced delirium has also been associated with the presence of basal ganglia lesions and severe white matter hyperintensities on MRI (Figiel et al. 1990). More recently, older adults with MDD who were treated with right unilateral (RUL) ultrabrief pulse ECT in combination with venlafaxine were found to have modest declines in performance across multiple neurocognitive measures at the group level (Lisanby et al. 2020, 2022). However, at the individual level, some older adults with MDD can show clinically significant impairment across many cognitive functions (Obbels et al. 2018).

Fourth, ECT results in highly characteristic cognitive changes. Anterograde amnesia that occurs in association with ECT is characterized by disrupted learning and rapid forgetting of new verbal and/or visuospatial information (Sackeim et al. 1993; Squire 1986; Steif et al. 1986; Weiner et al. 1986b). Following termination of ECT, the objective anterograde amnestic effects tend to resolve within a week to a few months (Sackeim et al. 1993, 2000, 2007, 2008; U.S. Food and Drug Administration 2018b; Weiner et al. 1986b).

ECT has also been found to be associated with retrograde amnesia, which is greatest in magnitude immediately after completion of an acute ECT treatment course. Difficulties in recalling both personal (autobiographical) and public information are usually greater for events that occurred temporally closest to the treatment (Lisanby et al. 2000; Sackeim et al. 1986, 1993, 2000; Weiner et al. 1986b). Although some patients do not exhibit or report problems with remembering remote events following ECT, others may have difficulty recalling events that transpired several months to years prior to ECT. When present, retrograde amnesia over the applicable time span is rarely complete. Rather, patients may have gaps or spottiness in their memories of personal and public events. In addition, patients who do develop profound or persistent retrograde amnesia may be more likely to have a preexisting neurological impairment or to have received ECT using methods associated with a greater magnitude of cognitive effects (e.g., sine wave stimulation, bilateral electrode placement, high electrical stimulus intensity) (Sackeim et al. 2007; Semkovska and McLoughlin 2013; Semkovska et al. 2011).

Inconsistencies in autobiographical memory (e.g., providing different answers to questions that are asked before the start of treatment and after the conclusion of treatment) have been found to persist for at least 6 months in some individuals (Sackeim et al. 2007). In addition, some individuals who have received ECT have reported more persistent loss of autobiographical memory. Although the timing and recency of the autobiographical event may affect the likelihood of forgetting autobiographical details (Daskalakis et al. 2020; Kopelman 2019), the emotional valence of events—that is, memories of pleasant or distressing events—appears to be unrelated to their likelihood of being forgotten (McElhiney et al. 1995). Because of the subjective nature of some reports of autobiographical retrograde amnesia, this issue is also discussed in section 20.2.1.

Relative to research on memory function after ECT, there is a paucity of research regarding the effects of ECT on other cognitive functions (McClintock et al. 2014; Semkovska and McLoughlin 2010). Impairments in attention and verbal fluency may be accentuated during the ECT course (Bayless et al. 2010; Calev et al. 1995; Miller et al. 2022; Sackeim et al. 1992; Semkovska and McLoughlin 2010), as can impairments of executive function (e.g., cognitive flexibility, complex planning) or skill acquisition, although, for the most part, such effects do not appear to be persistent (Ingram et al. 2008; Sackeim et al. 2007).

Information about cognitive effects of maintenance ECT is also more limited, although the available evidence suggests that such effects are less severe than with more frequent treatments administered during an acute ECT course (Barnes et al. 1997; Ezion et al. 1990; Grunhaus et al. 1990; Lisanby et al. 2022; Smith et al. 2010; Thienhaus et al. 1990; Thornton et al. 1990).

20.1.2. Typical Clinical Assessments of Objective Cognitive Side Effects

Assessment of cognitive function is important before the start of ECT to establish the patient's baseline level of functioning and should be repeated, at intervals determined by the treatment team, to identify and quantify changes in cognitive function as ECT treatment proceeds. As with the assessment of therapeutic change, it is suggested that, when possible, cognitive function assessments be conducted at least 24 hours after an ECT treatment so that acute postictal effects will have resolved. However, individuals who remain delirious or grossly disoriented an hour or more following a treatment should not be discharged home until recovery occurs or further assessment is carried out.

In its 2018 final reclassification action, the U.S. Food and Drug Administration (FDA) required that manufacturers of ECT devices include a warning that "ECT device use may be associated with: disorientation, confusion, and memory problems" (U.S. Food and Drug Administration 2018b). In addition, the FDA stated that ECT device manufacturers should recommend monitoring of cognitive status before and during

ECT treatment using a formal neuropsychological assessment for evaluating specific cognitive functions (e.g., orientation, attention, memory, executive function), although it did not specify the cognitive measures to be used or the timing of such evaluations (U.S. Food and Drug Administration 2018b).

In determining the best strategy for monitoring of cognitive changes with ECT, facilities should implement a standardized approach to assessing cognition using available, reliable, and valid instruments and assessment tools that match their practice setting and patient population. If significant cognitive changes are detected, more detailed testing can be pursued or the patient can be referred for comprehensive clinical neuropsychological assessment, as needed (McClintock et al. 2021; Roebuck-Spencer et al. 2017).

It should also be recognized that adjustments to this standardized approach may be needed for individual patients. Depending on the severity of psychiatric symptoms and the complexity and length of testing, some patients may be unable to tolerate a typical cognitive assessment and modifications may be needed to ensure tolerability and collection of useful cognitive information. Some individuals may not wish to participate in testing and testing may also be precluded in other individuals, such as those with catatonia, significant psychomotor retardation, or severe agitation (American Psychiatric Association 2016).

The clinical assessment of objective cognitive effects with ECT typically provides a brief overall assessment of cognitive functions so as to determine the presence or absence of global cognitive function impairment (Roebuck-Spencer et al. 2017). For bedside or informal assessments, orientation in three spheres (person, place, and time) should be determined. If indicated by the global clinical evaluation, a brief assessment of anterograde amnesia can be conducted by giving the patient several items to remember and by testing their recall of these items immediately and after approximately a short amount of time (e.g., ~5 minutes). Informal assessment of retrograde amnesia can be conducted by discussion with the patient of events in the recent and distant past (e.g., events associated with the day of the interview, food consumed at meals, recent trips or special occasions, memory for personal details such as home address or phone number) and corroboration with the patient's care partner (e.g., spouse, friend) if possible. Attention and processing speed can be assessed by asking the patient to recite the months of the year backward or count backward from 100 by sevens.

Multiple instruments are also available that can be administered by treatment team personnel at bedside, are easy to score and interpret, and can be used to assess global cognitive functioning and assist in clinical decision-making (Hermida et al. 2020a; Martin et al. 2020a; Moirand et al. 2018;). At present, for practical purposes, it is believed that instruments such as the Montreal Cognitive Assessment (MoCA), the Mini-Mental State Examination (MMSE), and the ElectroConvulsive Therapy Cognitive Assessment (ECCA) fulfill these criteria and meet the spirit of FDA recommendations (U.S. Food and Drug Administration 2018b). The MoCA (Nasreddine et al. 2005) is commonly used. In addition, one study found that certain tasks on the MoCA (e.g., phonemic fluency, five-word delayed recall) may be sensitive to ECT-induced cognitive effects (Moirand et al. 2018). The MMSE (Folstein et al. 1975, 2010) has also been frequently used but appears less sensitive to the neurocognitive effects of ECT (Kellner et al. 2016a; Semkovska and McLoughlin 2010). More recently, investigators developed a global cognitive measure specific for use in ECT practice, the ECCA (Hermida et al. 2020a). The initial study findings found it to be feasible, reliable, valid, and more sensitive to ECT-induced cognitive effects than is the MoCA. The ECCA assesses the domains of attention, autobiographical memory, and delayed verbal recall and includes global assessments of the patient's cognitive function by both the patient and the primary caregiver. synthesized other recommendations for cognitive assessment in ECT practice but also described the need to use cognitive measures and batteries that are not time-intensive and do not require substantial amounts of training to use.

20.1.3. Detailed Clinical Assessments of Objective Cognitive Side Effects

Suggestions have also been made in the literature for more extensive, but also more time-consuming, neurocognitive batteries to use before and after the ECT course that incorporate tests of other cognitive elements (Bayless et al. 2010; Martin et al. 2013, 2020a; Porter et al. 2008b). Many of these batteries require additional training to be administered with reliability. Martin and colleagues (2013) recommended a brief cognitive screening battery consisting of the modified MMSE and mental control items (e.g., saying the days of the week backward) that was found to be associated with cognitive outcomes using a comprehensive cognitive battery and, in addition, could be administered at the bedside.

Porter and colleagues (2008b) recommended a test battery that can be administered in under 1 hour by ECT treatment team members and includes an evaluation of depression symptom severity, global cognitive function, autobiographical memory consistency, word list learning and memory, and simple auditory attention and working memory, using the Montgomery-Åsberg Depression Rating Scale (MADRS), Modified Mini-Mental State Examination (3MSE), Autobiographical Memory Interview—Short Form (AMI-SF), Rey Auditory Verbal Learning Test (RAVLT), and Digit Span Forward and Backward, respectively. Bayless and colleagues (2010) recommended a neurocognitive battery for clinical use that comprised measures assessing comprehensive global cognitive function, verbal learning and memory, processing speed, visuospatial construction, phonemic fluency, and semantic fluency. Although these batteries are intended for clinical use, their length and level of detail may make them impractical to use in many settings and patient populations.

A number of specific tests are considered the gold standard in research studies to assess cognitive changes associated with ECT (e.g., Wechsler Memory Scale, 4th Edition [WMS-IV], Repeatable Battery for the Assessment of Neuropsychological Status, RAVLT). Some of the tests require a usage fee for each administration. In addition, they are not routinely used in clinical ECT practice because they typically require additional training to administer and considerable time for a patient to complete.

Multiple cognitive instruments are available that can identify anterograde amnesia by assessing learning, immediate recall, delayed recall, and recognition of newly learned information. For example, specific subtests of the WMS-IV (Wechsler 2009) provide age-adjusted normative information for immediate and delayed memory components. Unfortunately, there are no alternative versions of the WMS-IV, and repeated assessment may be confounded by practice effects. In contrast, the Randt Memory Test (Randt and Brown 1983; Randt et al. 1980) has five alternative forms. This instrument has subscales that assess delayed memory for verbal and pictorial material and is sensitive to the anterograde amnesia associated with ECT (Zervas and Jandorf 1993). When used with a delay recall procedure, the Buschke Selective Reminding Test (Hannay and Levin 1985) has been found to be useful for repeated assessment (Sackeim et al. 1993, 2000). Tasks involving delayed recall of simple and complex figures and delayed recognition memory for unfamiliar faces (Benton 1950; Lezak 1995; Sivan 1992) have shown sensitivity to ECT-associated anterograde amnesia for visuospatial information (Sackeim et al. 2000; Steif et al. 1986; Weiner et al. 1986b). Word list learning and memory measures such as the RAVLT (Rey 1964); California Verbal Learning Test, 3rd Edition (CVLT-3; Delis et al. 2017); and the Hopkins Verbal Learning Test-Revised (HVLT-R; Brandt and Benedict 2001) evaluate learning and recall of a word list immediately and after approximately a 20- to 30-minute delay. The RAVLT, CVLT-3, and HVLT-R have been shown to be sensitive to cognitive changes associated with ECT (Lisanby et al. 2020; Porter et al. 2008b; Semkovska and McLoughlin 2010; Vasavada et al. 2017). In fact, word list learning and recall memory tests, relative to paragraph memory tests, have been found to be more sensitive to ECT-induced cognitive effects (Semkovska and McLoughlin 2010).

Brief, reliable, and valid neuropsychological instruments that can gauge the extent of retrograde amnesia are less readily available. Tests have been used that formally assess recall or recognition of famous people or public events (Butters and Albert 1982; Goldberg and Barnett 1985; Squire 1986; Weiner et al. 1986b). However, most of these instruments categorize public events in relation to the decade of their prominence (e.g., 1970s, 1980s, 1990s), and as such require continual updating with new public events. The retrograde amnesia resulting from ECT tends to display a temporal gradient, such that events closest in time to the treatment course are most vulnerable to memory loss and remote events typically are spared (Sackeim 1992; Squire 1986). Consequently, available instruments may be insensitive and lack sufficient psychometric properties (e.g., test-retest reliability) to assess such retrograde amnesia.

An alternative approach has been to assess amnesia for autobiographical or personal memories, consistency of autobiographical memories, and specificity of autobiographical memory recall (Jelovac et al. 2016; Lisanby et al. 2000; Sackeim 2014; Sackeim et al. 2000; Semkovska and McLoughlin 2013, 2014; Weiner et al. 1986b). Memory loss for events in the patient's life is often the most distressing aspect of potential ECT-induced cognitive side effects. The AMI-SF (McElhiney et al. 1995; Sobin et al. 1995), which measures autobiographical memory recall consistency, has been used in ECT research and found to be sensitive to ECT technique (Sackeim et al. 2007). However, it is relatively lengthy and takes approximately 30–40 minutes to administer and score

(Sackeim et al. 2007). In addition, its psychometric properties have been called into question (Sackeim 2014; Semkovska and McLoughlin 2014), and an alternative administration and scoring method has been proposed (Semkovska et al. 2012).

In terms of more detailed global assessments of cognitive function, the Repeatable Battery for the Assessment of Neuropsychological Status provides coverage of five domains: immediate memory, visuospatial/constructional, language, attention, and delayed memory (Randolph et al. 1998). The Dementia Rating Scale, 2nd Edition (DRS-2; Jurica et al. 1988) has two forms available, was developed to assess changes in cognition over time with dementia, and includes subscores for attention, initiation/perseveration, construction, conceptualization, and memory. One study has reported on the use of the DRS-2 in older adults treated with ECT and found that the Initiation/Perseveration Index showed little change after completion of the ECT course relative to baseline performance (Lisanby et al. 2020).

20.1.4. Comprehensive Clinical and Research Assessments of Objective Cognitive Side Effects

More extensive comprehensive neurocognitive evaluations, which typically take multiple hours to administer, are not a standard part of clinical ECT practice (Weiner et al. 2013) and may not be readily available in all practice settings and geographic locations or suitable for the patient populations being treated. Nevertheless, they may be done as part of clinical research on ECT or if individuals experience cognitive effects of ECT that would benefit from comprehensive assessment. In addition, they can provide useful information to both the patient and ECT treatment team that can help guide decision-making as to changes in the treatment plan (Donders 2020), particularly for individuals who may be at increased risk for ECT-associated cognitive effects due to preexisting cognitive impairment or neurological illness. The complexity and lengthy administration time of such instruments may make it difficult for some patients to complete the assessment because of their psychiatric symptoms (e.g., severe psychomotor slowing or agitation, agitated psychosis). However, in research settings, a comprehensive neurocognitive evaluation can have multiple benefits that include identifying cognitive abilities, detecting cognitive strengths and weaknesses, informing contributions to cognitive weaknesses (e.g., demographic factors, clinical factors, treatment factors), clarifying diagnoses (e.g., intact cognitive function, mild cognitive impairment), and providing cognitive compensatory recommendations (Braun et al. 2011; Donders 2020; Temple et al. 2006).

Comprehensive neurocognitive evaluations are usually conducted by a clinical neuropsychologist and typically involve a neurodiagnostic interview, neurobehavioral status examination, and cognitive assessment using multiple measures to document abilities across multiple cognitive domains (McClintock et al. 2021; Roebuck-Spencer et al. 2017). As such, comprehensive neurocognitive evaluations require significant patient cooperation but provide a greater amount of information on the type and magnitude of ECT-induced cognitive adverse effects, including data on cognitive functions such as incidental learning, visuospatial learning and memory, and complex executive functions (Sackeim et al. 2000; Squire 1986).

20.2. Subjective Cognitive Side Effects

20.2.1. Characteristics of Subjective Cognitive Side Effects

Shortly after receiving ECT, some individuals may report that their cognitive function has improved or worsened relative to their pre-ECT cognitive baseline (Mattes et al. 1990; Sackeim et al. 1993, 2000; Weiner et al. 1986b). One study showed that 2 months after completion of ECT, self-reported memory function was improved relative to the pre-ECT baseline assessment of self-reported memory (Coleman et al. 1996). As in healthy individuals and individuals with neurological illnesses (Prudic et al. 2000; Sackeim and Stern 1997), memory self-ratings in those who have received ECT showed little to no association with objective neuropsychological testing results (Calev et al. 1991b; Coleman et al. 1996; Fischer et al. 2008; Squire and Slater 1983; Squire and Zouzounis 1988; Weiner et al. 1986b). In contrast, strong associations have been observed between mood state and subjective reports about memory among ECT recipients (Semkovska et al. 2023; Vann Jones and McCollum 2019) as well as in other patient populations (Mattes et al. 1990; Petersen et al. 2019; Potvin et al. 2016; Squire and Slater 1983; Squire and Zouzounis 1988; Weiner et al. 1986b). Furthermore, those with the greatest symptomatic benefit from ECT typically report the greatest improvement in subjective reports of cognitive function. Thus, when subjective memory impairment after ECT is reported, mood state, as well as cognition, should be assessed.

Uncommonly, some individuals treated with ECT later report profound cognitive impairment (Donahue 2000; Sackeim et al. 2007). Rarely, a dense amnesia for events of personal significance extending far into the past, or a broad and occupationally disabling impairment of cognitive function, has been reported (Sackeim 2000). Because these subjective impairments are unusual, determination of their absolute base rate is difficult. Nonetheless, when present, these profound subjective cognitive effects are distressing and concerning for the patients and their caregivers (Koopowitz et al. 2003; Rajagopal et al. 2013).

Multiple factors may contribute to such reports of severe cognitive impairment by ECT recipients. First, in some individuals, self-reports of profound ECT-induced cognitive impairment may reflect objective loss of function. In addition, in a community sample treated with ECT, subjective reports of adverse cognitive outcomes were correlated with the number of bitemporal (BT) ECT sessions, and persistent memory impairment was more common in women than in men (Sackeim et al. 2007). Second, some of the psychiatric conditions treated with ECT result in cognitive impairment as part of their natural history (see section 20.1.1). Third, as noted earlier, subjective evaluations of cognitive function typically show weak association with objective measurements but strong association with measures of mood state (Coleman et al. 1996; Petersen et al. 2019; Potvin et al. 2016; Serra-Blasco et al. 2019; Zlatar et al. 2018). One study recruited patients who expressed long-term concerns about ECT-associated cognitive effects and compared this sample with two control groups (Freeman et al. 1980). Objective neuropsychological differences among the groups were modest, but there were marked differences in assessments of mood state and medication status. Patients who reported persistent cognitive impairments with ECT were less likely to have benefited from the treatment and were more likely to have persistent psychiatric symptoms and treatment with psychotropic medication at the time of the study (Freeman et al. 1980; Frith et al. 1983). Fourth, discrepancies between objective neuropsychological test results and patient perceptions of pronounced cognitive impairment may also be related to factors such as patient selection bias in ECT follow-up studies or limitations in the sensitivity of objective cognitive function measures (Berman et al. 2008; Sackeim 2000). Finally, other factors may also play a role and require further study. For example, psychological factors unrelated to mood may be present (e.g., anxiety disorder, other secondary gain) (Fraser et al. 2008; Goodman and McCall 2015).

20.2.2. Typical Clinical Assessments of Subjective Cognitive Side Effects

Whether cognitive function is assessed formally or informally, the patient's perception of cognitive changes should be ascertained and documented (Eggleston and Porter 2021; Prudic et al. 2000). This assessment may be done by informally inquiring whether the patient has noticed any changes in the ability to concentrate (e.g., to follow a television program or read a magazine article), to remember visitors or events of the day, or to recall more remote events. It may be helpful to corroborate the patient's responses with a care partner. Also, as noted in section 20.1.2, the ECCA includes subjective cognitive change content.

20.2.3. Comprehensive Clinical and Research Assessments of Subjective Cognitive Side Effects

Patient perception of memory functioning may also be examined using quantitative instruments. The Squire Subjective Memory Questionnaire (SSMQ; Squire and Chace 1975; Squire and Slater 1983; Squire et al. 1979) has been used most often in studies of patients receiving ECT. Some questions have been raised about the reliability of the SSMQ because it requires patients to compare their current cognitive functioning with their functioning before the psychiatric episode, which can be a complex judgment (Coleman et al. 1996; Prudic et al. 2000). The Cognitive Failures Questionnaire (Broadbent et al. 1982) is a self-report instrument with a wider sampling of aspects of cognitive function. More recently, the National Institutes of Health Patient-Reported Outcomes Measurement Information System (PROMIS) created a brief self-report of applied cognition items that assesses perception of cognitive abilities and cognitive concerns that has been found to be psychometrically sound (Cella et al. 2010; Saffer et al. 2015). In addition, the items that assess cognitive abilities have been found to be associated with objective cognitive performance (Howland et al. 2017). Particularly in the case of severe reported cognitive deficits, comprehensive assessment should include determination of performance validity to evaluate effects of effort on performance (Harris and Merz 2021).

20.3. Addressing Cognitive Side Effects of ECT

During an ECT course, a clinically significant decrement in cognitive function scores may reflect the development of significant cognitive difficulties and should lead to consideration of modifications in ECT technique (see Table 20–1). In this regard, the FDA has also stated that if cognitive status declines during a course of ECT, then "steps should be taken to avoid further decline" (U.S. Food and Drug Administration 2018b). Adjustments such as using unilateral ECT in patients treated with a BT electrode placement, using more efficient waveforms (e.g., ultrabrief), assuring that dosing is not excessively suprathreshold, and increasing the time interval between treatments while maintaining clinical efficacy as much as possible can reduce the magnitude of short-term cognitive side effects and possibly shorten the duration of long-term cognitive adverse effects (Kolshus et al. 2017; McClintock et al. 2014; Miller et al. 2019; Prudic 2008; Sackeim et al. 2000; Semkovska et al. 2016).

When evaluating cognitive side effects of ECT, it is important to consider the individual's baseline cognitive function and the potential effects of their underlying psychiatric illness on cognition. For example, in those with MDD, short-term memory impairment is most marked for unstructured material that requires effortful processing in order to impose structure and organization (Butters et al. 2008; Elderkin-Thompson et al. 2011; Marazziti et al. 2010; McClintock et al. 2010). However, impairment in the recall of new information learned with assistance via structure, cues or hints, and recognition is less likely (Otto et al. 1994; Steif et al. 1986; Sternberg and Jarvik 1976; Turner et al. 2012; Zakzanis et al. 1998).

The possibility of other contributors to cognitive changes (e.g., medical, neurological, pharmacological) should also be considered, particularly if the onset of severe cognitive adverse effects is sudden. In addition, it may be necessary to discontinue or decrease the dose of medications that can exacerbate cognitive side effects, such as lithium carbonate (Patel et al. 2020; Sartorius et al. 2005), and medications with marked anticholinergic properties. A number of medications have been studied in an effort to reduce or prevent cognitive effects with ECT, but samples have been small. Most of these medications have not produced significant benefit (Alizadeh et al. 2015; Matthews et al. 2013; Niu et al. 2020; Pigot et al. 2008; Prakash et al. 2019), although acetylcholinesterase inhibitors, memantine, and liothyronine may warrant further research (Henstra et al. 2017; Verdijk et al. 2022).

Changes in cognitive function after an ECT course can also have implications for discharge planning and for the level of supervision and assistance required by the patient. Even in individuals with unchanged or improved performance on global cognitive function measures, other cognitive impairments, such as anterograde amnesia, may be present (Lisanby et al. 2020; Obbels et al. 2019; Semkovska and McLoughlin 2010). The extent and persistence of anterograde amnesia varies among ECT recipients and should be considered when making recommendations for the post-ECT convalescence period. Until this rapid forgetting of new information resolves, individuals may need restrictions, monitoring, or assistance with some instrumental activities of daily living (e.g., returning to work, making important financial decisions, driving).

Most commonly, cognitive functioning recovers markedly within a week to a month following the last ECT session (Sackeim et al. 1993), and patients and care partners should be reassured that this is generally the case. However, autobiographical memory inconsistency can show longer-term impairment with ECT, particularly for memories within 6 months of the treatment course (Fraser et al. 2008). If orientation or memory functioning show substantial deterioration with ECT that is unresolved at the end of the treatment course, a plan should be put in place to address it. Such a plan should include follow-up of cognitive function at specified intervals and might also include instruction about tools to enhance real-life cognitive performance, such as digital reminders or writing down items that need to be remembered (McClintock et al. 2014).

Recommendations

20.1. Objective Cognitive Side Effects

1. Assessment of cognitive function is important before the start of ECT to establish the patient's baseline level of cognitive functioning and should be repeated, at intervals determined by the treatment team, to identify and quantify changes in cognitive function as ECT treatment proceeds.
2. Informal bedside assessments of cognitive function can be supplemented with instruments such as the MoCA, MMSE, and ECCA that can be administered by treatment team personnel at bedside, are easy to score and interpret, and can be used to assess global cognitive functioning and assist in clinical decision-making.
3. The nature and magnitude of cognitive adverse effects of ECT can be influenced by factors related to treatment such as electrode place-

ment, stimulus waveform, stimulus intensity, frequency of ECT, anesthetic agents, and other concomitant medications.

4. Interpretation of cognitive effects with ECT can be confounded by cognitive changes that may occur with psychiatric diagnoses (e.g., MDD, schizophrenia, dementia) or concomitant neurological conditions.
5. Changes in psychiatric symptoms with treatment may influence performance on some cognitive measures.
6. Patients vary considerably in the extent and severity of cognitive side effects that develop following ECT.
7. Although the type and severity of cognitive alterations change rapidly with time following each treatment, patients typically experience a brief period of disorientation after each ECT.
8. Characteristic cognitive changes with ECT include

   a. Anterograde amnestic effects, characterized by disrupted learning and rapid forgetting of new verbal and/or visuospatial information, which tend to resolve within a week to a few months of an acute ECT course
   b. Retrograde amnesia, which may include difficulties in recalling personal (autobiographical) and public information and which is greatest in magnitude immediately after completion of an acute ECT course

20.2. Subjective Cognitive Side Effects

1. The patient's perception of cognitive changes with ECT should be ascertained, either formally or informally, with collateral information obtained from the patient's care partner when possible.
2. Shortly after ECT, patients may report that their cognitive function has improved or worsened relative to their pre-ECT cognitive baseline, and these subjective reports should be documented.
3. When subjective memory impairment is reported after ECT, mood state should be assessed as well as cognition because persistent depression has been associated with subjective memory concerns.
4. Although subjective reports of severe cognitive impairment are uncommon, further assessment is warranted to identify objective changes in cognitive function, persistent psychiatric symptoms, or other possible contributors.

20.3. Addressing Cognitive Side Effects of ECT

1. During an ECT course, a clinically significant decrement in cognitive function scores may reflect the development of cognitive difficulties and should lead to consideration of modifications in ECT technique.
2. If the onset of severe cognitive adverse effects is sudden, consideration of possible contributors (e.g., medical, neurological, pharmacological) is warranted, and medications that can exacerbate cognitive side effects (e.g., L-dopa, lithium) may need to be tapered or discontinued.
3. Most commonly, cognitive functioning recovers markedly within a week to a month following the last ECT session; however, autobiographical memory inconsistency can show longer-term impairment with ECT, particularly for memories within 6 months of the treatment course.
4. If severe cognitive adverse effects persist after completion of the ECT course, post-ECT referral for comprehensive clinical neuropsychological evaluation and the provision of potential compensatory strategies should be considered.
5. Decisions about discharge and levels of required supervision should incorporate information on changes in the patient's cognitive function, including anterograde amnesia.

CHAPTER 21

Management of Prolonged, Missed, Abortive, or Inadequate Seizures

Effective management of prolonged, missed, abortive, or inadequate seizures is dependent on proper motor and electroencephalogram (EEG) monitoring technique, as delineated in Chapter 15. The electroconvulsive therapy (ECT) psychiatrist should also be mindful of artifacts, inappropriately increased EEG amplification, and other factors that may interfere with accurate detection of seizure activity.

21.1. Prolonged and Tardive Seizures

Uncommonly, some patients experience prolonged seizures with ECT or may have a return of seizure activity after the initial seizure terminates (tardive seizures). As defined here, a prolonged seizure is one that is longer than 3 minutes by motor or EEG manifestations. Some practitioners use a more stringent definition of 2 minutes for a prolonged seizure (Abrams 2002; Royal College of Psychiatrists 1995). Status epilepticus can be defined as more than 30 minutes of either continuous seizure activity or two or more sequential seizures without an intervening full recovery of consciousness (Glauser et al. 2016). Each facility should develop standard protocols describing the steps to be taken in response to prolonged seizures, tardive seizures, and status epilepticus.

Because prolonged or tardive seizure activity may not be expressed in motor movements and may develop into nonconvulsive status epilepticus, EEG monitoring should be employed in all circumstances (Mayur et al. 1999; Parker et al. 2001; Scott and Riddle 1989). If the seizure is prolonged or hypoxia is evident, intubation may be needed to maintain an adequate level of oxygenation. Usually after 3 minutes of seizure activity, the seizure should be aborted pharmacologically using an anesthetic agent with anticonvulsant properties (e.g., methohexital, propofol) or a benzodiazepine. If an anesthetic agent with anticonvulsant properties has been used for the ECT anesthesia, the seizure can generally be terminated by administering the same anesthetic agent at the same dosage or half of the dosage used for the initial anesthesia. An alternative approach is intravenous administration of a benzodiazepine such as diazepam (5–10 mg) or midazolam (1–2 mg). If a single dose is not sufficient to interrupt the seizure activity, repeated and increasingly higher doses of benzodiazepine can be given. If the seizure activity is not terminated after administering two to three boluses of medication with anticonvulsant properties, the ECT team should consider transfer to an emergency medical setting. Generalized convulsive status epilepticus should be managed as a true medical emergency with aggressive treatments, including intravenous benzodiazepines (e.g., midazolam, lorazepam, diazepam) and other anticonvulsants (e.g., fosphenytoin, or alternatively phenytoin; valproic acid; levetiracetam; Glauser et al. 2016). While seizure activity is occurring, it is essential that the patient's airway and intravenous access are maintained and that vital signs are continuously monitored because prolonged seizures can be associated with periods of apnea, hypoxia, and metabolic acidosis, with an increased risk for neuronal damage (Betjemann and Lowenstein 2015).

After the seizure activity has been interrupted, patients should be monitored closely, particularly for cardiovascular instability and respiratory depression, until consciousness returns and vital signs are stable. Further evaluation may be advisable to identify any sequelae, determine the cause of the prolonged seizure, and outline steps that may be useful to prevent recurrence. When stimulus dose titration is used at the first treatment, patients often have the longest seizure of their ECT course. With an increment in stimulus intensity at subsequent treatments, seizure duration typically decreases. Children and adolescents typically have a lower seizure threshold than do adults and may have longer seizures, including more frequent prolonged seizures (Ghaziuddin et al. 2004, 2020) (see Chapter 9, section 9.5). Prolonged seizures and status epilepticus may also be more likely in patients receiving certain medications (e.g., theophylline, lithium, caffeine), even at therapeutic levels (Abrams 2002; Devanand et al. 1988a; Fink and Sackeim 1998; Peters et al. 1984). Although a case series suggested that the combination of lithium and ECT may be safe (Dolenc and Rasmussen 2005), other case reports suggested that concomitant lithium therapy may prolong seizures, particularly in combination with other psychotropic medications (Conway and Nelson 2001;

Rucker and Cook 2008; Weiner et al. 1980b). The second-generation antipsychotic clozapine, which is associated with an increased incidence of seizures, has been used with ECT without a significant increase in the seizure duration (Cardwell and Nakai 1995) or prolonged seizures (Grover et al. 2015). Preexisting electrolyte imbalance (Finlayson et al. 1989) and repeated induction of seizures within the same treatment session (e.g., multiple monitored ECT; Maletzky 1981; Strain and Bidder 1971) have also been reported to increase the likelihood of prolonged seizures. Although uncommon, nonconvulsive status epilepticus has also been reported with ECT (Aftab et al. 2018). It may be more likely in individuals who have conditions such as epilepsy or central nervous system abnormalities (e.g., frontal lobe disorders), who have had an abrupt taper of anticonvulsant medications, or who are receiving medications that lower the seizure threshold (Aftab et al. 2018).

Rarely, patients may have a spontaneous seizure that occurs within hours of an ECT treatment, which has been referred to as a tardive seizure (Warren et al. 2022). Tardive seizures occurring during the immediate postictal period are often not accompanied by motor manifestations, underscoring the need for EEG seizure monitoring (Parker et al. 2001; Rao et al. 1993). Although the causative factors for tardive seizures are unknown, the practitioner should investigate potential causes of a new onset of seizures.

Decisions about whether and how to continue an ECT series after a tardive or prolonged seizure, including status epilepticus, should be based on relevant risk-benefit considerations. In the case of easily manageable prolonged seizures, continuation of the ECT series is generally indicated, perhaps with prophylactic administration of the anticonvulsant agent of choice at the time where any subsequent seizures exceed 2 minutes. In addition, a decision to continue ECT should be made only following investigation and potential management of underlying causes of the event.

21.2. Missed Seizures

A *missed* seizure or subconvulsive stimulation occurs when no subsequent motor (tonic or clonic movements) or EEG seizure activity occurs after electrical stimulation. At times, some muscle groups will undergo a brief immediate contraction in response to stimulation, which should not be mistaken for a seizure.

After a missed seizure has occurred, it is important to review the causes, particularly when there is repeated difficulty in producing an ictal response. Factors that can lead to missed seizures include insufficient stimulus intensity, excessive dynamic impedance resulting from poor contact at the skin-electrode interface (see Chapter 14, section 14.6), premature stimulus termination, hypercarbia from inadequate ventilation, hypoxia, dehydration, and anticonvulsant actions of medications (including benzodiazepines and barbiturate anesthetic agents).

As an initial step, the practitioner should determine whether the dynamic impedance was excessive, if such information is available. If the impedance value was excessive, the preparation of the electrode sites, adequacy of electrode positioning, and integrity of the electrical circuit should be examined, and corrective measures should be taken. If excessive impedance was not an issue, vigorous hyperventilation should be attempted, and the patient should be restimulated at a higher stimulus dosage if possible. It is common practice to restimulate at 50%–100% above the original stimulus dosage. If the stimulus dosage is at the maximum level of the ECT device, augmentation strategies should be used as described below. It is preferable to wait at least 20 seconds between stimulations because some seizures may, rarely, be delayed by 20 seconds or more. This interval may also allow the effects of prior stimulation to dissipate.

Following a missed seizure, a number of additional strategies can be considered at subsequent treatments. Dehydrated patients should be examined for electrolyte imbalance, any indicated corrective measures should be taken, and vigorous hydration should be considered. Seizure induction can sometimes be facilitated by hyperventilating the patient prior to the ECT stimulus and maintaining an end tidal volume of at least 40 mm Hg (Sawayama et al. 2008). Using devices such as a laryngeal mask airway can help maintain the airway and provide more efficient ventilation. A shift in electrode placement (i.e., bilateral to right unilateral) or stimulus waveform (e.g., brief pulse to ultrabrief pulse) can also reduce the seizure threshold and facilitate seizure induction.

If possible, any medications with anticonvulsant properties should be reduced in dosage or discontinued (Virupaksha et al. 2010). For a patient who needs to continue an anticonvulsant medication, the medication dose can be held the night before and the morning of ECT. Patients who are receiving benzodiazepines may have difficulty reducing or holding doses because of anxiety or catatonia. Under these circumstances, flumazenil (0.5–1.0 mg IV) can be administered at the time of anesthetic induction (Bailine et al. 1994; Berigan et al. 1995; Doering and Ball 1995; Krystal et al. 1998b) (see Chapter 13, section 13.2.4).

Anesthetics vary in their effects on seizure threshold (Boylan et al. 2000; Gálvez et al. 2015; Krueger et al. 1993; Miller et al. 1985), and the anesthetic regimen may need modification to facilitate seizure elicitation (see Chapter 12). Etomidate and ketamine have the least effect on raising the seizure threshold, followed by methohexital, thiopental, and propofol (e.g., Stadtland et al. 2002). Thus, the practitioner may switch from a barbiturate anesthetic agent to etomidate (0.15–0.30 mg/kg IV) (Christensen et al. 1986; Saffer and Berk 1998; Trzepacz et al. 1993) or ketamine (2–3 mg/kg IV) (Krystal et al. 2003; Rasmussen et al. 1996) after considering the different side effects of the two agents. An alternative strategy is to lower the dose of the primary anesthetic agent (e.g., methohexital, propofol) and substitute or premedicate with short-acting narcotics (e.g., remifentanil, alfentanil) that have minimal effect on the seizure threshold (Loo et al. 2010). This strategy has the advantage of lowering the seizure threshold by allowing the barbiturate dose to be decreased and maintaining the patient on an anesthetic agent that they previously tolerated.

Less often, some clinicians have administered the adenosine antagonist caffeine sodium benzoate (500–2,000 mg IV, equivalent to 250–1,000 mg of pure caffeine) a few minutes before anesthetic induction to produce or lengthen generalized seizures (Calev et al. 1993; Coffey et al. 1987c, 1987d, 1990; Hinkle et al. 1987; Shapira et al. 1985, 1987). More rarely, theophylline has been administered, either intravenously at the time of ECT (Girish et al. 1996; Leentjens et al. 1996) or orally the night before ECT administration (Swartz and Lewis 1991). Each of these techniques will reliably increase seizure duration, perhaps by modulating seizure termination processes (Francis and Fochtmann 1994). However, most evidence suggests that caffeine or theophylline administration will not decrease seizure threshold or facilitate seizure induction in patients with repeated missed seizures (McCall et al. 1993), and, as discussed in Chapter 15, seizure duration per se may have little, if any, relationship to clinical outcome with ECT (Lalla and Milroy 1996; Nobler et al. 1993; Sackeim et al. 1991). Furthermore, standing regimens of theophylline may be associated with a high incidence of status epilepticus when combined with ECT, even when plasma levels are in the therapeutic range for the treatment of pulmonary disorder (10–20 ng/mL;

Devanand et al. 1988a; Fink and Sackeim 1998; Peters et al. 1984). Case reports also have described cardiac complications (Acevedo and Smith 1988; Beale et al. 1994c; Jaffe et al. 1990a). In addition, a rodent study raised the possibility that the combination of ECT and caffeine may result in neuropathological changes not observed with ECT alone (Enns et al. 1996). These concerns limit the circumstances in which caffeine and theophylline might be considered as augmentation agents in ECT.

Sometimes a missed seizure occurs at the maximal device settings that is not attributable to concurrent medications, excessive anesthetic dosage, or other modifiable factors (Krystal et al. 2000a; Lisanby et al. 1996). In this circumstance the practitioner may elect to use the technique of *double stimulation*. This technique involves delivering two electrical stimuli as close in time as possible to provide summation (Andrade 1991; Schneegans et al. 2019). If the interval between the stimuli is too great (e.g., more than a few seconds), it is unlikely that the two stimuli will summate to produce an effective seizure.

21.3. Abortive or Inadequate Seizures

At times, seizures will be elicited that are *abortive*—that is, too short in duration. Typically, such seizures will be less than 15 seconds by motor or EEG criteria. After an abortive seizure, the practitioner should first make a clinical judgment about its likely causes and whether restimulation will be conducted at the same session. Such decisions are not clear-cut because brief seizures may be due to either insufficient or markedly suprathreshold stimulus intensity (Riddle et al. 1993; Sackeim et al. 1991). Furthermore, there is no evidence to support a correlation between the length of the seizure and therapeutic efficacy (Rasmussen et al. 2006).

If a decision is made to restimulate the patient in the same session as an abortive seizure, the need for additional anesthetic and muscle relaxant agents should be determined on the basis of the patient's state of consciousness and degree of neuromuscular relaxation. Following an abortive seizure and the associated neuronal *refractory period*, a transient increase in seizure threshold is likely. Consequently, immediate restimulation may produce a missed seizure or another abortive seizure. Thus, it is advisable to use a longer time interval before restimulation than that used after a missed seizure. An interval of at least 45 seconds is generally sufficient.

Decisions about adjustments to the stimulus intensity will be informed by factors that may decrease seizure duration or increase seizure threshold as described for missed seizures as well as by the number of treatments given, the electrode placement, and the strategy used to determine stimulus dosing. If markedly suprathreshold stimulation is a possible cause of the abortive seizure, an increase in stimulus intensity is likely to increase risks of side effects without affecting seizure duration or therapeutic benefits. Ictal EEG characteristics may be helpful in this determination on the basis of evidence that significant increases in stimulus intensity above the seizure threshold are associated with a greater EEG amplitude and more postictal suppression (Krystal et al. 1993, 1995). On the other hand, seizure threshold increases with the number of treatments (Krystal et al. 1998a) and may be reflected by a decrement in ictal EEG expression or postictal suppression over the treatment course (Francis-Taylor et al. 2020; Krystal et al. 2000c) (see Chapter 15). Given the data indicating that treatment efficacy is linked to the degree to which the stimulus intensity exceeds the seizure threshold for some forms of ECT, repeating an empirical stimulus titration may help clarify whether adjustments in stimulus intensity are needed to maintain therapeutic adequacy (Abrams 2000; Kellner et al. 2016b; Krystal et al. 2000c; Lisanby et al. 1996; Loo et al. 2014; McCall et al. 2000; Sackeim et al. 1987a, 1993, 2000, 2008). Other strategies to address abortive or inadequate seizures include those discussed for management of missed seizures, such as addressing causes of increased dynamic impedance, hyperventilating prior to ECT, assuring adequate hydration, correcting electrolyte abnormalities, modifying the electrode placement, adjusting stimulus parameters, modifying the anesthetic agent (e.g., changing from methohexital to etomidate or ketamine, changing from propofol to another agent) (Luccarelli et al. 2021a), decreasing doses of the anesthetic agents or other medications with anticonvulsant properties, or administering flumazenil to counteract anticonvulsant effects of benzodiazepines.

It should also be emphasized that some patients consistently display short seizures (e.g., 15 seconds in motor manifestations) regardless of the adequacy of technique, and there is no evidence that such patients do not benefit from these treatments. This pattern is particularly likely to occur in older patients with high initial seizure thresholds (Sackeim et al. 1991) as well as later in the ECT course because seizure threshold rises and seizure duration declines with progressive treatment (Kales et al. 1997; Sackeim 1999; Sackeim et al. 1986).

As discussed in Chapter 15, the concept of seizure adequacy is still being delineated. Although it is clear that seizure duration is not the only pertinent criterion, studies continue to assess the clinical utility of other factors, including postictal suppression and measures of EEG seizure expression. In the absence of such clarity, ECT psychiatrists at many centers develop local consensus guidelines as to how an *adequate* seizure is defined. Such guidelines usually include a plan for management of inadequate seizures. A plan of this type commonly involves actions similar to those described above for abortive seizures.

Recommendations

21.1. Prolonged and Tardive Seizures

1. Each facility should have a procedure for identifying and treating prolonged seizures, tardive seizures, and status epilepticus.
2. Seizures lasting longer than 3 minutes should be terminated pharmacologically using an anesthetic agent with anticonvulsant properties (e.g., methohexital, propofol) or a benzodiazepine (e.g., midazolam, lorazepam, diazepam).
3. If the seizure has not terminated after administering two to three boluses of these medications, the ECT team should initiate more intensive interventions, including consideration of transfer to a higher level of emergency care.
4. While seizure activity is occurring, it is essential that vital signs are continuously monitored and that the patient's intravenous access and airway are maintained, recognizing that intubation may be needed to maintain oxygenation if the seizure does not readily terminate with initial management efforts.
5. EEG monitoring is important in identifying prolonged seizures (including nonconvulsive status epilepticus) and in distinguishing nonconvulsive status epilepticus from psychiatric syndromes that also present with clinical features such as unresponsiveness, agitation, or delirium.
6. Prolonged seizures and status epilepticus, including nonconvulsive status epilepticus, may be more likely in patients who have central nervous system abnormalities or preexisting electrolyte imbalance;

who have had an abrupt taper of anticonvulsant medication; or who are receiving medications that lower seizure threshold or interfere with seizure termination, such as theophylline.

7. Tardive seizures, which are defined as the rare occurrence of a spontaneous seizure within hours of an ECT treatment, may require EEG monitoring for identification.

8. Decisions about whether and how to continue an ECT series after a tardive or prolonged seizure, including status epilepticus, should be based on relevant risk-benefit considerations. In the case of easily manageable prolonged seizures, continuation of the ECT series is generally indicated, whereas with more difficult to manage prolonged seizures, tardive seizures, or status epilepticus, a decision to continue ECT should be made only following investigation and potential management of underlying causes of the event.

21.2. Missed Seizures

1. After a missed seizure, it is important to consider possible causes, such as insufficient stimulus intensity, poor contact at the skin-electrode interface, premature stimulus termination, hypercarbia from inadequate ventilation, hypoxia, dehydration, and anticonvulsant actions of medications (e.g., benzodiazepines, anesthetic agents).

2. Depending on the possible causes, strategies to address a missed seizure during the session or at subsequent sessions include the following:

   a. Assuring that electrode sites are well prepared, electrode positioning is adequate, and electrical continuity is intact from the patient to the ECT electrodes and the ECT device, particularly if the dynamic impedance during the stimulation was excessive

   b. Restimulating at 50%–100% above the original stimulus dose, after a delay of at least 20 seconds

   c. Hyperventilating prior to the ECT stimulus to maintain an end tidal volume of at least 40 mm Hg

   d. Modifying the electrode placement or stimulus parameters (e.g., change from bilateral ECT to right unilateral ECT, change from brief to ultrabrief pulse widths with right unilateral ECT)

   e. Assuring adequate hydration and correcting any electrolyte abnormalities

   f. Decreasing the dose of any anticonvulsant medications or, in the case of benzodiazepines, giving flumazenil just prior to anesthetic administration to counteract the anticonvulsant effect of these medications

   g. Lowering the dose of the primary anesthetic agent (e.g., methohexital, propofol) and substituting or premedicating with short-acting narcotics (remifentanil or alfentanil)

   h. Administering etomidate or ketamine as the anesthetic agent, with consideration given to the side effects of both medications

21.3. Abortive or Inadequate Seizures

1. After an abortive seizure, typically less than 15 seconds by motor or EEG criteria, the practitioner will need to decide its likely causes and whether to conduct restimulation at the same session.
2. Assessments of ictal EEG characteristics (ictal EEG expression, EEG amplitude, postictal suppression) and longitudinal changes in the ictal EEG can provide helpful information in assessing possible causes of an abortive seizure.
3. The patient's clinical status also influences decision-making because some patients show benefit from ECT despite consistently short seizures (e.g., 15 seconds of motor manifestations).
4. If markedly suprathreshold stimulation is a possible cause of the abortive seizure, restimulating at an increased stimulus intensity is likely to increase risks of side effects without affecting seizure duration or therapeutic benefits.
5. If a decision is made to restimulate the patient in the same session as an abortive seizure, the need for additional anesthetic and muscle relaxant agents should be determined on the basis of the patient's state of consciousness and degree of neuromuscular relaxation.
6. Following an abortive seizure and the associated neuronal refractory period, a transient increase in seizure threshold is likely, and an interval of at least 45 seconds prior to restimulation is suggested.
7. Repeating an empirical stimulus titration may help clarify whether adjustments in stimulus intensity are needed to maintain therapeutic adequacy.
8. Other strategies to address abortive seizures include those discussed for management of missed seizures.
9. The definition of an adequate seizure is still being delineated, but many centers develop local consensus guidelines; these typically include a plan for management of inadequate seizures that is similar to approaches for managing abortive seizures.

CHAPTER 22

Lack of Response to the Acute Electroconvulsive Therapy Course

Although most patients will respond to an acute course of electroconvulsive therapy (ECT), the initial ECT consultation should nevertheless consider the possibility of ECT nonresponse, as well as the need for post-ECT treatment alternatives. It is important that severely ill individuals who are referred for possible ECT understand that their disorder is indeed potentially treatable, be it with ECT or by other interventions. Discussion of the possibility of ECT nonresponse is an important element of informed consent (see Chapter 10) and will also provide safeguards against therapeutic nihilism related to the belief that ECT is a "treatment of last resort" (Iodice and McCall 2003).

Formal assessment of symptoms at fixed intervals can assist in identifying patients whose symptoms have not responded to or remitted with ECT (see Chapter 17). In addition, before concluding that a patient has had minimal or no response to ECT, it is important to assess the adequacy of the ECT trial. Specific considerations include whether adequate seizures were induced (see Chapter 15), whether the number of treatments was likely sufficient (see Chapter 18), and whether other modifications to ECT technique were made in an effort to optimize outcome (e.g., changing from right unilateral to bifrontal or bitemporal [BT] electrode placement, increasing the pulse width from ultrabrief to brief, increasing the delivered charge, repeating stimulus titration to ensure that stimulation dosages are sufficiently above seizure threshold, adding medications to augment efficacy; see Chapter 18). Premature discontinuation of the ECT series often results in incomplete symptom reduction and increased risk of relapse (Kellner et al. 2006; Prudic et al. 2004). Consequently, individuals who stop ECT because of side effects (e.g., cognitive impairment), patient preference, or other reasons may not have received an adequate acute ECT series.

When the response to an acute ECT series has been minimal or insufficient, the goal of post-ECT treatment will continue to be focused on treating the acute episode, which will depend on the diagnosis that is being treated. In addition to reevaluating the patient's diagnosis, it is important to reassess the patient's individualized treatment plan and review factors such as physical and psychiatric comorbidities, personality characteristics, psychosocial stressors, and history of treatment in current and prior episodes of illness.

A common approach is to modify the patient's pharmacological treatment regimen. For patients with depression, the timing of an ECT series typically occurs after several antidepressant trials from different classes (Kraus et al. 2019), most often selective serotonin reuptake inhibitors (SSRIs) and serotonin-norepinephrine reuptake inhibitors (SNRIs). Although some evidence suggests that previously ineffective medications may become effective after ECT (Shapira et al. 1988), this strategy has been challenged, and continued treatment with an ineffective medication is not recommended (Sackeim et al. 1990). Switching medication class (e.g., pre-ECT SSRI to post-ECT SNRI) may be a more effective strategy (Iodice and McCall 2003).

Consideration of tricyclic antidepressants (TCAs) and monoamine oxidase inhibitor (MAOI) antidepressants is also warranted. TCAs and MAOIs, including transdermal selegiline, can often be effective even when other treatments have not worked (Cipriani et al. 2018; Gillman 2018; Kriston et al. 2014; Meister et al. 2016; Ricken et al. 2017; Thomas et al. 2015; Ulrich et al. 2017). Although prescription data show that the majority of MAOI recipients have a history of ECT (Shulman et al. 2009), earlier consideration of MAOIs in treatment-resistant depression has been suggested (Van den Eynde et al. 2022). Most patients find that side effects are manageable, particularly when compared with persistent symptoms of depression. In addition, the dietary interactions with MAOIs have been reduced by modern food production and hygiene standards (Van den Eynde et al. 2022).

Combination treatment or augmentation strategies can also be considered. In particular, combining antidepressants with different mechanisms may be more effective than use of a single antidepressant (Henssler et al. 2016). For example, a combination of the MAOI antidepressant tranylcypromine with the TCA amitriptyline was well tolerated and was associated with clinical benefit in an open-label trial for individuals with no symptom improvement after an acute ECT series

(Ferreira-Garcia et al. 2018). Use of lithium as an antidepressant augmentation strategy is another consideration (Nelson et al. 2014), as are antidepressant augmentation strategies for treatment-resistant depression in general (Nuñez et al. 2022; Taylor et al. 2020).

Ketamine, a noncompetitive high-affinity N-methyl-D-aspartate (NMDA) receptor antagonist, has been associated with an antidepressant response within hours when it is administered as an intravenous infusion (Zarate et al. 2006). With repeated administration, ketamine also appears to be beneficial in individuals who might otherwise be referred for ECT (Anand et al. 2023; de A Simoes Moreira et al. 2023; Ekstrand et al. 2022; Menon et al. 2023; Rhee et al. 2022). In individuals with no symptom improvement during an acute ECT course, an open-label trial of ketamine infusions demonstrated moderate effect sizes, but the degree of response was less robust than in ECT naïve subjects (Ibrahim et al. 2011). Esketamine, the ketamine S-enantiomer, has a higher affinity for the NMDA receptor than the R-enantiomer does and is approved by the U.S. Food and Drug Administration in an intranasal formulation for treatment-resistant nonpsychotic depressive episodes (Popova et al. 2019). Even though individuals with a recent ECT series were excluded from the esketamine trial, this medication may be an option if not initiated prior to the ECT series.

Psychotherapy should also be considered after insufficient response to ECT to target ongoing psychosocial stressors or concomitant psychiatric disorders. Depressed patients with concomitant personality disorders may have diminished improvement from an ECT series (Feske et al. 2004; McClintock et al. 2011a) and can benefit from a multifaceted treatment plan that includes pharmacotherapy and psychotherapy. Cognitive-behavioral therapy (CBT) has reduced the risk of relapse in the maintenance phase of treatment (Brakemeier et al. 2014). If not already implemented, CBT or interpersonal psychotherapy may have synergistic effects with post-ECT pharmacotherapy for depressive episodes (Li et al. 2018; van Bronswijk et al. 2019).

Other neuromodulation treatments may also be considered after ECT nonresponse (see Chapter 24). In addition, a second ECT series may be an option for individuals who have not responded to ECT (Sackeim et al. 2020). After the initial course, one of the aforementioned treatment options should be used, and the second ECT series should occur after a sufficient delay to permit full recovery from cognitive side effects of the initial ECT course. Before initiating a second ECT course, the medical records from the initial series should be carefully reviewed. If not used during the initial series, ECT optimization strategies can be considered for the second ECT series. For example, if midseries parameter adjustments were not made during the initial ECT series, the second series may be initiated with the more effective brief pulse width and BT electrode placement. Adjustments to concomitant medications can also be considered. For example, concurrent medications that have adverse impacts on seizure threshold should be discontinued, and the dose of the induction agent should be optimized to reduce the impact on seizure threshold and promote seizure adequacy (Kronsell et al. 2021). Specific psychotropic medications may also be added that could act synergistically with ECT. For depressive episodes, all antidepressant classes enhance the efficacy of the ECT series with equivalent effect sizes (Pluijms et al. 2021), whereas for psychotic disorders, clozapine provides synergistic benefit with ECT (Petrides et al. 2015).

Recommendations

1. Discussion of the possibility of ECT nonresponse is an important element of informed consent, but patients should understand that their disorder is potentially treatable, be it with ECT or by other interventions.
2. Formal assessment of symptoms at fixed intervals can help identify patients whose symptoms have not responded to or remitted with ECT.
3. Patients who stop ECT prematurely because of side effects (e.g., cognitive impairment), patient preference, or other reasons may have an increased risk of relapse as well as incomplete symptom reduction.
4. Before concluding that a patient has had minimal or no response to ECT, the adequacy of the ECT trial should be determined, including whether the number of treatments was likely sufficient, adequate seizures were induced, and modifications to ECT technique were made in an effort to optimize outcome.
5. When there has been minimal or no response to an acute ECT series, it is important to reassess the patient's diagnosis and individualized treatment plan, including review of factors such as physical and psychiatric comorbidities, personality characteristics, psychosocial stressors, and treatment during current and prior episodes of illness.

6. Following a lack of response to an acute ECT course, subsequent treatment will be dependent on the patient's diagnosis and other clinical factors as delineated in the individualized treatment plan.

7. Strategies that can be considered in depressed patients who have not remitted to an acute ECT series include

    a. An antidepressant from a different class than was used prior to ECT

    b. A TCA, MAOI, or a combination of TCA plus an MAOI antidepressant

    c. Augmenting an antidepressant with a second antidepressant with a different mechanism, lithium, or a second-generation antipsychotic

    d. Ketamine or esketamine

    e. An evidence-based form of psychotherapy for depression, such as CBT or interpersonal psychotherapy

    f. Other neuromodulation treatments, including transcranial magnetic stimulation and vagus nerve stimulation

8. After recovery from the initial ECT series, a second optimized ECT series can be considered with concurrent pharmacotherapy (e.g., antidepressant with depression, clozapine with schizophrenia) and more effective ECT parameters (e.g., brief pulse waveform, BT electrode placement).

CHAPTER 23

Management of Patients Following an Electroconvulsive Therapy Course

23.1. General Considerations

For individuals with a response or remission of symptoms during the acute electroconvulsive therapy (ECT) series, the goals of pharmacotherapy are to reduce the risk of relapse or recurrence. Continuation and maintenance treatments have become the norm in contemporary psychiatric practice (American Psychiatric Association 2002, 2010, 2021). Continuation treatment is traditionally defined as the provision of somatic treatment over the 6-month period after the onset of remission in an acute episode of psychiatric illness to prevent relapse, whereas treatment that extends beyond that time and aims to prevent a recurrent episode of illness is defined as maintenance treatment (American Psychiatric Association 2010; Bauer et al. 2017; Elias et al. 2018). However, many patients who receive ECT have nonepisodic illnesses such as schizophrenia or catatonia due to medical conditions. In addition, in many patients, the boundaries of relapse and remission are unclear, making it difficult to determine the starting points for continuation or maintenance phases of treatment. Thus, for the purposes of simplicity and clarity, in this chapter we use the term *maintenance* for all treatments administered after the completion of an acute course of ECT, which occurs over 2–4 weeks in most but not all patients.

Because individuals referred for ECT are particularly likely to have symptoms that have been resistant to medication and other treatments, there is a high risk of relapse, particularly during the first few weeks and months after ECT (Aronson et al. 1987; Bourgon and Kellner 2000; Grunhaus et al. 1995; Jelovac et al. 2013; Kellner et al. 2006; Sackeim et al. 1990, 1993, 2001a; Spiker et al. 1985; Stoudemire et al. 1994). In the absence of maintenance treatment, relapse rates approach 80% at 6 months (Sackeim et al. 2001a; van den Broek et al. 2006). For this reason, maintenance pharmacotherapy should be instituted as soon as possible after completion of an acute ECT course, if not during the ECT course itself. Furthermore, unless limited by adverse effects, maintenance therapy should be maintained for a minimum of 6 months and could be extended for longer periods on the basis of individual history and disease characteristics. Maintenance therapy may consist of pharmacotherapy and/or continued ECT. Other neurostimulation therapies also can be considered alone or in conjunction with pharmacotherapy. In addition, there is a role for adjunctive psychotherapy in many patients.

23.2. Maintenance Pharmacotherapy

On the basis of earlier studies (Imlah et al. 1965; Kay et al. 1970; Seager and Bird 1962) and clinical experience, traditional practice has suggested that maintenance pharmacotherapy should vary with the patient's clinical diagnosis. For example, patients with major depressive disorder generally receive maintenance therapy with antidepressant agents, patients with bipolar disorder receive a mood-stabilizing medication, and patients with schizophrenia receive antipsychotic medications (Braga et al. 2019; Chanpattana et al. 1999b; Sackeim 1994). Patients with a mood disorder may also receive an antipsychotic medication, if indicated on the basis of their clinical symptoms. Typically, medication dosages are maintained at the clinically effective dose range for acute treatment, with adjustment up or down depending on response (American Psychiatric Association 2002, 2010, 2021). Other factors that will determine choice of maintenance pharmacotherapy include the patient's history of response to treatment and consideration of adverse effects.

The optimal approach to maintenance pharmacotherapy after a course of ECT continues to undergo active study. However, evidence suggests that a combination of an antidepressant and lithium reduces the risk of relapse for patients with major depressive disorder (Atiku et al. 2015; Brus et al. 2019; Kellner et al. 2006, 2016b, 2016a; Sackeim 1994; Sackeim et al. 2001a; Tew et al. 2007). In addition, when clinically feasible, practitioners should consider a class of pharmacological agents to which the patient's symptoms did not manifest resistance during treatment of the acute episode.

23.3. Maintenance ECT

Although maintenance therapy with psychotropic medications is the prevailing practice following an acute course of ECT, high relapse rates (Aronson et al. 1987; Kellner et al. 2006; Sackeim et al. 1990, 1993, 2001a; Spiker et al. 1985; Stoudemire et al. 1994; Tew et al. 2007) have often led practitioners to recommend maintenance ECT (Decina et al. 1987; Jaffe et al. 1990b; Kramer 1987; McCall et al. 1992), especially in patients whose symptoms have not responded to medication during the index episode (Flint and Rifat 1998; Meyers 1992; Sackeim et al. 1990; Shapira et al. 1995). Practice guidelines describe maintenance ECT as a viable option for long-term management of patients with major depression, bipolar disorder, and schizophrenia (American Psychiatric Association 2002, 2010, 2021). Thus, facilities should offer maintenance ECT as a treatment choice.

Maintenance ECT was first mentioned in the 1940s (Geoghegan and Stevenson 1949; Kalinowsky 1943; Kerman 1945; Moore 1943), and the first comprehensive description of the practice was published by Wolff in 1957. Early literature on maintenance ECT consists primarily of retrospective series in patients with major depression (Beale et al. 1996; Clarke et al. 1989; Decina et al. 1987; Dubin et al. 1992; Ezion et al. 1990; Grunhaus et al. 1990; Kramer 1990, 1999; Lôo et al. 1990; Matzen et al. 1988; Petrides et al. 1994; Puri et al. 1992; Schwarz et al. 1995; Thienhaus et al. 1990; Thornton et al. 1990; Vanelle et al. 1994), mania (Abrams 1990; Godemann and Hellweg 1997; Husain et al. 1993; Jaffe et al. 1991; Kellner et al. 1990; Vanelle et al. 1994), schizophrenia (Braga et al. 2019; Chanpattana 1998; Chanpattana et al. 1999b; Höflich et al. 1995; Lohr et al. 1994; Sajatovic and Meltzer 1993; Uçok and Uçok 1996), and Parkinson's disease (Aarsland et al. 1997; Friedman and Gordon 1992; Höflich et al. 1995; Jeanneau 1993; Wengel et al. 1998; Zervas and Fink 1991). Review articles have also tended to report good results among patients receiving maintenance ECT treatment (Abrams 2002; Escande et al. 1992; Jarvis et al. 1992; Monroe 1991; Rabheru and Persad 1997; Sackeim 1994; Stephens et al. 1993), and there are suggestions that this approach may be cost-effective (Bonds et al. 1998; Schwarz et al. 1995; Steffens et al. 1995; Vanelle et al. 1994).

Some studies have included comparison groups not receiving maintenance ECT or have compared use of mental health resources before and after implementation of maintenance ECT. One large controlled study of maintenance treatment involved 201 patients with major depressive disorder who were randomly assigned to receive maintenance ECT or combination pharmacotherapy with lithium carbonate plus nortriptyline hydrochloride following a successful course of ECT (Kellner et al. 2006). Both strategies were successful in sustaining remission in 46% of patients (Kellner et al. 2006). In the Prolonging Remission in Depressed Elderly (PRIDE) study, all patients received pharmacotherapy with a combination of lithium and venlafaxine, and a portion of the sample was randomly assigned to receive four maintenance ECT treatments at approximately 1-week intervals plus additional ECT for emerging symptoms (Kellner et al. 2016b, 2016a). The latter group had better outcomes, with fewer relapses (13% vs. 20%) and lower depression ratings during the entire 6-month study period (Kellner et al. 2016a). A small randomized controlled trial in geriatric patients with psychotic depression also suggested that maintenance therapy with a combination of antidepressant and ECT may delay relapse more effectively than use of pharmacotherapy alone (Navarro et al. 2008).

The specific frequency and timing of treatments has been the subject of considerable discussion (Abrams 2002; Atashnama et al. 2020; Bailine et al. 2019; Fink et al. 1996; Gill and Kellner 2019; Kramer 1987; Longcope and Fink 1990; Monroe 1991; Petrides 1998; Petrides et al. 1994; Rabheru and Persad 1997; Sackeim 1994; Scott et al. 1991), but studies have not yet compared the efficacy of specific regimens. In practice, the intensity of the maintenance ECT regimen will depend on the patient's likelihood of early relapse. Typically, however, treatments are started on a weekly basis, with the interval between treatments gradually extended to a month, depending on the clinical response. A schedule of 10 ECT sessions in a 6-month period was successful in sustaining remission in 46% of patients (Kellner et al. 2006). Attempts to improve outcomes by individualizing the timing of ECT sessions have been described (Odeberg et al. 2008). The possibility that a more intensive and individualized schedule of maintenance ECT could be even more effective in sustaining remission was proposed (Kellner and Lisanby 2008; Lisanby et al. 2008) and then validated (Kellner et al. 2016b, 2016a) in the PRIDE study.

Before embarking on maintenance treatment with ECT, individuals should meet the following criteria: 1) response to acute course of ECT; 2) either a patient preference for maintenance ECT or resistance or intolerance to pharmacotherapy alone; and 3) an ability and willingness of the patient (or surrogate consenter) to receive maintenance ECT, provide informed consent, and adhere to the overall treatment plan, including any necessary behavioral and dietary restrictions. Because maintenance ECT is typically administered to patients who are in clinical remission and because relatively long intertreatment intervals are used, it is most often given on an outpatient basis. Thus, the requirements for receiving outpatient treatment should also be fulfilled (see Chapter 8).

In individuals who are to receive maintenance ECT, informed consent should be obtained initially and renewed on the basis of the number of treatments or a specified duration of time as dictated by local or state requirements (see Chapter 10). The risks and benefits of maintenance ECT should be discussed with the patient (or surrogate consenter) at regular intervals as an integral part of their care plan. If the total duration of ECT (i.e., acute ECT course plus maintenance ECT) is more than 3 months, a rationale should be provided to the consenter and documented in the medical record. The overall clinical treatment plan should also be updated at least every 6 months and include an assessment of whether maintenance ECT continues to be indicated. Coordination of the treatment plan should also occur between the ECT treatment team and the mental health team that provides ongoing care to the patient (if different from the ECT treatment team).

Before each maintenance ECT treatment, the ECT psychiatrist should 1) assess the patient's clinical status and current medications, 2) determine whether the treatment is indicated, 3) verify the presence of a consent for treatment, and 4) decide the timing of the next treatment. To provide an ongoing assessment of risk factors, an interval medical history focusing on specific organ systems at risk with ECT and a focused physical examination with vital signs should be done before each treatment, with further assessment as clinically indicated. Particular attention should be paid to recent falls or head trauma, cardiorespiratory or neurological symptoms, medication changes, and emergency visits or hospitalizations. Typically, this brief evaluation is accomplished by the ECT psychiatrist and the anesthesia provider on the day of the treatment. In patients receiving maintenance ECT, the frequency of routine repeated anesthesia preoperative evaluations and laboratory testing varies with clinical need as well as local and national guidelines. To detect evidence of relapse or recurrence, it is useful to obtain outcome measures on a regular basis, such as ratings of clinical global impression and disorder-specific symptoms (see Chapter

17). Although cognitive effects appear to be less severe with maintenance ECT than with more frequent treatments administered during an acute ECT course (Barnes et al. 1997; Ezion et al. 1990; Grunhaus et al. 1990; Lisanby et al. 2022; Smith et al. 2010; Thienhaus et al. 1990; Thornton et al. 1990; Yoldi-Negrete et al. 2022), brief objective and subjective assessment of cognitive function should be conducted at regular intervals, with more formal testing (e.g., simple bedside assessment of memory function) when clinically indicated (see Chapter 20).

At present, no applicable data indicate how long maintenance therapy should be sustained after acute ECT. Assuming that the treatment is well tolerated, a prolonged period of maintenance therapy may be prudent because many patients referred for ECT have severe illness and frequent recurrences. The duration of maintenance ECT and the precise timing of treatment tapering should be determined on the basis of risk-benefit considerations, taking into account factors such as prior responses to treatment tapering, prior episodes of illness (including their number, frequency, and severity), prior response to other maintenance treatments, benefits and tolerability of maintenance ECT, family history, patient preference, and the ability of the patient to adhere to the treatment plan (including treatment accessibility, patient reliability, cognitive functioning, and support of significant others). Abrupt discontinuation of maintenance treatment should be avoided because of the potential risk of triggering a recurrence (Braithwaite et al. 2022; Ghaziuddin et al. 2021; Lambrichts et al. 2021; Methfessel et al. 2021; Van de Velde et al. 2021).

23.4. Maintenance Treatment With Other Somatic Therapies

Evidence for the effectiveness of maintenance transcranial magnetic stimulation (TMS) after a successful course of ECT is limited. In one case series, six depressed patients remained without relapse for 6 months (Cristancho et al. 2013). A retrospective review showed that TMS treatment outcomes were not related to prior ECT response (Yuan et al. 2020). Other data on the efficacy of TMS as a maintenance treatment (i.e., after initial TMS treatment) are limited and equivocal (Benadhira et al. 2017; d'Andrea et al. 2023; Matsuda et al. 2023; Pridmore and May 2018; Pridmore et al. 2018; Sargent and Allen 2023; Wang et al. 2017; Wilson et al. 2022). There has been a suggestion that ketamine infusions may be used for maintenance therapy after a successful course of ECT; however, the one randomized trial that aimed to study this approach was unable to obtain a sufficient number of subjects, and of the subjects who did participate, none completed the 4-week post-ECT trial of ketamine or midazolam (Finnegan et al. 2019). Evidence for maintenance ketamine therapy after initial ketamine treatment has been limited because samples have been small, with short durations of follow-up (Barenboim and Lafer 2018; Phillips et al. 2019; Vande Voort et al. 2016).

23.5. Maintenance Psychotherapy

For many patients, individual, group, or family psychotherapy after ECT may be useful in helping to resolve residual symptoms, prevent relapse, facilitate better ways to cope with stressors, assist the patient in reorganizing their social and vocational activities, and encourage a return to normal life. Patients with major depressive disorder may benefit from the combination of maintenance psychotherapy and ECT, as shown by data for cognitive-behavioral therapy, supportive psychotherapy, and group psychotherapy (Brakemeier et al. 2014; McClintock et al. 2011a; Rogan and Wilkinson 2023; Wilkinson et al. 2017).

Recommendations

23.1. General Considerations

1. Maintenance therapy, typically consisting of psychotropic medication and/or maintenance ECT, is indicated for all patients because of a high rate of relapse in its absence.
2. Maintenance therapy should begin immediately on completion of the acute ECT course.
3. Unless limited by adverse effects, maintenance therapy should be provided for a minimum of 6 months and could be extended for longer periods on the basis of individual history and disease characteristics.

23.2. Maintenance Pharmacotherapy

1. The choice of psychotropic medication should be determined by the patient's psychiatric diagnosis, history of treatment response, and consideration of adverse effects.

2. When clinically feasible, practitioners should consider a class of pharmacological agents to which the patient's symptoms did not manifest resistance during treatment of the acute episode.
3. In patients treated with ECT for major depressive episodes, evidence suggests that combination pharmacotherapy with an antidepressant and lithium is more effective than either modality alone.

23.3. Maintenance ECT

1. Maintenance ECT should be available in programs administering ECT.
2. Maintenance ECT is most often given on an outpatient basis, but the choice of treatment setting will depend on the patient's level of psychiatric and medical risk and their ability to adhere to the requirements of treatment on an outpatient basis.
3. Maintenance ECT may be combined with pharmacotherapy.
4. Patients referred for maintenance ECT should meet the following criteria:
   a. A history of response to an acute course of ECT
   b. Either a patient preference for maintenance ECT or resistance to or intolerance of pharmacotherapy alone
   c. An ability and willingness of the patient (or surrogate consenter) to provide informed consent to receive maintenance ECT
   d. Ability (with the assistance of others) to adhere to the overall treatment plan, including any necessary behavioral restrictions
5. Maintenance ECT treatments should be administered at the minimum frequency compatible with sustained remission and should be adjusted as necessary, with timing of treatments individualized for each patient, considering both beneficial and adverse effects.
6. Consent for ECT should be obtained at least every 6 months.
7. If the total duration of ECT (i.e., acute ECT course plus maintenance ECT) is more than 3 months, a rationale should be provided to the consenter and documented in the medical record.
8. The consent should be reviewed with the patient at regular intervals, and the risks and benefits of maintenance ECT should be discussed with the patient as an integral part of their care plan.
9. The overall clinical treatment plan should be updated at least every 6 months and should include an assessment of whether maintenance ECT continues to be indicated.

10. Coordination of the treatment plan should also occur between the ECT treatment team and the mental health team that provides ongoing care to the patient (if different from the ECT treatment team).

11. Before each maintenance ECT treatment, the ECT psychiatrist and the mental health team caring for the patient (if different from the ECT psychiatrist) should

    a. Assess the patient's current medications and clinical status, with particular attention paid to a focused physical examination with vital signs, recent medication changes, falls or head trauma, cardiorespiratory or neurological symptoms, and emergency visits or hospitalizations
    b. Determine whether the treatment is indicated
    c. Verify the presence of a consent for treatment
    d. Decide the timing of the next treatment

12. Other suggested evaluations during the maintenance ECT course include

    a. Clinical outcome measures such as ratings of clinical global impression and disorder-specific symptoms, which should be obtained at regular intervals to detect relapse or recurrence
    b. Brief objective and subjective assessment of cognitive function conducted at regular intervals, with more formal testing (e.g., simple bedside assessment of memory function) when clinically indicated
    c. Anesthesiology preoperative evaluation and laboratory testing when clinically indicated or required by local or national guidelines

13. The duration of maintenance ECT and the precise timing of treatment tapering should be determined on the basis of risk-benefit considerations, taking into account factors such as prior responses to treatment tapering, prior episodes of illness (including their number, frequency, and severity), prior response to other maintenance treatments, benefits and tolerability of maintenance ECT, family history, patient preference, and the ability of the patient to adhere to the treatment plan (including treatment accessibility, patient reliability, cognitive functioning, and support of significant others).

14. Abrupt discontinuation of maintenance treatment should be avoided because of the potential risk of triggering a recurrence.

23.4. Maintenance Treatment With Other Somatic Therapies

Maintenance treatment with TMS and with ketamine have been suggested as options following treatment with ECT, but evidence is currently minimal.

23.5. Maintenance Psychotherapy

After an acute ECT course, individual, group, or family psychotherapy can be a useful component of maintenance treatment for many patients.

CHAPTER 24

New and Emerging Neuromodulation Techniques

24.1. Overview

Electroconvulsive therapy (ECT) was the first intervention to achieve regular clinical use in psychiatry in the 1930s before the development of modern psychiatric medications in the late 1950s. Research on ECT has focused on approaches to maintaining the efficacy of ECT in psychiatric disorders while minimizing potential ECT side effects, particularly cognitive side effects. In this chapter, we review the increasing number of neuromodulation techniques that could potentially have antidepressant efficacy comparable to that of ECT while minimizing side effects, including device-based approaches that do not involve inducing seizures. Familiarity with the present research on the indications, contraindications, risks, and benefits associated with these treatment approaches provides additional options for patients with treatment-resistant depression (TRD) and new insights into the neuroanatomical basis of TRD.

24.2. Devices Cleared by the FDA for Treatment-Resistant Depression

At the time of this writing, devices that are cleared by the U.S. Food and Drug Administration (FDA) for clinical use in TRD include transcranial magnetic stimulation (TMS) and vagus nerve stimulation (VNS) (Table 24–1). Both TMS and VNS are approved by the FDA as safe and effective for the treatment of depression that has not responded to prior treatment. As discussed in this chapter, TMS and VNS differ in their mechanisms of action, speed of response, overall response rates, and side effect profiles.

Table 24–1. *FDA-cleared and emerging neuromodulation approaches*

Technology	FDA-cleared indications	Mode of delivery	Form of energy	Seizure induced	Anesthesia required
Deep brain stimulation (DBS)	OCD, movement disorders	Surgical implant	Electrical	No	Yes[a]
External trigeminal nerve stimulation (eTNS)	ADHD	Transcutaneous	Electrical	No	No
Focal electrically administered seizure therapy (FEAST)		Transcranial	Electrical	Yes	Yes
Individualized low-amplitude seizure therapy (iLAST)		Transcranial	Electrical	Yes	Yes
Low-amplitude ECT		Transcranial	Electrical	Yes	Yes
Low-field magnetic stimulation (LFMS)		Transcranial	Magnetic	No	No
Low-intensity focused ultrasound (LIFU)		Transcranial	Ultrasound	No	No
Magnetic seizure therapy (MST)		Transcranial	Magnetic	Yes	Yes
Synchronized transcranial magnetic stimulation (sTMS)		Transcranial	Magnetic	No	No
Temporal interference (TI)		Transcranial	Electrical	No	No
Transcranial alternating current stimulation (tACS)	Class II when used to treat insomnia or anxiety; Class I when used to treat MDD	Transcranial	Electrical	No	No
Transcranial direct current stimulation (tDCS)		Transcranial	Electrical	No	No

Table 24–1. FDA-cleared and emerging neuromodulation approaches *(continued)*

Technology	FDA-cleared indications	Mode of delivery	Form of energy	Seizure induced	Anesthesia required
Transcranial electric stimulation therapy (TEST)		Transcranial	Electrical	No	Yes
Transcranial magnetic stimulation (TMS)	MDD, OCD, smoking cessation	Transcranial	Magnetic	No	No
Transcranial photobiomodulation (t-PBM)		Transcranial	Light	No	No
Transcutaneous auricular vagus nerve stimulation (taVNS)	Opioid withdrawal symptoms	Transcutaneous	Electrical	No	No
Transcutaneous cervical VNS (tcVNS)	Cluster and migraine headache	Transcutaneous	Electrical	No	No
Vagus nerve stimulation (VNS)	MDD, epilepsy	Surgical implant	Electrical	No	Yes[a]

Note. ADHD=attention-deficit/hyperactivity disorder; MDD=major depressive disorder; OCD=obsessive-compulsive disorder.
[a]For surgical implantation only.

24.2.1. Transcranial Magnetic Stimulation

TMS devices apply rapidly alternating magnetic fields to the head using an electromagnetic coil placed on the scalp (Fitzgerald and Daskalakis 2023; Higgins and George 2019; Rossi et al. 2021). The applied magnetic fields induce weak electrical currents in the brain underneath the coil. Those weak electrical currents stimulate neurons and, when applied repeatedly over the course of weeks, can change the functioning of brain circuits in a lasting fashion. Two basic coil shapes are in clinical use today: the figure 8 coil and the deep TMS coil (also referred to as dTMS or H-coil). The H-coil has different variations targeting different brain regions, and these variations are designed for specific indications. TMS is an outpatient procedure and is often given in a clinic setting, either in a medical facility or in the community. A series of treatment sessions is administered, typically 5 days per week over 4–6 weeks.

TMS is FDA cleared in adults for the treatment of major depressive disorder using the figure 8 coil (O'Reardon et al. 2007) or the H-1 dTMS coil (Levkovitz et al. 2015) targeting the prefrontal cortex. The H-7 dTMS coil is FDA cleared for the treatment of adults with obsessive-compulsive disorder (Carmi et al. 2019). The H-ADD coil is FDA cleared for smoking cessation in adults (Dinur-Klein et al. 2014).

TMS has a relatively benign side effect profile in comparison with ECT (Fitzgerald and Daskalakis 2023; Higgins and George 2019; Rossi et al. 2021; Wang et al. 2022). TMS does not require sedation, and thus it lacks the risks associated with anesthesia. Unlike ECT, TMS does not have a reported risk of memory loss. TMS is not known to affect driving, so there are no driving restrictions during the treatment course. Common side effects of TMS include headache and scalp pain. These are typically mild to moderate and usually can be managed effectively with over-the-counter analgesics. There is a risk of hearing loss due to the loud clicking noise the coil generates, but this is effectively prevented by properly inserted earplugs for both the patient and the coil operator. In rare circumstances, hearing loss may be associated with tinnitus, which can be severe. Induction of a seizure during a TMS session is a more serious but rare side effect. Following established safety guidelines for the use of TMS reduces, but does not eliminate, the risk of a TMS-associated seizure (McClintock et al. 2018; Rossi et al. 2021).

Although ECT has a greater efficacy rate than TMS does, using currently approved dosing parameters (Chen et al. 2017), the favorable safety profile of TMS often leads to it being considered prior to referring a patient for ECT. Recent work has demonstrated that image-guided and accelerated protocols can significantly speed response to TMS (Cole et al. 2020, 2022; U.S. Food and Drug Administration 2023). Some studies also have suggested that suicidal ideation can be reduced with TMS (Cui et al. 2022; Mehta et al. 2022; Wilkening et al. 2022). Nevertheless, prompt referral for ECT is typically indicated in patients with a high degree of clinical severity, especially those with catatonia, the psychotic subtype of major depression, or acute suicide risk or those otherwise in need of a rapid treatment response. Investigational work is underway to optimize dosing to accelerate response and enhance the effectiveness of TMS (Cole et al. 2020), but these approaches to dosing were not FDA cleared at the time of this writing.

TMS can also be considered in the context of persisting depressive symptoms following an acute course of ECT (Cristancho et al. 2013), and a retrospective review demonstrated that ECT responsivity was not related to subsequent TMS treatment outcomes (Yuan et al. 2020). Some preliminary studies suggested that dTMS and accelerated theta burst protocols for TMS may be particularly useful following nonresponse to ECT; however, these were open-label studies with small sample sizes (Rosenberg et al. 2010; Smesny et al. 2001; Williams et al. 2018), and additional research is needed.

24.2.2. Vagus Nerve Stimulation

With VNS, electrode leads are surgically implanted and attached to ascending afferents in the cervical region of the vagus nerve in the neck. The electrode leads are connected to a stimulator unit, resembling a pacemaker, which delivers a weak electrical current and is implanted in the superficial tissues of the chest. The device is programmed using a wand held on the chest over the stimulator device. This wand can be used to turn the device on and off, as well as to adjust the parameters of stimulation. As a surgical implant, VNS carries risks not seen with ECT, including the risk of bleeding and infection, although these risks are relatively low. VNS does not carry the risk of cognitive side effects seen with ECT (Sackeim et al. 2001b). VNS also differs from ECT in the time needed for therapeutic response, which can be months or longer with VNS (Rush et al. 2000; Rush et al. 2005b; Sackeim et al. 2001c).

VNS was initially approved for the treatment of medication-refractory epilepsy and later gained FDA clearance in 2005 for the adjunctive treatment of chronic or recurrent treatment-resistant nonpsychotic depression in adults that has not responded to at least four antidepressant treatments of adequate dosage and duration (Austelle et al. 2022). Although the acute phase randomized controlled trial (RCT) did not find definitive evidence of efficacy in TRD (Rush et al. 2005a), a nonrandomized comparison of active VNS compared with treatment as usual found significant benefit of adjunctive VNS therapy over 1 year (George et al. 2005). Persistent benefits of VNS have also been observed at longer follow-up intervals (Aaronson et al. 2013; Kumar et al. 2019; Marangell et al. 2002; Nahas et al. 2005). A large double-blind randomized placebo-controlled trial sponsored by the Centers for Medicare and Medicaid Services is currently underway to provide additional evidence regarding the safety and efficacy of VNS in TRD (U.S. Centers for Medicare and Medicaid Services 2022).

VNS may be considered as an option following nonresponse to ECT, on the basis of the evidence for long-term benefit in a sample of patients with highly treatment resistant depression, many of whom had not responded to ECT (Rush et al. 2000, 2005b; Sackeim et al. 2001c). Use of VNS could also be considered prior to ECT in patients whose depression has not responded to at least four antidepressant treatments but who have contraindications to ECT or do not require a rapid treatment response. With the different response trajectories for ECT and VNS, some patients with TRD may benefit from ECT during the acute phase of the episode, with use of VNS for maintenance treatment (O'Reardon et al. 2006). However, the evidence for this approach is limited and comes from small case series and open-label reports (Aaronson et al. 2021; Burke and Husain 2006; Warnell and Elahi 2007).

In situations where ECT is given following VNS implantation, the manufacturer recommends turning off the VNS pulse generator prior to ECT (Burke and Husain 2006). This is also wise given the anticonvulsant properties of VNS that may interfere with seizure induction with ECT. After ECT, the VNS pulse generator should be interrogated, and stimulation parameters should be reset to their pre-ECT values.

24.3. Emerging Nonconvulsive Neuromodulation Devices

A growing number of devices are under investigation for TRD or are cleared for other indications (see Table 24–1). Additional RCT evidence and evaluation of safety and efficacy by regulatory bodies will be needed before these experimental approaches can be recommended for routine clinical use in patients, including patients referred for ECT because of TRD. Access to these interventions may be available through approved research studies (see https://clinicaltrials.gov). This is a rapidly changing field, so it is useful to check the latest literature and updates on FDA approval status.

24.3.1. Deep Brain Stimulation

Patients receiving deep brain stimulation (DBS) undergo the surgical implantation of electrodes in the brain, attached to a pulse generator implanted in the chest. Unlike ECT, DBS carries the risks of intracerebral hemorrhage and infection. DBS received humanitarian use exemption from the FDA for the treatment of refractory obsessive-compulsive disorder on the basis of evidence from clinical trials supporting its efficacy (Vicheva et al. 2020). DBS remains experimental in the treatment of depression (Coffey and Caroff 2022). A number of studies showed promising response and remission rates at long-term open-label follow-up in patients with highly treatment resistant symptoms (Aibar-Durán et al. 2022; Alemany et al. 2023; Bergfeld et al. 2022; Crowell et al. 2019; Fenoy et al. 2022; Hitti et al. 2021). However, two randomized sham-controlled trials failed to find efficacy of DBS targeting the subcallosal cingulate (Holtzheimer et al. 2017) or the ventral capsule/ventral striatum (Dougherty et al. 2015). Other DBS targets, including the median forebrain bundle (Coenen et al. 2019) and the lateral habenula (Wang et al. 2021), are also under investigation.

Novel approaches that are showing promise, but remain at a very preliminary stage, have targeted the patient's personalized distributed networks related to depression rather than focusing on specific neuroanatomic sites such as the anterior cingulate (Sullivan et al. 2021). Other studies have used brain-machine interfaces to decode and modulate mood states from intracerebral recordings in real time (Rao et al. 2018; Scangos et al. 2021; Shanechi 2019).

24.3.2. Low-Intensity Transcranial Electrical Stimulation

A variety of transcranial electrical stimulation devices, including transcranial direct current stimulation (tDCS) and transcranial alternating current stimulation (tACS), administer weak electrical currents to the scalp in an attempt to modulate brain function. These devices are battery-operated, portable, and inexpensive, and they carry minimal side effects when administered within established safety guidelines (Antal et al. 2017). Some versions are adapted for at-home use. Variations of these devices are available over the counter as lifestyle products without claims of health benefits and without proven efficacy in treating serious mental disorders.

For tDCS, a weak constant current is applied to the scalp, in contrast to tACS, which uses alternating currents; tDCS alters neuronal excitability by redistributing the neuronal membrane potential. Although tDCS has an excellent safety profile, RCT evidence has been mixed regarding its efficacy in the treatment of depression. A recent meta-analysis described tDCS as effective for the treatment of major depressive disorder when applied with the anode on the left dorsolateral prefrontal cortex (Fregni et al. 2021). Among the largest of the RCTs of tDCS in depression, the Electrical Current Therapy for Treating Depression Clinical Study (ELECT-TDCS) trial could not confirm that tDCS was noninferior to escitalopram (Brunoni et al. 2017), although it was superior to placebo. A second multicenter RCT found that active tDCS was not more effective than placebo (Loo et al. 2018). These results suggest that tDCS, at least as currently administered, has not shown superior efficacy when compared with antidepressant medication. In addition, when given as an augmentation therapy, the combination of tDCS plus cognitive-behavioral therapy (CBT) was no better than CBT alone or CBT plus sham tDCS (Aust et al. 2022). However, in an individual participant data meta-analysis, better response was associated with longer treatment duration, lower depression severity, and less treatment resistance (Nikolin et al. 2023). These findings suggest that more research is needed to establish the most effective dosing strategy, treatment duration, and characteristics of patients who may benefit from tDCS.

Cranial electrotherapy stimulators (CESs) are defined by the FDA as a prescription device that applies electrical currents to the head to treat psychiatric conditions without inducing a seizure (Code of Federal Regulations 2022). These devices are considered Class II (special controls) when used to treat insomnia and/or anxiety and Class III (premarket approval) when intended to treat depression. The CES devices that are currently on the market deliver a form of tACS, which is thought to alter neural oscillations. The literature on the therapeutic efficacy of tACS for depression is largely anecdotal, and evidence from sham-controlled RCTs is limited at present (Alexander et al. 2019).

24.3.3. High-Intensity Transcranial Electric Stimulation

Although elicitation of a seizure has been thought to be essential to the antidepressant action of ECT, the antidepressant action of nonconvulsive interventions such as TMS has prompted a reexamination of whether high-intensity electrical stimulation might have antidepressant effects in the absence of a seizure. In an open-label study of 11 patients, antidepressant effects were seen when an electrical current was delivered under anesthesia with a bifrontal electrode placement and the same pulse amplitude as ECT but at a frequency and duration below the seizure threshold (Regenold et al. 2015). Previously called *nonconvulsive electrotherapy* and now referred to as *transcranial electric stimulation therapy* (TEST), this nonconvulsive approach seeks to retain the antidepressant efficacy of ECT but without the side effects associated with seizure induction. RCT evidence will be needed to evaluate this approach further and to shed light on the relative contributions of the electrical stimulation and the seizure in driving the antidepressant effects of ECT.

24.3.4. Transcutaneous Electrical Stimulation

Transcutaneous electrical stimulators use weak electrical currents to target cranial nerves in the subcutaneous tissues rather than targeting the brain directly as done with transcranial approaches. With transcutaneous cervical VNS (tcVNS), the cervical branch of the vagus nerve is accessed by placing electrodes on the neck. The FDA has cleared tcVNS for adjunctive use in the preventive treatment of cluster headaches and the acute treatment of pain associated with episodic cluster headache as well as migraine headache in adults (Silberstein et al. 2016; U.S. Food and Drug Administration 2022). In a similar fashion, with transcutaneous auricular vagus nerve stimulation (taVNS), the auricular branch of the vagus nerve is accessed by placing electrodes on the concha of the ear. Use of taVNS is being studied for a range of conditions, including depression and posttraumatic stress disorder. Auricular neural stimulation is also thought to engage several other cranial nerves, in addition to the vagus nerve, and has been FDA cleared to aid in the reduction of symptoms associated with opioid withdrawal. The trigeminal nerve can be stimulated by placing electrodes on the forehead. A device to deliver external trigeminal nerve stimulation (eTNS) at home during sleep was granted de novo classification by the FDA for the treatment of attention-deficit/hyperactivity disorder in children (U.S. Food and Drug Administration 2018a).

24.3.5. Low-Intensity Transcranial Magnetic Stimulation

A number of approaches to deliver TMS with intensities lower than those of conventional TMS are currently in various stages of development. Low-field magnetic stimulation (LFMS) is based on the finding that some patients reported rapid mood elevation after a brain magnetic resonance imaging scan using specific time-varying gradient magnetic fields that induce electrical currents in broad regions of the brain. A double-blind proof-of-concept trial in 84 patients with TRD failed to replicate the rapid antidepressant response reported in earlier smaller studies (Fava et al. 2018).

Similar to tACS, synchronized transcranial magnetic stimulation (sTMS) was developed in an attempt to entrain neural oscillations. It uses LFMS generated by static electromagnets placed on the head that spin at a frequency matching the individual's endogenous alpha frequency. A double-blind sham-controlled trial of sTMS did not find significant benefit in the intent to treat sample of 202 patients with depression, although the per protocol sample of 120 patients showed greater reduction in depression scores in the active group compared with the sham group (Leuchter et al. 2015).

24.3.6. Focusing Transcranial Stimulation at Depth

The electrical fields generated in the brain by tDCS and tACS can be made more focal through the use of multielectrode arrays, but they cannot be focused at depth (i.e., inducing currents in deep brain structures without stimulating the overlying cortex). Temporal interference is a potential technology that attempts to circumvent this limitation (Esmaeilpour et al. 2021; Grossman et al. 2017). It uses a multielectrode array that delivers electrical currents with small differences in frequency (e.g., 2 and 2.05 kHz). The high frequency currents act as carrier waves, which generate a lower frequency current (in this case, 50 Hz) in deeper brain structures. The kHz frequencies are theorized to be biologically inactive, allowing a virtual focusing in deeper brain structures with the lower frequency. Optimizing dosing and procedures for applying temporal interference in humans are active areas of research.

Low-intensity focused ultrasound (LIFU), also known as transcranial focused ultrasound, is another approach to stimulation of deeper brain structures. At high intensities, focused ultrasound is a noninvasive way of targeting specific brain structures for therapeutic purposes, either by inducing focal lesions or by opening the blood-brain barrier to allow drug delivery to specific brain regions. At low intensities, focused ultrasound has been reported to modulate neuronal activity (Legon et al. 2014). Recent evidence suggests that targeting deep structures with LIFU in humans is possible and, with further development, may hold therapeutic potential for a variety of conditions (Badran et al. 2020; Fomenko et al. 2018).

24.3.7. Transcranial Photobiomodulation

Transcranial photobiomodulation (t-PBM) refers to the use of various forms of light to affect brain activity. These devices use lasers applied through the scalp to deliver wavelengths of light that are absorbed by cytochrome c oxidase, an enzyme involved in mitochondrial function. Saucedo et al. (2021) reported that t-PBM influences cerebrovascular function and may exert neurocognitive effects. Some studies suggest that t-PBM may have antidepressant effects, but results from one RCT (Iosifescu et al. 2022) showed no difference between t-PBM and sham treatment. Thus, findings on use of this experimental technique in treating severe psychiatric disorders remain preliminary (Cassano et al. 2018; Zaizar et al. 2023).

24.4. Emerging Convulsive Neuromodulation Devices

A variety of approaches are under investigation to reduce the side effects of ECT yet preserve therapeutic benefits by inducing seizures with more focused stimulation (Figure 24–1). The premise is that seizures could be induced in brain regions that are responsible for ECT's antidepressant efficacy, but stimulation of regions linked to side effects would be minimal, yielding an improved safety profile. These techniques fall into three general categories: 1) inducing weaker and more focused electrical fields in the brain using electromagnetic induction (as in the case of magnetic seizure therapy [MST]), 2) applying lower-amplitude electrical pulses with conventional ECT electrode placements, and 3) combining individualized amplitudes with modified electrode configurations in an attempt to better focus the electrical field, as with focal electrically administered seizure therapy (FEAST) and individualized low-amplitude seizure therapy (iLAST).

24.4.1. Magnetic Seizure Therapy

MST uses high-intensity TMS, applied under anesthesia, to induce therapeutic seizures for the treatment of depression (Lisanby et al. 2001b). MST takes advantage of the ability of high-dose TMS to induce seizures, coupled with the relative focality of TMS-induced electrical currents in the brain as compared with direct electrical stimulation of the scalp

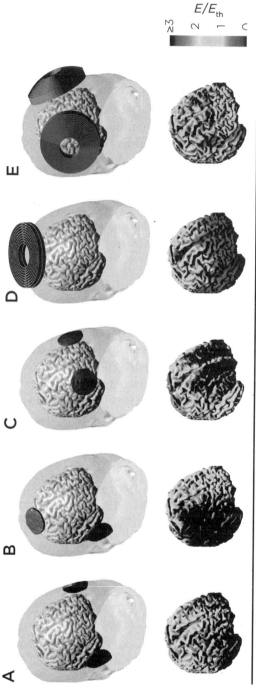

Figure 24–1. Simulation models of (A) bitemporal ECT, (B) right unilateral ECT, (C) bifrontal ECT, (D) MST with circular coil placed over vertex, and (E) MST with twin coil placed over midline prefrontal cortex. Stimulation strength (E-field magnitude relative to neural activation threshold, E/E_{th}; see Deng et al. 2011) on the cortical surface at current of 800 mA for ECT and 100% of maximum stimulator output for MST. See Plate 2 to view this figure in color.

ECT=electroconvulsive therapy; MST=magnetic seizure therapy.
Source. Zhi-De Deng. Used with permission.

(Figures 24–1D and 24–1E). In contrast to ECT, MST induces weak and superficial electrical currents in the brain (Lee et al. 2017). MST induces less cognitive impairment than ECT while preserving its antidepressant effects (Daskalakis et al. 2020; McClintock et al. 2011d). A randomized double-blind confirmatory efficacy study is currently underway to evaluate whether the antidepressant efficacy of MST is noninferior to ECT (National Institutes of Health 2022a).

24.4.2. Lower-Amplitude ECT

The observation that MST can induce therapeutic seizures with low-current amplitudes challenged the dogma that the pulse amplitude on ECT devices needs to be kept at the maximum of 0.8–0.9 A. Although a pilot study showed that right unilateral (RUL) ECT could induce seizures with a current amplitude of 0.5 A (Rosa et al. 2011), it is not clear that adopting this strategy with conventional ECT electrode placements will retain the therapeutic efficacy of ECT. For example, a double-blind RCT that used RUL ECT and 0.3 ms pulse width stimuli found that lower pulse amplitudes may reduce some cognitive side effects, but they were also associated with less antidepressant efficacy (Abbott et al. 2021) (see Chapter 14).

24.4.3. Individualized Amplitude Coupled With Novel Electrode Configurations

FEAST couples individualized pulse amplitude with a novel electrode configuration that seeks to focus electrical current in the prefrontal cortex (see Figure 24–1C) (Spellman et al. 2009). An open-label nonrandomized trial of FEAST found that it had similar efficacy to RUL ECT without a difference in side effects (Sahlem et al. 2020; Youssef et al. 2021b). Frontomedial ECT is an experimental electrode placement that attempts to achieve better focusing of electrical current in the frontal pole and medial prefrontal cortex with less spread to other cortical areas than with FEAST (see Figure 24–1B) (W. H. Lee et al. 2016).

With iLAST, an individualized pulse amplitude is coupled with an array of smaller electrodes to better focus the electrical field and adjust for individual differences in anatomy (Peterchev et al. 2015). The safety and feasibility of this approach is currently under study (National Institutes of Health 2022b).

24.5. Conclusions and Future Directions

An expanding array of new technologies offers potential therapeutic options for patients with TRD who may present for ECT (see Table 24–1). These interventions are at various stages of development. At present, only two of these approaches—TMS and VNS—are FDA cleared for TRD, and each has distinct risks and benefits as reviewed in this chapter. Current literature suggests that ECT is more effective than TMS in patients who need rapid relief, who are psychotic, or who have symptoms of catatonia. ECT also has a larger evidence database for patients with TRD and is more rapidly acting than VNS.

Because of its favorable side effect profile, TMS is often tried before ECT in patients with mild to moderate depression, whereas ECT remains the treatment of choice in patients with severe major depression, especially when there is a need for rapid therapeutic response, as in the case of acute suicide risk, psychosis, and/or catatonia. New developments in TMS dosing hold promise in improving its efficacy and speed of response. As research progresses with these novel tools, the field is learning more about the mechanisms underlying the efficacy and side effects of ECT. This emerging knowledge base may inform the development of more targeted treatments in the future, which can further refine the risk-benefit ratio of ECT.

Appendix

Sample Consent Forms and List of Acronyms and Abbreviations

The consent forms in this appendix are provided as samples. Appropriate modifications should be made to reflect local requirements. In addition, clinicians should be sure that warnings shared by the manufacturer are included in the written consent form and in the discussion of risks and benefits with patients.

Electroconvulsive Therapy (ECT) Consent Form: Acute Treatment Course

Name of Patient: _____

    Dr. _____ has recommended that _____ receive treatment with a series of electroconvulsive therapy (ECT) for treatment of _____. The nature of this treatment has been described to me, as well as why it is being recommended and its potential risks and benefits.

    ECT is most often used to treat severe episodes of depression or catatonia. If ECT is recommended for a condition other than a severe depressive episode or catatonia, or if the patient is younger than 13 years old, a rationale for ECT use has been given based on available evidence.

    Whether ECT or an alternative treatment such as medication; psychotherapy; or some other type of brain stimulation treatment, such as transcranial magnetic stimulation (TMS), is most appropriate at the present time has also been described and depends on prior experience with these treatments; the illness features; and other considerations, including likelihood of improvement and relative risks.

    ECT involves a series of treatments that may be given on an inpatient or outpatient basis. The treatments are administered in a specially equipped area and are usually given in the morning. Because the treatments involve general anesthesia, the patient will have had nothing to eat or drink for at least several hours before each treatment. Additional instructions may also be given based on specific patient needs or circumstances.

    To prepare for the treatment, adhesive electrode pads will be placed on the head and body to record heart wave (electrocardiogram [ECG]) and brain wave (electroencephalogram [EEG]) activity during the treatment, and a sensor will be placed around one of the fingers to record blood oxygen saturation. A blood pressure cuff will be placed on an arm and, usually, on a leg. This monitoring involves no pain or discomfort other than that generally associated with blood pressure monitoring.

    Before the treatment, a small catheter will be placed in a vein so that intravenous medications can be given. As part of the treatment, an anesthetic medication will be administered through the catheter and will quickly produce sleep. Next, another medication is given that will quickly cause muscles to relax. Additional medications may also be given, if needed. Throughout the procedure, the patient is provided pure oxygen to breathe. Because individuals receiving ECT will be asleep after receiving the anesthetic medication, they should not experience pain or discomfort or remember the procedure itself.

The stimulus electrodes that are used for ECT can be placed on the head in several different ways. The most common such approaches are bilateral ECT, in which one stimulus electrode is placed over the left temple area and the other over the right temple area, and unilateral ECT, in which both electrodes are placed on the same side of the head, usually the right side. Right unilateral ECT (electrodes on the right side) is likely to produce less memory difficulty than bilateral ECT. However, for some patients, bilateral ECT may be a more rapid or effective treatment. The choice of stimulus electrode placement has been discussed with me, and _____ electrode placement has been recommended. The possibility of a change in electrode placement has also been discussed with me.

After the individual receiving ECT is asleep and muscular relaxation has taken place, a brief and carefully controlled amount of electricity will be passed between the two stimulus electrodes that have been placed on the head. The electrical current delivered to the stimulus electrodes produces a seizure in the brain. The features of this electrical stimulus will be adjusted to the patient's individual needs. The medication used to provide muscle relaxation will greatly soften the body movements that would ordinarily accompany the seizure, and the body should move very little. The seizure will be monitored by EEG and typically lasts for about 1 minute. The anesthetic medications typically wear off within a few minutes after they are given, and the patient awakens and is moved to a recovery area. Individuals receiving ECT may be temporarily confused and/or agitated on awakening, but these effects usually disappear rapidly. Continuous monitoring and observation is maintained until the treatment team determines that the patient can either return to the inpatient unit or leave for home (if receiving outpatient ECT).

The number of treatments received during an acute series of ECT will depend on a patient's response and cannot be known ahead of time. A typical acute course of ECT involves 6–12 treatments, but some patients may need fewer, and some may require more treatments. Treatments are usually given three times a week, but the frequency may vary depending on individual needs.

Although ECT is being recommended for its benefits as compared with other possible treatments, there is no guarantee of improvement, and recovery may be complete, partial, or not at all. The likelihood and extent of expected improvements with ECT depends on a number of factors, including the disorder being treated, and have been discussed with me. If another mental disorder is present in addition to that for which ECT is being provided, that disorder should not be expected to improve with ECT, and there is a small chance that it might temporarily become worse.

During the weeks and months after an acute ECT course, there is a high risk that symptoms of the disorder being treated will return, although we cannot predict when this might occur. To make the return of symptoms less likely after ECT, treatment with medication, psychotherapy, and/or additional ECT treatments or other types of brain stimulation will be needed. Recommendations for treatment to prevent return of symptoms will be discussed when the acute ECT series is completed or before that time. If intermittent ECT is recommended to prevent return of symptoms, a separate consent form for maintenance ECT will need to be signed before that treatment begins.

People who receive ECT differ considerably in the extent to which they experience side effects of treatment. If any factors exist that would substantially increase the risk of ECT, this information has been taken into account before recommending ECT, and the details of these risk factors have been discussed. To reduce the risk of complications, an individual will receive an assessment by a member of the facility's anesthesiology team before the initial ECT, including any needed laboratory tests or clinical consultations. To further increase treatment safety, psychiatric and medical medications may be adjusted. However, in spite of all such preparations, it is possible that medical complications can still occur.

Possible side effects and cautions associated with ECT are listed below:

- **Frequent side effects include** headache, muscle soreness, and nausea. These side effects usually respond to simple treatment. A brief period of confusion and disorientation when awakening from anesthesia is also common, as are problems with memory, which will be covered in detail later in this consent form.
- **Less common side effects include** irregularities or other abnormalities in heart rate and rhythm, most of which are mild and short-lasting.
- **Rare side effects include** dental complications; bone fractures or dislocations; skin burns; heart attack; stroke; severe respiratory difficulty; prolonged or recurrent seizure activity; and, in very rare instances, death.

This is not an all-inclusive list but is representative of items of potential clinical significance. The possibility of other types of medical complications cannot be ruled out, and risks of complications are likely to be higher in individuals with severe medical conditions.

An acute ECT series can affect cognitive processes, such as attention, concentration, memory, and other aspects of thinking. Because of these possible problems with confusion and memory, no important personal or business decisions should be made during or immediately after the acute ECT series. In addition, a patient receiving ECT should refrain from driving or engaging in other activities for which memory difficulties may be troublesome over this time period.

In terms of cognitive effects of ECT, memory problems are reported most often. When they occur, the severity of memory problems is often related to the number and type of ECT treatments given in the acute series. A smaller number of treatments is likely to produce less memory difficulty than a larger number, whereas bilateral ECT is more likely than right unilateral ECT to lead to memory difficulty. Difficulties in remembering new information and past events tend to be spotty, with small and inconsistent gaps in recall. Following completion of an acute ECT series, the patient's performance on standardized memory tests typically will return to pre-ECT levels within several weeks. Ability to recall events from before ECT also tends to improve over several months following the ECT course. Nevertheless, some individuals may report having memory problems that remain for months or years, or even permanently. These problems are usually, but not always, related to remembering events occurring during or shortly before the acute ECT series. Individuals may also report difficulty remembering information that was learned in the past. In spite of such problems, research shows that most patients whose symptoms have otherwise improved with ECT believe that those benefits outweigh any problems with memory.

If a medical emergency arises while the patient is at the facility, emergency interventions will be instituted. Consent for ECT includes a willingness for such emergency treatment to be provided and a recognition that any do not resuscitate orders will be placed on hold during the ECT procedure and recovery period. It is also understood that neither the institution providing treatment nor the treating physicians are required to provide long-term medical treatment and that the cost of such treatment must be covered personally or through medical insurance or other medical coverage. In addition, no compensation will be paid for a patient's lost wages or other consequential damages.

I understand all of the information in this form, and by signing this form, I give my consent for up to ___ treatments. I will be asked to provide consent again if a larger number of ECT treatments is recommended. This decision is being made voluntarily, and I may withdraw my consent for further treatment at any time. I understand that I may ask members of the treatment team any questions regarding ECT prior to providing consent or if any questions arise during this treatment series. In addition, I understand that I may contact Dr. _____, who is in charge of ECT at this facility, if I have questions or concerns during the ECT treatment series.

I have been or will be given a copy of this consent form to keep.

_____

Signature   Date   Time

Relationship to patient: _____

Person obtaining consent: _____

_____

Signature   Date   Time

Electroconvulsive Therapy (ECT) Consent Form: Maintenance Treatment Course

Name of Patient: _____

Dr. _____ has recommended that _____ receive maintenance electroconvulsive therapy (ECT) to potentially decrease the likelihood of relapse or the return of significant or severe symptoms of the psychiatric condition for which an acute course of ECT was recently administered. The rationale for maintenance ECT, including why it is being recommended, as well as potential risks and benefits, has been described to me.

ECT is most often used to treat severe episodes of depression or catatonia. If maintenance ECT is recommended for a condition other than a severe depressive episode or catatonia or if the patient is younger than 13 years old, a rationale for ECT use has been given based on available evidence.

Maintenance ECT can be given either on its own or in addition to other treatment, such as medication; psychotherapy; or some other type of brain stimulation treatment, such as transcranial magnetic stimulation (TMS). The recommended approach at the present time has also been described to me and will depend on prior experience with these treatments, the illness features, and other considerations, including likelihood of benefits and relative risks.

Although maintenance ECT is expected to decrease the likelihood of relapse in the psychiatric condition for which the acute course of ECT was administered, this outcome cannot be guaranteed, and there may be a partial or complete return of psychiatric symptoms despite receiving maintenance ECT. The likelihood and extent of benefits with maintenance ECT depend on a number of factors, including the disorder being treated, and have been discussed with me. If another mental disorder is present in addition to that for which ECT is being provided, that disorder should not be expected to improve with maintenance ECT, and there is a small chance that it might temporarily become worse.

Maintenance ECT involves a series of ECT treatments, typically on an outpatient basis, with the treatments usually separated in time by 1 or more weeks. If the patient continues to do well, the interval between treatments may often be gradually increased to a month or more. The number and frequency of maintenance treatments provided will depend on the clinical course, including past treatment history and the type and severity of the episode of illness for which an acute series of ECT was given. For some individuals, maintenance ECT may continue over a period of months or even years. However, if the total duration of ECT (i.e., acute ECT course plus maintenance ECT) is more than 3 months, a rationale should be provided to the consenter and documented in the medical record.

The administration of each maintenance ECT treatment is typically identical to that of the acute ECT series that has recently been completed. The treatments are administered in a specially equipped area and are usually given in the morning. Because the treatments involve general anesthesia, the patient will have had nothing to eat or drink for at least several hours before each treatment. Additional instructions may also be given based on specific patient needs or circumstances.

To prepare for the treatment, adhesive electrode pads will be placed on the head and body to record heart wave (electrocardiogram [ECG]) and brain wave (electroencephalogram [EEG]) activity during the treatment, and a sensor will be placed around one of the fingers to record blood oxygen saturation. A blood pressure cuff will be placed on an arm and, usually, on a leg. This monitoring involves no pain or discomfort other than that generally associated with blood pressure monitoring.

Before the treatment, a small catheter will be placed in a vein so that intravenous medications can be given. As part of the treatment, an anesthetic medication will be administered through the catheter and will quickly produce sleep. Next, another medication is given that will quickly cause muscles to relax. Additional medications may also be given, if needed. Throughout the procedure, the patient is provided pure oxygen to breathe. Because individuals receiving ECT will be asleep after receiving the anesthetic medication, they should not experience pain or discomfort or remember the procedure itself.

The stimulus electrodes that are used for ECT can be placed on the head in several different ways. The most common such approaches are bilateral ECT, in which one stimulus electrode is placed over the left temple area and the other over the right temple area, and unilateral ECT, in which both electrodes are placed on the same side of the head, usually the right side. Right unilateral ECT (electrodes on the right side) is likely to produce less memory difficulty than bilateral ECT. However, for some patients, bilateral ECT may be a more rapid or effective treatment. The choice of stimulus electrode placement has been discussed with me, and _____ electrode placement has been recommended. The possibility of a change in electrode placement has also been discussed with me.

After the individual receiving ECT is asleep and muscular relaxation has taken place, a brief and carefully controlled amount of electricity will be passed between the two stimulus electrodes that have been placed on the head. The electrical current delivered to the stimulus electrodes produces a seizure in the brain. The features of this electrical stimulus will be adjusted to the patient's individual needs. The medication used to provide muscle relaxation will greatly soften the body movements that would ordinarily accompany the seizure, and the body should move very little. The seizure will be monitored by EEG and typically lasts for about 1 minute. The anesthetic medications typically wear off within a few minutes after they are given, and the patient awakens and is moved to a recovery area. Individuals receiving ECT may be temporarily confused and/or agitated on awakening, but these effects usually disappear rapidly. Continuous monitoring and observation is maintained until the treatment team determines that the patient can either return to the inpatient unit or leave for home (if receiving outpatient ECT).

People who receive ECT differ considerably in the extent to which they experience side effects of treatment. If any factors exist that would substantially increase the risk of ECT, this information has been taken into account before recommending ECT, and the details of these risk factors have been discussed. To reduce the risk of complications, an individual will have received an assessment by a member of the facility's anesthesiology team, including any needed laboratory tests or clinical consultations. To further increase treatment safety, psychiatric and medical medications may be adjusted. However, in spite of all such preparations, it is possible that medical complications can still occur.

Possible side effects and cautions associated with ECT are listed below:

- **Frequent side effects include** headache, muscle soreness, and nausea. These side effects usually respond to simple treatment. A brief period of confusion and disorientation when awakening from anesthesia is also common, as are problems with memory, which will be covered in detail later in this consent form.
- **Less common side effects include** irregularities or other abnormalities in heart rate and rhythm, most of which are mild and short-lasting.

- **Rare side effects include** dental complications; bone fractures or dislocations; skin burns; heart attack; stroke; severe respiratory difficulty; prolonged or recurrent seizure activity; and, in very rare instances, death.

This is not an all-inclusive list but is representative of items of potential clinical significance. The possibility of other types of medical complications cannot be ruled out, and risks of complications are likely to be higher in individuals with severe medical conditions.

Maintenance ECT can affect cognitive processes, such as attention, concentration, memory, and other aspects of thinking. However, any such problems are typically less severe than with an acute ECT series because of the increased spacing between the treatments over time. When difficulties in remembering new information and past events do occur, they tend to be spotty, with small and inconsistent gaps in recall. Nevertheless, on the day that a maintenance ECT treatment is given, the patient should refrain from driving, making important personal or business decisions, or engaging in other activities for which confusion or memory difficulties may be troublesome. The ECT psychiatrist will also advise whether these recommendations would apply over a longer period if maintenance ECT is being given frequently with a shorter interval between each treatment.

As discussed in the consent form signed prior to the acute ECT series, the patient's performance on standardized memory tests typically returns to pre-ECT levels within several weeks after completion of an acute ECT series. While the patient is receiving maintenance ECT, cognitive difficulties (including memory problems) associated with the acute ECT course will usually decrease over several months, similar to what would occur if maintenance ECT was not being administered. Nevertheless, some individuals may report having memory problems that remain for months or years, or even permanently. These problems are usually, but not always, related to remembering events occurring during or shortly before the acute ECT series. Individuals may also report difficulty remembering information that was learned in the past.

If a medical emergency arises while the patient is at the facility, emergency interventions will be instituted immediately. Consent for ECT includes a willingness for such emergency treatment to be provided and a recognition that any do not resuscitate orders will be placed on hold during the ECT procedure and recovery period. It is also understood that neither the institution providing treatment nor the treating physicians are required to provide long-term medical treatment and that the cost of such treatment must be covered personally or through medical insurance or other medical coverage. In addition, no compensation will be paid for a patient's lost wages or other consequential damages.

I understand all of the information in this form and that, by signing this form, I am giving consent for an additional ___ treatments. I will be asked to provide consent again if a larger number of ECT treatments is recommended. This decision is being made voluntarily, and I may withdraw my consent for further treatment at any time. I understand that I may ask members of the treatment team any questions regarding ECT prior to providing consent or if any questions arise during this treatment series. In addition, I understand that I may contact Dr. _____, who is in charge of ECT at this facility, if I have questions or concerns during the ECT treatment series.

I have been or will be given a copy of this consent form to keep.

_____
Signature   Date   Time

Relationship to patient: _____

Person obtaining consent: _____

_____
Signature   Date   Time

List of Acronyms and Abbreviations

A	ampere
AA	anesthesiologist assistant
AAA	abdominal aortic aneurysm
ACLS	advanced cardiac life support
ADHD	attention-deficit/hyperactivity disorder
AMBU	artificial manual breathing unit
AMI-SF	Autobiographical Memory Interview–Short Form
APA	American Psychiatric Association
ASA	American Society of Anesthesiologists
ASQ	Anxiety Symptoms Questionnaire
ASRM	Altman Self-Rating Mania Scale
BAI	Beck Anxiety Inventory
BCRS	Braunig Catatonia Rating Scale
BDI-II	Beck Depression Inventory II
BF	bifrontal
BFCRS	Bush-Francis Catatonia Rating Scale
BL	bifrontal
BMI	body mass index
BPD	bipolar disorder
BPRS	Brief Psychiatric Rating Scale
BPRS-E	Brief Psychiatric Rating Scale–Expanded
BRMRS	Bech-Rafaelsen Mania Rating Scale
BSDS	Bipolar Spectrum Disorder Scale
BT	bitemporal
CABG	coronary artery bypass graft
CARS-M	Clinician-Administered Rating Scale for Mania
CCRN	critical care registered nurse
CES	cranial electrotherapy stimulator
CGI	Clinical Global Impression
CI	confidence interval
CME	continuing medical education
COPD	chronic obstructive pulmonary disease
COVID-19	coronavirus disease 2019
CRNA	certified registered nurse anesthetist
CVLT-3	California Verbal Learning Test, 3rd Edition
DBS	deep brain stimulation

List of Acronyms and Abbreviations (continued)

DNR	do not resuscitate
DOACs	direct oral anticoagulants
DRS-2	Dementia Rating Scale, 2nd Edition
DSM	*Diagnostic and Statistical Manual of Mental Disorders*
dTMS	deep TMS coil
DVT	deep vein thrombosis
ECCA	ElectroConvulsive Therapy Cognitive Assessment
ECG	electrocardiogram
ECT	electroconvulsive therapy
EEG	electroencephalogram
ERAQ	ECT-Related Anxiety Questionnaire
eTNS	external trigeminal nerve stimulation
FDA	United States Food and Drug Administration
FEAST	focal electrically administered seizure therapy
FM	frontomedial ECT
GAD-7	Generalized Anxiety Disorder Scale
HARS	Hamilton Anxiety Rating Scale
HCL-32	Hypomania Checklist 32
HIV	human immunodeficiency virus
HR	hazard ratio
HRQOL	health-related quality of life
HRSD	Hamilton Rating Scale for Depression
$HRSD_{17ANX}$	$HRSD_{17}$ Anxiety Subscale
HVLT-R	Hopkins Verbal Learning Test–Revised
ICD	International Classification of Diseases
IDS-C, IDS-SR	Inventory of Depressive Symptomatology, Clinician-Rated and Self-Report versions
$IDS-C_{ANX}$	Inventory of Depressive Symptomatology Anxiety Subscale
iLAST	individualized low-amplitude seizure therapy
INR	international normalized ratio
ISS	Internal State Scale
IV	intravenous
LFMS	low-field magnetic stimulation
LIFU	low-intensity focused ultrasound
LMA	laryngeal mask airway

List of Acronyms and Abbreviations (continued)

mA	milliampere
MacCAT-T	MacArthur Competence Assessment Tool for Treatment
MADRS	Montgomery-Åsberg Depression Rating Scale
MAOI	monoamine oxidase inhibitor
mA-sec	milliampere-second
mC	millicoulomb
MDD	major depressive disorder
MDE	major depressive episode
MDQ	Mood Disorder Questionnaire
MI	myocardial infarction
MMECT	multiple monitored ECT
MMSE	Mini-Mental State Examination
3MSE	Modified Mini-Mental State Examination
MoCA	Montreal Cognitive Assessment
MRI	magnetic resonance imaging
MSQ	Mood Swings Questionnaire
MST	magnetic seizure therapy
NCRS	Northoff Catatonia Rating Scale
NCSE	nonconvulsive status epilepticus
NET	nonconvulsive electrotherapy
NIH	National Institutes of Health
NIMH	National Institute of Mental Health
NINDS	National Institute of Neurological Disorders and Stroke
NMDA	N-methyl-D-aspartate
NMS	neuroleptic malignant syndrome
NPO	nil per os (nothing by mouth)
NSAIDs	nonsteroidal anti-inflammatory drugs
OCD	obsessive-compulsive disorder
PAA	physician assistant anesthetist
PACU	postanesthesia care unit
PANSS	Positive and Negative Syndrome Scale
PCP	phencyclidine
PDAS	Psychotic Depression Assessment Scale
PE	pulmonary embolism
PGI	Patient Global Impression

List of Acronyms and Abbreviations (continued)

PHQ	Patient Health Questionnaire
PICC	peripherally inserted central catheter
PPE	personal protective equipment
PROMIS	Patient-Reported Outcomes Measurement Information System
QIDS-C, QIDS-SR	Quick Inventory of Depressive Symptomatology, Clinician-rated and Self-Report
QOL	quality of life
RAVLT	Rey Auditory Verbal Learning Test
RBANS	Repeatable Battery for the Assessment of Neuropsychological Status
RCT	randomized controlled trial
RUL	right unilateral
SCAARED	Screen for Adult Anxiety Related Disorders
SF-36	Medical Outcomes Study Short Form Survey
SMDDS	Symptoms of Major Depressive Disorder Scale
SNRI	serotonin-norepinephrine reuptake inhibitor
SRMI	Self-Report Manic Inventory
SSMQ	Squire Subjective Memory Questionnaire
SSRI	selective serotonin reuptake inhibitor
STAI	State Trait Anxiety Inventory
STAR*D	Sequenced Treatment Alternatives to Relieve Depression
sTMS	synchronized transcranial magnetic stimulation
tACS	transcranial alternating current stimulation
taVNS	transcutaneous auricular vagus nerve stimulation
TCA	tricyclic antidepressant
tcVNS	transcutaneous cervical VNS
tDCS	transcranial direct current stimulation
TEST	transcranial electric stimulation therapy
tFUS	transcranial focused ultrasound
TMS	transcranial magnetic stimulation
t-PBM	transcranial photobiomodulation
TRD	treatment-resistant depression
VNS	vagus nerve stimulation
WHO	World Health Organization

List of Acronyms and Abbreviations (continued)

WHODAS 2.0	World Health Organization Disability Assessment Schedule 2.0
WHOQOL	WHO Quality of Life
WHOQOL-BREF	WHO Quality of Life BREF
WMS-IV	Wechsler Memory Scale, 4th Edition
YMRS	Young Mania Rating Scale

References

Aaronson ST, Carpenter LL, Conway CR, et al: Vagus nerve stimulation therapy randomized to different amounts of electrical charge for treatment-resistant depression: acute and chronic effects. Brain Stimul 6(4):631–640, 2013 23122916

Aaronson ST, Goldwaser EL, Kutzer DJ, et al: Vagus nerve stimulation in patients receiving maintenance therapy with electroconvulsive therapy: a series of 10 cases. J ECT 37(2):84–87, 2021 34029305

Aarsland D, Larsen JP, Waage O, et al: Maintenance electroconvulsive therapy for Parkinson's disease. Convuls Ther 13(4):274–277, 1997 9437571

Abbott CC, Miller J, Lloyd M, et al: Electroconvulsive therapy electrode placement for bipolar state-related targeted engagement. Int J Bipolar Disord 7(1):11, 2019 31053985

Abbott CC, Quinn D, Miller J, et al: Electroconvulsive therapy pulse amplitude and clinical outcomes. Am J Geriatr Psychiatry 29(2):166–178, 2021 32651051

Abboud T, Raya J, Sadri S, et al: Fetal and maternal cardiovascular effects of atropine and glycopyrrolate. Anesth Analg 62(4):426–430, 1983 6829946

Abdallah CG, Fasula M, Kelmendi B, et al: Rapid antidepressant effect of ketamine in the electroconvulsive therapy setting. J ECT 28(3):157–161, 2012 22847373

Abdi S, Fishman SM, Messner E: Acute exacerbation of depression after discontinuation of monoamine oxidase inhibitor prior to cardiac surgery. Anesth Analg 83(3):656–657, 1996 8780301

Abeysundera H, Campbell A, Sarma S: Worsening of movement disorder following treatment with electroconvulsive therapy in a patient with Huntington's disease. BMJ Case Rep 12(8):e230389, 2019 31401578

Abraham KR, Kulhara P: The efficacy of electroconvulsive therapy in the treatment of schizophrenia: a comparative study. Br J Psychiatry 151:152–155, 1987 3318990

Abrams R: Is unilateral electroconvulsive therapy really the treatment of choice in endogenous depression? Ann N Y Acad Sci 462:50–55, 1986 3518574

Abrams R: ECT as prophylactic treatment for bipolar disorder. Am J Psychiatry 147(3):373–374, 1990 2309965

Abrams R: Electroconvulsive therapy in the medically compromised patient. Psychiatr Clin North Am 14(4):871–885, 1991 1771152

Abrams R: The mortality rate with ECT. Convuls Ther 13(3):125–127, 1997 9342128

Abrams R: Electroconvulsive therapy requires higher dosage levels: Food and Drug Administration action is required. Arch Gen Psychiatry 57(5):445–446, 2000 10807484

Abrams R: Electroconvulsive Therapy. New York, Oxford University Press, 2002

Abrams R, Fink M: The present status of unilateral ECT: some recommendations. J Affect Disord 7(3–4):245–247, 1984 6241207

Abrams R, Swartz CM: ECT Instruction Manual for the Thymatron DG. Chicago, IL, Somatics, 1989

Abrams R, Taylor MA: Anterior bifrontal ECT: a clinical trial. Br J Psychiatry 122(570):587–590, 1973 4717031

Abrams R, Fink M, Feldstein S: Prediction of clinical response to ECT. Br J Psychiatry 122(569):457–460, 1973 4718282

Abrams R, Swartz CM, Vedak C: Antidepressant effects of high-dose right unilateral electroconvulsive therapy. Arch Gen Psychiatry 48(8):746–748, 1991 1883258

Accreditation Council for Graduate Medical Education: ACGME Program Requirements for Graduate Medical Education in Psychiatry. July 1, 2022. Available at: www.acgme.org/globalassets/pfassets/programrequirements/400_psychiatry_2022v2.pdf. Accessed October 10, 2022.

Acevedo AG, Smith JK: Adverse reaction to use of caffeine in ECT. Am J Psychiatry 145(4):529–530, 1988 3348458

Acharya D, Harper DG, Achtyes ED, et al: Safety and utility of acute electroconvulsive therapy for agitation and aggression in dementia. Int J Geriatr Psychiatry 30(3):265–273, 2015 24838521

Adam LA, Crowe RR: Use of ECT in idiopathic intracranial hypertension. J ECT 19(4):234–237, 2003 14657778

Adrissi J, Nadkarni NA, Gausche E, et al: Electroconvulsive therapy (ECT) for refractory psychiatric symptoms in Huntington's disease: a case series and review of the literature. J Huntingtons Dis 8(3):291–300, 2019 31322579

Aftab A, VanDercar A, Alkhachroum A, et al: Nonconvulsive status epilepticus after electroconvulsive therapy: a review of literature. Psychosomatics 59(1):36–46, 2018 28802513

Agüera-Ortiz L, García-Ramos R, Grandas Pérez FJ, et al: Focus on depression in Parkinson's disease: a Delphi consensus of experts in psychiatry, neurology, and geriatrics. Parkinsons Dis 2021:6621991, 2021 33628415

Ahern E, Semkovska M: Cognitive functioning in the first-episode of major depressive disorder: a systematic review and meta-analysis. Neuropsychology 31(1):52–72, 2017 27732039

Ahmed J, Metrick M, Gilbert A, et al: Electroconvulsive therapy for super refractory status epilepticus. J ECT 34(1):e5–e9, 2018 28937549

Ahmed S, Khan AM, Mekala HM, et al: Combined use of electroconvulsive therapy and antipsychotics (both clozapine and non-clozapine) in treatment resistant schizophrenia: a comparative meta-analysis. Heliyon 3(11):e00429, 2017 29264404

Ahmed SK, Stein GS: Negative interaction between lithium and ECT. Br J Psychiatry 151:419–420, 1987 3427307

Aibar-Durán JÁ, Rodríguez Rodríguez R, de Diego Adeliño FJ, et al: Long-term results of deep brain stimulation for treatment-resistant depression: outcome analysis and correlation with lead position and electrical parameters. Neurosurgery 90(1):72–80, 2022 34982873

Akcaboy ZN, Akcaboy EY, Yigitbaşl B, et al: Effects of remifentanil and alfentanil on seizure duration, stimulus amplitudes and recovery parameters during ECT. Acta Anaesthesiol Scand 49(8):1068–1071, 2005 16095445

Albertsen LN, Lauridsen JK: A review: electroconvulsive therapy in cochlear implant patients. J ECT 38(1):10–12, 2022 34699392

Albin SM, Stevens SR, Rasmussen KG: Blood pressure before and after electroconvulsive therapy in hypertensive and nonhypertensive patients. J ECT 23(1):9–10, 2007 17435564

Alemany C, Puigdemont D, Martín-Blanco A, et al: Response and safety outcomes in treatment-resistant depression after subcallosal cingulate gyrus deep brain stimulation: long-term follow-up study. J Clin Psychiatry 84(4):22m14622, 2023 37378475

Alexander ML, Alagapan S, Lugo CE, et al: Double-blind, randomized pilot clinical trial targeting alpha oscillations with transcranial alternating current stimulation (tACS) for the treatment of major depressive disorder (MDD). Transl Psychiatry 9(1):106, 2019 30837453

Alexopoulos GS, Frances RJ: ECT and cardiac patients with pacemakers. Am J Psychiatry 137(9):1111–1112, 1980 7425169

Alexopoulos GS, Meyers BS, Young RC, et al: The course of geriatric depression with "reversible dementia": a controlled study. Am J Psychiatry 150(11):1693–1699, 1993 8105707

Ali M, Malathesh BC, Chatterjee SS, et al: Delirium with concurrent use of lithium and ECT and the safety implications: case reports and review of the literature. Case Rep Psychiatry 2023:9117292, 2023 37200983

Ali S, Welch CA, Park LT, et al: Encephalitis and catatonia treated with ECT. Cogn Behav Neurol 21(1):46–51, 2008 18327024

Ali SA, Mathur N, Malhotra AK, et al: Electroconvulsive therapy and schizophrenia: a systematic review. Mol Neuropsychiatry 5(2):75–83, 2019 31192220

Ali-Melkkilä T, Kaila T, Kanto J, et al: Pharmacokinetics of glycopyrronium in parturients. Anaesthesia 45(8):634–637, 1990 2400072

Alizadeh NS, Maroufi A, Jamshidi M, et al: Effect of memantine on cognitive performance in patients under electroconvulsive therapy: a double-blind randomized clinical trial. Clin Neuropharmacol 38(6):236–240, 2015 26536019

Allen RM: Pseudodementia and ECT. Biol Psychiatry 17(12):1435–1443, 1982 7159640

Al-Qadhi SA, Chawla T, Seabrook JA, et al: Competency by design for electroconvulsive therapy in psychiatry postgraduate training: face and content validation study. J ECT 36(1):18–24, 2020 31990735

Altman E: Rating scales for mania: is self-rating reliable? J Affect Disord 50(2-3):283–286, 1998 9858088

Altman EG, Hedeker DR, Janicak PG, et al: The Clinician-Administered Rating Scale for Mania (CARS-M): development, reliability, and validity. Biol Psychiatry 36(2):124–134, 1994 7948445

Altman EG, Hedeker D, Peterson JL, et al: The Altman Self-Rating Mania Scale. Biol Psychiatry 42(10):948–955, 1997 9359982

Amanullah S, Delva N, McRae H, et al: Electroconvulsive therapy in patients with skull defects or metallic implants: a review of the literature and case report. Prim Care Companion CNS Disord 14(2):14, 2012 22943035

American Academy of Pediatrics Committee on Drugs: Transfer of drugs and other chemicals into human milk. Pediatrics 108(3):776–789, 2001 11533352

American College of Obstetricians and Gynecologists: ACOG Committee Opinion No. 775: nonobstetric surgery during pregnancy. Obstet Gynecol 133(4):e285–e286, 2019 30913200

American Medical Association: Code of Medical Ethics: Privacy, Confidentiality, and Medical Records. Available at: www.ama-assn.org/delivering-care/ethics/code-medical-ethics-privacy-confidentiality-medical-records. Accessed October 11, 2020.

American Nurses Association: Psychiatric-Mental Health Nursing: Scope and Standards of Practice, 2nd Edition. Silver Spring, MD, American Nurses Association, 2014

American Psychiatric Association: Electroconvulsive Therapy (Task Force Report #14). Washington, DC, American Psychiatric Association, 1978

American Psychiatric Association: The Practice of ECT: Recommendations for Treatment, Training, and Privileging. Washington, DC, American Psychiatric Press, 1990

American Psychiatric Association: Diagnostic and Statistical Manual of Mental Disorders, 4th Edition. Washington, DC, American Psychiatric Association Publishing, 1994

American Psychiatric Association: Diagnostic and Statistical Manual of Mental Disorders, 4th Edition, Text Revision. Washington, DC, American Psychiatric Association Publishing, 2000

American Psychiatric Association: The Practice of Electroconvulsive Therapy: Recommendations for Treatment, Training, and Privileging (A Task Force Report of the American Psychiatric Association), 2nd Edition. Washington, DC, American Psychiatric Association, 2001

American Psychiatric Association: Practice Guideline for the Treatment of Patients With Bipolar Disorder. Washington, DC, American Psychiatric Publishing, 2002

American Psychiatric Association: Practice Guideline for the Treatment of Patients With Major Depressive Disorder, 3rd Edition. Arlington, VA, American Psychiatric Association, 2010

American Psychiatric Association: Diagnostic and Statistical Manual of Mental Disorders, 5th Edition. Arlington, VA, American Psychiatric Association Publishing, 2013

American Psychiatric Association: American Psychiatric Association Practice Guidelines for the Psychiatric Evaluation of Adults, 3rd Edition. Arlington, VA, American Psychiatric Association Publishing, 2016

American Psychiatric Association: The American Psychiatric Association Practice Guideline for the Treatment of Patients With Schizophrenia, 3rd Edition. Washington, DC, American Psychiatric Association, 2021

American Psychiatric Association: Diagnostic and Statistical Manual of Mental Disorders, 5th Edition, Text Revision. Washington, DC, American Psychiatric Association Publishing, 2022

American Psychiatric Association Council on Psychiatry and Law: American Psychiatric Association resources document on principles of informed consent in psychiatry. J Am Acad Psychiatry Law 25(1):121–125, 1997 9148888

American Society of Anesthesiologists: Practice guidelines for preoperative fasting and the use of pharmacologic agents to reduce the risk of pulmonary aspiration: application to healthy patients undergoing elective procedures: an updated report by the American Society of Anesthesiologists task force on preoperative fasting and the use of pharmacologic agents to reduce the risk of pulmonary aspiration. Anesthesiology 126(3):376–393, 2017 28045707

American Society of Anesthesiologists: Statement on ASA Physical Status Classification System. Washington, DC, American Society of Anesthesiologists, 2020a. Available at: www.asahq.org/standards-and-practice-parameters/statement-on-asa-physical-status-classification-system. Accessed April 29, 2022.

American Society of Anesthesiologists: Committee on Standards and Practice Parameters Standards for Basic Anesthetic Monitoring. Washington, DC, American Society of Anesthesiologists, 2020b. Available at: www.asahq.org/standards-and-guidelines/standards-for-basic-anesthetic-monitoring. Accessed January 3, 2021.

Amritwar A, Karia S, De Sousa A, et al: Electroconvulsive therapy in a patient with glaucoma. Natl Med J India 29(2):85–86, 2016 27586212

Anand A, Mathew SJ, Sanacora G, et al: Ketamine versus ECT for nonpsychotic treatment-resistant major depression. N Engl J Med 388(25):2315–2325, 2023 37224232

Anastasian ZH, Khan N, Heyer EJ, et al: Effect of atropine dose on heart rate during electroconvulsive therapy. J ECT 30(4):298–302, 2014 24755728

Andersen FA, Arsland D, Holst-Larsen H: Effects of combined methohexitone-remifentanil anaesthesia in electroconvulsive therapy. Acta Anaesthesiol Scand 45(7):830–833, 2001 11472282

Andersen K, Balldin J, Gottfries CG, et al: A double-blind evaluation of electroconvulsive therapy in Parkinson's disease with "on-off" phenomena. Acta Neurol Scand 76(3):191–199, 1987 2446463

Anderson EL, Reti IM: ECT in pregnancy: a review of the literature from 1941 to 2007. Psychosom Med 71(2):235–242, 2009 19073751

Anderson IM: Does electroconvulsive therapy damage the brain? Lancet Psychiatry 5(4):294–295, 2018 29523430

Anderson IM, Blamire A, Branton T, et al: Ketamine augmentation of electroconvulsive therapy to improve neuropsychological and clinical outcomes in depression (Ketamine-ECT): a multicentre, double-blind, randomised, parallel-group, superiority trial. Lancet Psychiatry 4(5):365–377, 2017 28359862

Andrade C: Double stimulation to elicit an adequate treatment. Convuls Ther 7(4):300–302, 1991 11941139

Andrade C, Bolwig TG: Electroconvulsive therapy, hypertensive surge, blood-brain barrier breach, and amnesia: exploring the evidence for a connection. J ECT 30(2):160–164, 2014 24800688

Andrade C, Gangadhar BN, Subbakrishna DK, et al: A double-blind comparison of sinusoidal wave and brief-pulse electroconvulsive therapy in endogenous depression. Convuls Ther 4(4):297–305, 1988a 11940979

Andrade C, Gangadhar BN, Swaminath G, et al: Mania as a side effect of electroconvulsive therapy. Convuls Ther 4(1):81–83, 1988b 11940945

Andrade C, Gangadhar BN, Channabasavanna SM: Further characterization of mania as a side effect of ECT. Convuls Ther 6(4):318–319, 1990 11941087

Andrews M, Hasking P: Effect of two educational interventions on knowledge and attitudes towards electroconvulsive therapy. J ECT 20(4):230–236, 2004 15591856

Aneja J, Grover S, Agarwal M, et al: Use of electroconvulsive therapy in the presence of glaucoma: a case report and review of literature. Indian J Psychol Med 35(1):80–83, 2013 23833347

Angst J, Angst K, Baruffol I, et al: ECT-induced and drug-induced hypomania. Convuls Ther 8(3):179–185, 1992 11941168

Angst J, Adolfsson R, Benazzi F, et al: The HCL-32: towards a self-assessment tool for hypomanic symptoms in outpatients. J Affect Disord 88(2):217–233, 2005 16125784

Angulo M, Rooks BT, Gill M, et al: Psychometrics of the screen for adult anxiety related disorders (SCAARED): a new scale for the assessment of DSM-5 anxiety disorders. Psychiatry Res 253:84–90, 2017 28359032

Antal A, Alekseichuk I, Bikson M, et al: Low intensity transcranial electric stimulation: safety, ethical, legal regulatory and application guidelines. Clin Neurophysiol 128(9):1774–1809, 2017 28709880

Aoki N, Suwa T, Kawashima H, et al: Sevoflurane in electroconvulsive therapy: a systematic review and meta-analysis of randomised trials. J Psychiatr Res 141:16–25, 2021 34171759

Apfelbaum JL, Hagberg CA, Caplan RA, et al: Practice guidelines for management of the difficult airway: an updated report by the American Society of Anesthesiologists Task Force on Management of the Difficult Airway. Anesthesiology 118(2):251–270, 2013 23364566

Appelbaum PS: Clinical practice: assessment of patients' competence to consent to treatment. N Engl J Med 357(18):1834–1840, 2007 17978292

Appelbaum PS, Lidz CW, Meisel A: Informed Consent: Legal Theory and Clinical Practice. New York, Oxford University Press, 1987

Applegate RJ: Diagnosis and management of ischemic heart disease in the patient scheduled to undergo electroconvulsive therapy. Convuls Ther 13(3):128–144, 1997 9342129

Arkan B, Üstün B: Examination of the effect of education about electroconvulsive therapy on nursing practice and patient satisfaction. J ECT 24(4):254–259, 2008 18708947

Aronson TA, Shukla S, Hoff A: Continuation therapy after ECT for delusional depression: a naturalistic study of prophylactic treatments and relapse. Convuls Ther 3(4):251–259, 1987 11940926

Aronson TA, Shukla S, Hoff A, et al: Proposed delusional depression subtypes: preliminary evidence from a retrospective study of phenomenology and treatment course. J Affect Disord 14(1):69–74, 1988 2892870

Askew G, Pearson KW, Cryer D: Informed consent: can we educate patients? J R Coll Surg Edinb 35(5):308–310, 1990 2283610

Atashnama A, Aly H, Krishnan V, et al: Naturalistic outcomes of continuation right unilateral ultrabrief ECT in major depression: a retrospective chart review. Australas Psychiatry 28(3):286–290, 2020 32391725

Atiku L, Gorst-Unsworth C, Khan BU, et al: Improving relapse prevention after successful electroconvulsive therapy for patients with severe depression: completed audit cycle involving 102 full electroconvulsive therapy courses in West Sussex, United Kingdom. J ECT 31(1):34–36, 2015 25029538

Augoustides JG, Greenblatt E, Abbas MA, et al: Clinical approach to agitation after electroconvulsive therapy: a case report and literature review. J ECT 18(4):213–217, 2002 12468998

Auriacombe M, Rénéric JP, Usandizaga D, et al: Post-ECT agitation and plasma lactate concentrations. J ECT 16(3):263–267, 2000 11005048

Auron M, Duran Castillo MY, Garcia OFD: Perioperative management of pregnant women undergoing nonobstetric surgery. Cleve Clin J Med 88(1):27–34, 2021 33384312

Aust S, Brakemeier EL, Spies J, et al: Efficacy of augmentation of cognitive behavioral therapy with transcranial direct current stimulation for depression: a randomized clinical trial. JAMA Psychiatry 79(6):528–537, 2022 35442431

Austelle CW, O'Leary GH, Thompson S, et al: A comprehensive review of vagus nerve stimulation for depression. Neuromodulation 25(3):309–315, 2022 35396067

Austgen G, Meyers MS, Gordon M, et al: The use of electroconvulsive therapy in neuropsychiatric complications of coronavirus disease 2019: a systematic literature review and case report. J Acad Consult Liaison Psychiatry 63(1):86–93, 2022 34358726

Avery D, Lubrano A: Depression treated with imipramine and ECT: the DeCarolis study reconsidered. Am J Psychiatry 136(4B):559–562, 1979 426143

Avery D, Winokur G: Mortality in depressed patients treated with electroconvulsive therapy and antidepressants. Arch Gen Psychiatry 33(9):1029–1037, 1976 962487

Avramov MN, Husain MM, White PF: The comparative effects of methohexital, propofol, and etomidate for electroconvulsive therapy. Anesth Analg 81(3):596–602, 1995 7653829

Ayres CM: The relative value of various somatic therapies in schizophrenia. J Neuropsychiatry 1:154–162, 1960 13795367

Azuma H, Fujita A, Sato K, et al: Postictal suppression correlates with therapeutic efficacy for depression in bilateral sine and pulse wave electroconvulsive therapy. Psychiatry Clin Neurosci 61(2):168–173, 2007 17362434

Azuma H, Yamada A, Shinagawa Y, et al: Ictal physiological characteristics of remitters during bilateral electroconvulsive therapy. Psychiatry Res 185(3):462–464, 2011 20605640

Babigian HM, Guttmacher LB: Epidemiologic considerations in electroconvulsive therapy. Arch Gen Psychiatry 41(3):246–253, 1984 6703844

Babu GN, Thippeswamy H, Chandra PS: Use of electroconvulsive therapy (ECT) in postpartum psychosis: a naturalistic prospective study. Arch Womens Ment Health 16(3):247–251, 2013 23568390

Bachu AK, Kotapati VP, Kainth T, et al: Electroconvulsive therapy in individuals with dementia/major NCD presenting with behavioral symptoms: a systematic review. Int Psychogeriatr 12:1–16, 2023 37170574

Bader GM, Silk KR, Dequardo JR, et al: Electroconvulsive therapy and intracranial aneurysm. Convuls Ther 11(2):139–143, 1995 7552055

Badran BW, Caulfield KA, Stomberg-Firestein S, et al: Sonication of the anterior thalamus with MRI-guided transcranial focused ultrasound (tFUS) alters pain thresholds in healthy adults: a double-blind, sham-controlled study. Brain Stimul 13(6):1805–1812, 2020 33127579

Bagadia VN, Dave KP, Shah LP: A comparative study of physical treatments in schizophrenia. Int J Psychiatry 12:190–204, 1970

Bagadia VN, Abhyankar RR, Doshi J, et al: A double blind controlled study of ECT vs chlorpromazine in schizophrenia. J Assoc Physicians India 31(10):637–640, 1983 6671932

Bagadia VN, Abhyankar R, Pradhan PV, et al: Reevaluation of ECT in schizophrenia: right temporoparietal versus bitemporal electrode placement. Convuls Ther 4(3):215–220, 1988 11940967

Baghai TC, Marcuse A, Brosch M, et al: The influence of concomitant antidepressant medication on safety, tolerability and clinical effectiveness of electroconvulsive therapy. World J Biol Psychiatry 7(2):82–90, 2006 16684680

Bailine S, Kremen N, Kohen I, et al: Bitemporal electroconvulsive therapy for depression in a Parkinson disease patient with a deep-brain stimulator. J ECT 24(2):171–172, 2008 18580566

Bailine SH, Safferman A, Vital-Herne J, et al: Flumazenil reversal of benzodiazepine-induced sedation for a patient with severe pre-ECT anxiety. Convuls Ther 10(1):65–68, 1994 7914463

Bailine SH, Rifkin A, Kayne E, et al: Comparison of bifrontal and bitemporal ECT for major depression. Am J Psychiatry 157(1):121–123, 2000 10618025

Bailine SH, Petrides G, Doft M, et al: Indications for the use of propofol in electroconvulsive therapy. J ECT 19(3):129–132, 2003 12972980

Bailine SH, Sanghani SN, Petrides G: Maintenance electroconvulsive therapy is not acute electroconvulsive therapy. J ECT 35(1):1–2, 2019 30045170

Bainbridge D, Martin J, Arango M, et al: Perioperative and anaesthetic-related mortality in developed and developing countries: a systematic review and meta-analysis. Lancet 380(9847):1075–1081, 2012 22998717

Baker A, Simon N, Keshaviah A, et al: Anxiety Symptoms Questionnaire (ASQ): development and validation. Gen Psychiatr 32(6):e100144, 2019 31922090

Baker AA, Game JA, Thorpe JG: Physical treatment for schizophrenia. J Ment Sci 104(436):860–864, 1958 13588346

Baker AA, Bird G, Lavin NI, et al: E.C.T. in schizophrenia. J Ment Sci 106:1506–1511, 1960 13686065

Bali IM: The effect of modified electroconvulsive therapy on plasma potassium concentration. Br J Anaesth 47(3):398–401, 1975 1138748

Balon R: Rating scales for anxiety/anxiety disorders. Curr Psychiatry Rep 9(4):271–277, 2007 17880857

Balsamo M, Romanelli R, Innamorati M, et al: The State-Trait Anxiety Inventory: shadows and lights on its construct validity. J Psychopathol Behav Assess 35:475–486, 2013

Barekatain M, Jahangard L, Haghighi M, et al: Bifrontal versus bitemporal electroconvulsive therapy in severe manic patients. J ECT 24(3):199–202, 2008 18772704

Barenboim I, Lafer B: Maintenance use of ketamine for treatment-resistant depression: an open-label pilot study. Br J Psychiatry 40(1):110, 2018 29590266

Barnes RC, Hussein A, Anderson DN, et al: Maintenance electroconvulsive therapy and cognitive function. Br J Psychiatry 170:285–287, 1997 9229039

Bassa A, Sagués T, Porta-Casteràs D, et al: The neurobiological basis of cognitive side effects of electroconvulsive therapy: a systematic review. Brain Sci 11(10):11, 2021 34679338

Battersby M, Ben-Tovim D, Eden J: Electroconvulsive therapy: a study of attitudes and attitude change after seeing an educational video. Aust N Z J Psychiatry 27(4):613–619, 1993 8135686

Bauer J, Hageman I, Dam H, et al: Comparison of propofol and thiopental as anesthetic agents for electroconvulsive therapy: a randomized, blinded comparison of seizure duration, stimulus charge, clinical effect, and cognitive side effects. J ECT 25(2):85–90, 2009 19092676

Bauer M, Severus E, Möller HJ, et al: Pharmacological treatment of unipolar depressive disorders: summary of WFSBP guidelines. Int J Psychiatry Clin Pract 21(3):166–176, 2017 28367707

Bauer MS, Crits-Christoph P, Ball WA, et al: Independent assessment of manic and depressive symptoms by self-rating. Scale characteristics and implications for the study of mania. Arch Gen Psychiatry 48(9):807–812, 1991 1929771

Baweja R, Singareddy R: Concomitant use of maintenance ECT and vagus nerve stimulation for more than 10 years in treatment-resistant depression. Am J Psychiatry 170(9):1059–1061, 2013 24030616

Baxter LRJr, Roy-Byrne P, Liston EH, et al: Informing patients about electroconvulsive therapy: effects of a videotape presentation. Convuls Ther 2(1):25–29, 1986 11940842

Bayless JD, McCormick LM, Brumm MC, et al: Pre- and post-electroconvulsive therapy multidomain cognitive assessment in psychotic depression: relationship to premorbid abilities and symptom improvement. J ECT 26(1):47–52, 2010 19710624

Bazoukis G, Yeung C, Wui Hang Ho R, et al: Association of QT dispersion with mortality and arrhythmic events: a meta-analysis of observational studies. J Arrhythm 36(1):105–115, 2019 32071628

Beale MD, Kellner CH: ECT in treatment algorithms: no need to save the best for last. J ECT 16(1):1–2, 2000 10735326

Beale MD, Kellner CH, Lemert R, et al: Skeletal muscle relaxation in patients undergoing electroconvulsive therapy. Anesthesiology 80(4):957, 1994a 7848406

Beale MD, Kellner CH, Pritchett JT, et al: Stimulus dose-titration in ECT: a 2-year clinical experience. Convuls Ther 10(2):171–176, 1994b 8069643

Beale MD, Pritchett JT, Kellner CH: Supraventricular tachycardia in a patient receiving ECT, clozapine, and caffeine. Convuls Ther 10(3):228–231, 1994c 7834261

Beale MD, Bernstein HJ, Kellner CH: Maintenance electroconvulsive therapy for geriatric depression: a one year follow-up. Clin Gerontol 16:86–90, 1996

Beale MD, Kellner CH, Gurecki P, et al: ECT for the treatment of Huntington's disease: a case study. Convuls Ther 13(2):108–112, 1997a 9253530

Beale MD, Kellner CH, Parsons PJ: ECT for the treatment of mood disorders in cancer patients. Convuls Ther 13(4):222–226, 1997b 9437566

Bean G, Nishisato S, Rector NA, et al: The assessment of competence to make a treatment decision: an empirical approach. Can J Psychiatry 41(2):85–92, 1996 8705968

Bech P, Rafaelsen OJ, Kramp P, et al: The mania rating scale: scale construction and inter-observer agreement. Neuropharmacology 17(6):430–431, 1978 673161

Beck AT, Epstein N, Brown G, et al: An inventory for measuring clinical anxiety: psychometric properties. J Consult Clin Psychol 56(6):893–897, 1988 3204199

Beck AT, Steer RA, Brown GK: Beck Depression Inventory Manual, 2nd Edition. San Antonio, TX, Psychological Corporation, 1996

Belz M, Methfessel I, Spang M, et al: Overlooking the obvious? Influence of electrolyte concentrations on seizure quality parameters in electroconvulsive therapy. Eur Arch Psychiatry Clin Neurosci 270(2):263–269, 2020 31317265

Benadhira R, Thomas F, Bouaziz N, et al: A randomized, sham-controlled study of maintenance rTMS for treatment-resistant depression (TRD). Psychiatry Res 258:226–233, 2017 28844559

Benatov R, Sirota P, Megged S: Neuroleptic-resistant schizophrenia treated with clozapine and ECT. Convuls Ther 12(2):117–121, 1996 8744173

Benton AL: A multiple choice type of the visual retention test. AMA Arch Neurol Psychiatry 64(5):699–707, 1950 14770617

Beresford BJ, Glick D, Dinwiddie SH: Combination propofol-alfentanil anesthesia for electroconvulsive therapy in patients receiving monoamine oxidase inhibitors. J ECT 20(2):120–122, 2004 15167430

Bergfeld IO, Ooms P, Lok A, et al: Efficacy and quality of life after 6–9 years of deep brain stimulation for depression. Brain Stimul 15(4):957–964, 2022 35772671

Berigan TR, Harazin J, Williams HL II: Use of flumazenil in conjunction with electroconvulsive therapy. Am J Psychiatry 152(6):957, 1995 7755138

Berlim MT, Van den Eynde F, Daskalakis ZJ: Efficacy and acceptability of high frequency repetitive transcranial magnetic stimulation (rTMS) versus electroconvulsive therapy (ECT) for major depression: a systematic review and meta-analysis of randomized trials. Depress Anxiety 30(7):614–623, 2013 23349112

Berman RM, Prudic J, Brakemeier EL, et al: Subjective evaluation of the therapeutic and cognitive effects of electroconvulsive therapy. Brain Stimul 1(1):16–26, 2008 20633366

Besse M, Belz M, Folsche T, et al: Serum neurofilament light chain (NFL) remains unchanged during electroconvulsive therapy. World J Biol Psychiatry 21(2):148–154, 2020 31818180

Betjemann JP, Lowenstein DH: Status epilepticus in adults. Lancet Neurol 14(6):615–624, 2015 25908090

Bhanushali MJ, Tuite PJ: The evaluation and management of patients with neuroleptic malignant syndrome. Neurol Clin 22(2):389–411, 2004 15062519

Bhat RS, Mayur P, Chakrabarti I: ECT-donepezil interaction: a single case report. Int J Geriatr Psychiatry 19(6):594–595, 2004 15211544

Bhatia SC, Bhatia SK, Gupta S: Concurrent administration of clozapine and ECT: a successful therapeutic strategy for a patient with treatment-resistant schizophrenia. J ECT 14(4):280–283, 1998 9871852

Bica BE, Moro AL, Hax V, et al: Electroconvulsive therapy as a treatment for refractory neuropsychiatric lupus with catatonia: three case studies and literature review. Lupus 24(12):1327–1331, 2015 25972366

Bikson M, Esmaeilpour Z, Adair D, et al: Transcranial electrical stimulation nomenclature. Brain Stimul 12(6):1349–1366, 2019 31358456

Birmaher B, Brent D, Bernet W, et al: Practice parameter for the assessment and treatment of children and adolescents with depressive disorders. J Am Acad Child Adolesc Psychiatry 46(11):1503–1526, 2007 18049300

Björck S, Palaszewski B, Friberg L, et al: Atrial fibrillation, stroke risk, and warfarin therapy revisited: a population-based study. Stroke 44(11):3103–3108, 2013 23982711

Black DW, Winokur G, Nasrallah A: ECT in unipolar and bipolar disorders: a naturalistic evaluation of 460 patients. Convuls Ther 2(4):231–237, 1986 11940870

Black DW, Winokur G, Nasrallah A: Treatment and outcome in secondary depression: a naturalistic study of 1087 patients. J Clin Psychiatry 48(11):438–441, 1987a 3680184

Black DW, Winokur G, Nasrallah A: The treatment of depression: electroconvulsive therapy v antidepressants: a naturalistic evaluation of 1,495 patients. Compr Psychiatry 28(2):169–182, 1987b 3829660

Black DW, Winokur G, Nasrallah A: Treatment of mania: a naturalistic study of electroconvulsive therapy versus lithium in 438 patients. J Clin Psychiatry 48(4):132–139, 1987c 3104316

Black DW, Hulbert J, Nasrallah A: The effect of somatic treatment and comorbidity on immediate outcome in manic patients. Compr Psychiatry 30(1):74–79, 1989a 2494019

Black DW, Winokur G, Mohandoss E, et al: Does treatment influence mortality in depressives? A follow-up of 1076 patients with major affective disorders. Ann Clin Psychiatry 1:165–173, 1989b

Black DW, Winokur G, Nasrallah A: A multivariate analysis of the experience of 423 depressed inpatients treated with electroconvulsive therapy. Convuls Ther 9(2):112–120, 1993 11941200

Blaj A, Worrall A, Chaplin R: Electroconvulsive therapy: the practice and training needs of referring psychiatrists in the United Kingdom and Republic of Ireland. J ECT 23(2):78–81, 2007 17548975

Bloch M, Admon D, Bonne O, et al: Electroconvulsive therapy in a depressed heart transplant patient. Convuls Ther 8(4):290–293, 1992 11941181

Bloch Y, Pollack M, Mor I: Should the administration of ECT during clozapine therapy be contraindicated? Br J Psychiatry 169(2):253–254, 1996 8871811

Blumberger DM, Seitz DP, Herrmann N, et al: Low medical morbidity and mortality after acute courses of electroconvulsive therapy in a population-based sample. Acta Psychiatr Scand 136(6):583–593, 2017 28922451

Bodley PO, Halwax K, Potts L: Low serum pseudocholinesterase levels complicating treatment with phenelzine. BMJ 3(5669):510–512, 1969 5801348

Boeke A, Pullen B, Coppes L, et al: Catatonia associated with systemic lupus erythematosus (SLE): a report of two cases and a review of the literature. Psychosomatics 59(6):523–530, 2018 30270156

Boere E, Birkenhäger TK, Groenland TH, et al: Beta-blocking agents during electroconvulsive therapy: a review. Br J Anaesth 113(1):43–51, 2014 24942714

Bøg FK, Jørgensen MB, Andersen ZJ, Osler M: Electroconvulsive therapy and subsequent epilepsy in patients with affective disorders: a register-based Danish cohort study. Brain Stimul 11(2):411–415, 2018 29203131

Boland X, Dratcu L: Electroconvulsive therapy and COVID-19 in acute inpatient psychiatry: more than clinical issues alone. J ECT 36(3):223–224, 2020 32826545

Bolwig TG, Hertz MM, Paulson OB, et al: The permeability of the blood-brain barrier during electrically induced seizures in man. Eur J Clin Invest 7(2):87–93, 1977 404164

Bond ED: Results of treatment in psychoses—with a control series. IV. General data and summary. Am J Psychiatry 110(12):885–887, 1954 13158622

Bonds C, Frye MA, Coudreaut MF, et al: Cost reduction with maintenance ECT in refractory bipolar disorder. J ECT 14(1):36–41, 1998 9661092

Borgatta L, Jenny RW, Gruss L, et al: Clinical significance of methohexital, meperidine, and diazepam in breast milk. J Clin Pharmacol 37(3):186–192, 1997 9089420

Borisovskaya A, Bryson WC, Buchholz J, et al: Electroconvulsive therapy for depression in Parkinson's disease: systematic review of evidence and recommendations. Neurodegener Dis Manag 6(2):161–176, 2016 27033556

Boronow J, Stoline A, Sharfstein SS: Refusal of ECT by a patient with recurrent depression, psychosis, and catatonia. Am J Psychiatry 154(9):1285–1291, 1997 9286190

Borowitz AH: An investigation into combined electroconvulsive and chlorpromazine therapy in the treatment of schizophrenia. S Afr Med J 33:836–840, 1959 13802929

Botto F, Alonso-Coello P, Chan MT, et al: Myocardial injury after noncardiac surgery: a large, international, prospective cohort study establishing diagnostic criteria, characteristics, predictors, and 30-day outcomes. Anesthesiology 120(3):564–578, 2014 24534856

Bourgon LN, Kellner CH: Relapse of depression after ECT: a review. J ECT 16(1):19–31, 2000 10735328

Bowie CR, Best MW, Depp C, et al: Cognitive and functional deficits in bipolar disorder and schizophrenia as a function of the presence and history of psychosis. Bipolar Disord 20(7):604–613, 2018 29777563

Boylan LS, Haskett RF, Mulsant BH, et al: Determinants of seizure threshold in ECT: benzodiazepine use, anesthetic dosage, and other factors. J ECT 16(1):3–18, 2000 10735327

Braga RJ, John M, Schooler NR, et al: Continuation electroconvulsive therapy for patients with clozapine-resistant schizophrenia: a pilot study. J ECT 35(3):156–160, 2019 30973454

Braghiroli KS, Einav S, Heesen MA, et al: Perioperative mortality in older patients: a systematic review with a meta-regression analysis and meta-analysis of observational studies. J Clin Anesth 69:110160, 2021 33338975

Braithwaite R, McKeown HL, Lawrence VJ, et al: Successful electroconvulsive therapy in a patient with confirmed, symptomatic COVID-19. J ECT 36(3):222–223, 2020 32453191

Braithwaite R, Chaplin R, Sivasanker V: Effects of the COVID-19 pandemic on provision of electroconvulsive therapy. BJPsych Bull 46(3):137–140, 2022 33977894

Brakemeier EL, Merkl A, Wilbertz G, et al: Cognitive-behavioral therapy as continuation treatment to sustain response after electroconvulsive therapy in depression: a randomized controlled trial. Biol Psychiatry 76(3):194–202, 2014 24462229

Brandon S, Cowley P, McDonald C, et al: Electroconvulsive therapy: results in depressive illness from the Leicestershire trial. Br Med J (Clin Res Ed) 288(6410):22–25, 1984 6418300

Brandon S, Cowley P, McDonald C, et al: Leicester ECT trial: results in schizophrenia. Br J Psychiatry 146:177–183, 1985 3884080

Brandt J, Benedict RHB: Hopkins Verbal Learning Test-Revised (HVLT-R) Professional Manual. Lutz, FL, Psychological Assessment Resources, 2001

Braun M, Tupper D, Kaufmann P, et al: Neuropsychological assessment: a valuable tool in the diagnosis and management of neurological, neurodevelopmental, medical, and psychiatric disorders. Cogn Behav Neurol 24(3):107–114, 2011 21945982

Bräunig P, Krüger S, Shugar G, et al: The catatonia rating scale I: development, reliability, and use. Compr Psychiatry 41(2):147–158, 2000 10741894

Breakey WR, Kala AK: Typhoid catatonia responsive to ECT. BMJ 2(6083):357–359, 1977 890296

Briggs GG, Towers CV, Forinash AB: Briggs Drugs in Pregnancy and Lactation: A Reference Guide to Fetal and Neonatal Risk, 12th Edition. Philadelphia, PA, Wolters Kluwer Health, 2022

Briggs MC, Pasculli RM, Bryson EO, et al: Troponins and electroconvulsive therapy (ECT): caution in reporting results. Am J Med 124(11):e11, author reply e13, 2011 21722866

Bright-Long LE, Fink M: Reversible dementia and affective disorder: the Rip Van Winkle syndrome. Convuls Ther 9(3):209–216, 1993 11941215

Brill NQ, Crumpton E, Eiduson S, et al: An experimental study of the relative effectiveness of various components of electro-convulsive therapy. Am J Psychiatry 115(8):734–735, 1959a 13617504

Brill NQ, Crumpton E, Eiduson S, et al: Predictive and concomitant variables related to improvement with actual and simulated ECT. AMA Arch Gen Psychiatry 1:263–272, 1959b 13804440

Brill NQ, Crumpton E, Eiduson S, et al: Relative effectiveness of various components of electroconvulsive therapy; an experimental study. AMA Arch Neurol Psychiatry 81(5):627–635, 1959c 13636530

Brimacombe JR, Berry AM: Cricoid pressure. Can J Anaesth 44(4):414–425, 1997 9104526

Broadbent DE, Cooper PF, FitzGerald P, et al: The cognitive failures questionnaire (CFQ) and its correlates. Br J Clin Psychol 21(1):1–16, 1982 7126941

Bross RB: Near fatality with combined ECT and reserpine. Am J Psychiatry 113(10):933, 1957 13402992

Brown JC: An Interventional Psychiatry Track. Am J Psychiatry Resid J 15(1):11–14, 2019 32467864

Brown NI, Mack PF, Mitera DM, et al: Use of the ProSeal laryngeal mask airway in a pregnant patient with a difficult airway during electroconvulsive therapy. Br J Anaesth 91(5):752–754, 2003 14570805

Brown SK, Nowlin RB, Sartorelli R, et al: Patient experience of electroconvulsive therapy: a retrospective review of clinical outcomes and satisfaction. J ECT 34(4):240–246, 2018 29613943

Bruce BB, Henry ME, Greer DM: Ischemic stroke after electroconvulsive therapy. J ECT 22(2):150–152, 2006 16801834

Bruce EM, Crone N, Fitzpatrick G, et al: A comparative trial of ECT and tofranil. Am J Psychiatry 117:76–80, 1960 13805124

Brunoni AR, Moffa AH, Sampaio-Junior B, et al: Trial of electrical direct-current therapy versus escitalopram for depression. N Engl J Med 376(26):2523–2533, 2017 28657871

Brus O, Cao Y, Gustafsson E, et al: Self-assessed remission rates after electroconvulsive therapy of depressive disorders. Eur Psychiatry 45:154–160, 2017 28865389

Brus O, Cao Y, Hammar Å, et al: Lithium for suicide and readmission prevention after electroconvulsive therapy for unipolar depression: population-based register study. BJPsych Open 5(3):e46, 2019 31189487

Bryden M: Laterality: Functional Asymmetry in the Intact Brain. New York, Academic Press, 1982

Bryden MP, Steenhuis RE: Issues in the assessment of handedness, in Cerebral Laterality: Theory and Research. Edited by Kitterle FL. Hillsdale, NJ, Erlbaum, 1991, pp 35–51

Bryson A, Gardner H, Wilson I, et al: Temporal lobe epilepsy following maintenance electroconvulsive therapy: electrical kindling in the human brain? Epilepsia 57(11):e216–e220, 2016 27666327

Bryson EO, Aloysi AS: A strategy for management of ECT patients during the COVID-19 pandemic. J ECT 36(3):149–151, 2020 32826544

Bryson EO, Aloysi AS, Popeo DM, et al: Methohexital and succinylcholine dosing for electroconvulsive therapy (ECT): actual versus ideal. J ECT 28(3):e29–e30, 2012a 22914634

Bryson EO, Popeo DM, Kellner CH: Electroconvulsive therapy (ECT) after pulmonary edema. J ECT 28(2):e25–e26, 2012b 22622302

Bryson EO, Popeo D, Briggs M, et al: Electroconvulsive therapy (ECT) in patients with cardiac disease: hemodynamic changes. J ECT 29(1):76–77, 2013 23422523

Bryson EO, Aloysi AS, Farber KG, et al: Individualized anesthetic management for patients undergoing electroconvulsive therapy: a review of current practice. Anesth Analg 124(6):1943–1956, 2017 28277323

Buchan H, Johnstone E, McPherson K, et al: Who benefits from electroconvulsive therapy? Combined results of the Leicester and Northwick Park trials. Br J Psychiatry 160:355–359, 1992 1562861

Buday J, Albrecht J, Mareš T, et al: Brain tumors and electroconvulsive therapy: a literature overview of the last 80 years. Front Neurol 11:723, 2020a 32849199

Buday J, Albrecht J, Mareš T, et al: A case report of pulmonary embolism during electroconvulsive therapy and its further application after somatic stabilization. Brain Stimul 13(1):250–252, 2020b 31558373

Bukowski N, Laurin A, Laforgue EJ, et al: Efficacy and safety of electroconvulsive therapy in patients with deep brain stimulation: literature review, case report for patient with essential tremor, and practical recommendations. J ECT 38(3):e29–e40, 2022 36018735

Bulbena A, Berrios GE: Pseudodementia: facts and figures. Br J Psychiatry 148:87–94, 1986 3955324

Burke MJ, Husain MM: Concomitant use of vagus nerve stimulation and electroconvulsive therapy for treatment-resistant depression. J ECT 22(3):218–222, 2006 16957540

Burke WJ, Rutherford JL, Zorumski CF, et al: Electroconvulsive therapy and the elderly. Compr Psychiatry 26(5):480–486, 1985 4028698

Burke WJ, Rubin EH, Zorumski CF, et al: The safety of ECT in geriatric psychiatry. J Am Geriatr Soc 35(6):516–521, 1987 3571804

Burns CM, Stuart GW: Nursing care in electroconvulsive therapy. Psychiatr Clin North Am 14(4):971–988, 1991 1771158

Bush G, Fink M, Petrides G, et al: Catatonia. I. Rating scale and standardized examination. Acta Psychiatr Scand 93(2):129–136, 1996a 8686483

Bush G, Fink M, Petrides G, et al: Catatonia. II. Treatment with lorazepam and electroconvulsive therapy. Acta Psychiatr Scand 93(2):137–143, 1996b 8686484

Bushnell DM, McCarrier KP, Bush EN, et al: Symptoms of Major Depressive Disorder Scale: performance of a novel patient-reported symptom measure. Value Health 22(8):906–915, 2019 31426932

Butterfield NN, Graf P, Macleod BA, et al: Propofol reduces cognitive impairment after electroconvulsive therapy. J ECT 20(1):3–9, 2004 15087989

Butters MA, Becker JT, Nebes RD, et al: Changes in cognitive functioning following treatment of late-life depression. Am J Psychiatry 157(12):1949–1954, 2000 11097959

Butters MA, Young JB, Lopez O, et al: Pathways linking late-life depression to persistent cognitive impairment and dementia. Dialogues Clin Neurosci 10(3):345–357, 2008 18979948

Butters N, Albert M: Processes underlying failures to recall remote events, in Human Memory and Amnesia. Edited by Cermak L. Hillsdale, NJ, Erlbaum, 1982, pp 257–274

Cabrera JL, Auerbach JS, Merelman AH, et al: The high-risk airway. Emerg Med Clin North Am 38(2):401–417, 2020 32336333

Calarge CA, Crowe RR: Electroconvulsive therapy in myasthenia gravis. Ann Clin Psychiatry 16(4):225–227, 2004 15702571

Calarge CA, Crowe RR, Gergis SD, et al: The comparative effects of sevoflurane and methohexital for electroconvulsive therapy. J ECT 19(4):221–225, 2003 14657775

Calaway K, Coshal S, Jones K, et al: A systematic review of the safety of electroconvulsive therapy use during the first trimester of pregnancy. J ECT 32(4):230–235, 2016 27327556

Calev A, Cohen R, Tubi N, et al: Disorientation and bilateral moderately suprathreshold ECT. Convuls Ther 7(2):99–110, 1991a 11941109

Calev A, Kochav-Lev E, Tubi N, et al: Change in attitude toward electroconvulsive therapy: effects of treatment, time since treatment, and severity of depression. Convuls Ther 7(3):184–189, 1991b 11941121

Calev A, Fink M, Petrides G, et al: Caffeine pretreatment enhances clinical efficacy and reduces cognitive effects of electroconvulsive therapy. Convuls Ther 9(2):95–100, 1993 11941197

Calev A, Gaudino EA, Squires NK, et al: ECT and non-memory cognition: a review. Br J Clin Psychol 34(4):505–515, 1995 8563658

Caliyurt O, Tuglu C, Vardar E: Aortic aneurysm and electroconvulsive therapy in elderly depressive patient. J ECT 19(4):242–244, 2003 14657780

Canbek O, Ipekcıoglu D, Menges OO, et al: Comparison of propofol, etomidate, and thiopental in anesthesia for electroconvulsive therapy: a randomized, double-blind clinical trial. J ECT 31(2):91–97, 2015 25268043

Caracci G, Decina P: Fluoxetine and prolonged seizure. Convuls Ther 7(2):145–147, 1991 11941116

Cardwell BA, Nakai B: Seizure activity in combined clozapine and ECT: a retrospective view. Convuls Ther 11(2):110–113, 1995 7552049

Carmi L, Tendler A, Bystritsky A, et al: Efficacy and safety of deep transcranial magnetic stimulation for obsessive-compulsive disorder: a prospective multicenter randomized double-blind placebo-controlled trial. Am J Psychiatry 176(11):931–938, 2019 31109199

Carney MW, Roth M, Garside RF: The diagnosis of depressive syndromes and the prediction of ECT response. Br J Psychiatry 111:659–674, 1965 14337413

Carney MW, Rogan PA, Sebastian J, et al: A controlled comparative trial of unilateral and bilateral sinusoidal and pulse E.C.T. in endogenous depression. PDM 7(1–8):77–79, 1976 1052834

Carr ME Jr, Woods JW: Electroconvulsive therapy in a patient with unsuspected pheochromocytoma. South Med J 78(5):613–615, 1985 3992309

Carroll BT, Graham KT, Thalassinos AJ: A common pathogenesis of the serotonin syndrome, catatonia, and neuroleptic malignant syndrome. J Neuropsychiatry 13:150, 2001

Carrozzino D, Patierno C, Fava GA, et al: The Hamilton Rating Scales for Depression: a critical review of clinimetric properties of different versions. Psychother Psychosom 89(3):133–150, 2020 32289809

Cassano P, Petrie SR, Mischoulon D, et al: Transcranial photobiomodulation for the treatment of major depressive disorder: the ELATED-2 Pilot Trial. Photomed Laser Surg 36(12):634–646, 2018 30346890

Castaneda-Ramirez S, Becker TD, Bruges-Boude A, et al: Systematic review: electroconvulsive therapy for treatment-resistant mood disorders in children and adolescents. Eur Child Adolesc Psychiatry 32(9):1529–1560, 2023 34999973

Caudill GB, Rosenquist P, McCall WV: Could monoamine oxidase inhibitors promote asystole in electroconvulsive therapy patients? J ECT 27(3):264–265, 2011 21865961

Cella D, Riley W, Stone A, et al: The Patient-Reported Outcomes Measurement Information System (PROMIS) developed and tested its first wave of adult self-reported health outcome item banks: 2005–2008. J Clin Epidemiol 63(11):1179–1194, 2010 20685078

Centanni NR, Craig WY, Whitesell DL, et al: Safety of ECT in patients receiving an oral anticoagulant. Ment Health Clin 11(4):254–258, 2021 34316422

Centers for Disease Control and Prevention: Infection Control: Guidelines and Guidance Library. Available at: www.cdc.gov/infectioncontrol/guidelines/index.html. Accessed April 25, 2022.

Chacko M, Job A, Caston F III, et al: COVID-19-induced psychosis and suicidal behavior: case report. SN Compr Clin Med 2(11):2391–2395, 2020 33015547

Chai-Adisaksopha C, Crowther M, Isayama T, et al: The impact of bleeding complications in patients receiving target-specific oral anticoagulants: a systematic review and meta-analysis. Blood 124(15):2450–2458, 2014 25150296

Chakrabarti N, Basu A, Das D, et al: Attitudes towards electroconvulsive therapy among nonpsychiatrist medical graduates and postgraduates. J ECT 19(3):177–178, 2003 12972990

Chan P, Waxman RE, Woo S, et al: Electroconvulsive therapy for neuropsychiatric symptoms due to major neurocognitive disorder: a prospective, observational study. J ECT 38(2):81–87, 2022 35613007

Chang JC, Davis AM, Klein-Gitelman MS, et al: Impact of psychiatric diagnosis and treatment on medication adherence in youth with systemic lupus erythematosus. Arthritis Care Res (Hoboken) 73(1):30–38, 2021 32937032

Chanpattana W: Maintenance ECT in schizophrenia: a pilot study. J Med Assoc Thai 81(1):17–24, 1998 9470317

Chanpattana W: Combined ECT and clozapine in treatment-resistant mania. J ECT 16(2):204–207, 2000 10868331

Chanpattana W, Andrade C: ECT for treatment-resistant schizophrenia: a response from the far East to the UK. NICE report. J ECT 22(1):4–12, 2006 16633199

Chanpattana W, Sackeim HA: Electroconvulsive therapy in treatment-resistant schizophrenia: prediction of response and the nature of symptomatic improvement. J ECT 26(4):289–298, 2010 20375701

Chanpattana W, Chakrabhand ML, Kongsakon R, et al: Short-term effect of combined ECT and neuroleptic therapy in treatment-resistant schizophrenia. J ECT 15(2):129–139, 1999a 10378152

Chanpattana W, Chakrabhand ML, Sackeim HA, et al: Continuation ECT in treatment-resistant schizophrenia: a controlled study. J ECT 15(3):178–192, 1999b 10492856

Chathanchirayil SJ, Bhat R: Post-electroconvulsive therapy status epilepticus and tardive seizure in a patient with rapid cycling bipolar disorder, epilepsy, and intellectual disability. J ECT 28(3):183–184, 2012 22868490

Chawla N: Anesthesia for electroconvulsive therapy. Anesthesiol Clin 38(1):183–195, 2020 32008651

Chen JJ, Zhao LB, Liu YY, et al: Comparative efficacy and acceptability of electroconvulsive therapy versus repetitive transcranial magnetic stimulation for major depression: a systematic review and multiple-treatments meta-analysis. Behav Brain Res 320:30–36, 2017 27876667

Chen L, Peterson E, Wong G, et al: Safe and successful treatment of depression with electroconvulsive therapy in a patient with implanted spinal cord stimulators. Brain Stimul 13(4):955–956, 2020 32278713

Chen P, Ganguli M, Mulsant BH, et al: The temporal relationship between depressive symptoms and dementia: a community-based prospective study. Arch Gen Psychiatry 56(3):261–266, 1999 10078504

Cheney CO, Drewry PH: Results of nonspecific treatment in dementia praecox. Am J Psychiatry 95:203–217, 1938

Chessen DH, Geha DG, Salzman C: ECT, glaucoma, and prolonged apnea. Dis Nerv Syst 35(4):152–153, 1974 17894110

Chiao S, Isenberg K, North CS: Psychotropic medication effects on seizure threshold and seizure duration during electroconvulsive therapy stimulus titration. J ECT 36(2):115–122, 2020 31609275

Childers RT Jr: Comparison of four regimens in newly admitted female schizophrenics. Am J Psychiatry 120:1010–1011, 1964 14138834

Chou KL, Hurtig HI, Jaggi JL, et al: Electroconvulsive therapy for depression in a Parkinson's disease patient with bilateral subthalamic nucleus deep brain stimulators. Parkinsonism Relat Disord 11(6):403–406, 2005 15994113

Christensen P, Kragh-Sørensen P, Sørensen C, et al: EEG-monitored ECT: a comparison of seizure duration under anesthesia with etomidate and thiopentone. Convuls Ther 2(3):145–150, 1986 11940860

Christensen STJ, Staalsø JM, Jørgensen A, et al: Electro convulsive therapy: modification of its effect on the autonomic nervous system using anti-cholinergic drugs. Psychiatry Res 271:239–246, 2019 30504059

Christopher EJ: Electroconvulsive therapy in the medically ill. Curr Psychiatry Rep 5(3):225–230, 2003 12773277

Chrobak AA, Siwek M, Dudek D, et al: Content overlap analysis of 64 (hypo)mania symptoms among seven common rating scales. Int J Methods Psychiatr Res 27(3):e1737, 2018 30058102

Ciapparelli A, Dell'Osso L, Tundo A, et al: Electroconvulsive therapy in medication-nonresponsive patients with mixed mania and bipolar depression. J Clin Psychiatry 62(7):552–555, 2001 11488367

Cicala G, Barbieri MA, Spina E, et al: A comprehensive review of swallowing difficulties and dysphagia associated with antipsychotics in adults. Expert Rev Clin Pharmacol 12(3):219–234, 2019 30700161

Cinderella MA, Nichols NA, Munjal S, et al: Antiepileptics in electroconvulsive therapy: a mechanism-based review of recent literature. J ECT 38(2):133–137, 2022 34739420

Cipriani A, Furukawa TA, Salanti G, et al: Comparative efficacy and acceptability of 21 antidepressant drugs for the acute treatment of adults with major depressive disorder: a systematic review and network meta-analysis. Lancet 391(10128):1357–1366, 2018 29477251

Clarke TB, Coffey CE, Hoffman GW Jr, et al: Continuation therapy for depression using outpatient electroconvulsive therapy. Convuls Ther 5(4):330–337, 1989 11941031

Clinical Research Centre: The Northwick Park ECT trial: predictors of response to real and simulated ECT. Clinical Research Centre, Division of Psychiatry. Br J Psychiatry 144:227–237, 1984 6367874

Cloutier AA, Seiner SJ, Solomon HV, et al: Treatment of electroconvulsive therapy-emergent hypomania and mania: a systematic review of the literature. J Clin Psychiatry 83(1):21r13911, 2021 34792870

Cochlear: Cochlear: Nucleus Hybrid L24 Cochlear Implant (CI24REH): Patient Information. Available at: https://mss-p-007-delivery.sitecorecontenthub.cloud/api/public/content/82db5a4a1d58481fa44a01bbaa15ceee?v=62698c39. Accessed May 12, 2022.

Cochran M, DeBattista C, Schmiesing C, et al: Negative-pressure pulmonary edema: a potential hazard in patients undergoing ECT. J ECT 15(2):168–170, 1999 10378160

Code of Federal Regulations: 21 CFR 882.5800. September 29, 2022. Available at: www.ecfr.gov/current/title-21/chapter-I/subchapter-H/part-882/subpart-F/section-882.5800. Accessed October 1, 2022.

Coenen VA, Bewernick BH, Kayser S, et al: Superolateral medial forebrain bundle deep brain stimulation in major depression: a gateway trial. Neuropsychopharmacology 44(7):1224–1232, 2019 30867553

Coffey CE: Brain morphology in primary mood disorders: implications for electroconvulsive therapy. Psychiatr Ann 26:713–716, 1996

Coffey CE: The Institute of Medicine's "Quality Chasm" Report: implications for ECT care. J ECT 19(1):1–3, 2003 12621269

Coffey CE, Weiner RD, Kalayjian R, et al: Electroconvulsive therapy in osteogenesis imperfecta: issues of muscular relaxation. Convuls Ther 2(3):207–211, 1986 11940868

Coffey CE, Hinkle PE, Weiner RD, et al: Electroconvulsive therapy of depression in patients with white matter hyperintensity. Biol Psychiatry 22(5):629–636, 1987a 3580437

Coffey CE, Hoffman G, Weiner RD, et al: Electroconvulsive therapy in a depressed patient with a functioning ventriculoatrial shunt. Convuls Ther 3(4):302–306, 1987b 11940933

Coffey CE, Weiner RD, Hinkle PE, et al: Augmentation of ECT seizures with caffeine. Biol Psychiatry 22(5):637–649, 1987c 3580438

Coffey CE, Weiner RD, McCall WV, et al: Electroconvulsive therapy in multiple sclerosis: a magnetic resonance imaging study of the brain. Convuls Ther 3(2):137–144, 1987d 11940906

Coffey CE, Figiel GS, Weiner RD, et al: Caffeine augmentation of ECT. Am J Psychiatry 147(5):579–585, 1990 2183632

Coffey CE, Lucke J, Weiner RD, et al: Seizure threshold in electroconvulsive therapy: I. Initial seizure threshold. Biol Psychiatry 37(10):713–720, 1995a 7640326

Coffey CE, Lucke J, Weiner RD, et al: Seizure threshold in electroconvulsive therapy (ECT) II. The anticonvulsant effect of ECT. Biol Psychiatry 37(11):777–788, 1995b 7647162

Coffey RJ, Caroff SN: Commentary on the continued investigational status of DBS for psychiatric indications. Stereotact Funct Neurosurg 100(3):156–167, 2022 35104827

Cohen D, Paillère-Martinot ML, Basquin M: Use of electroconvulsive therapy in adolescents. Convuls Ther 13(1):25–31, 1997 9152585

Cohen D, Taieb O, Flament M, et al: Absence of cognitive impairment at long-term follow-up in adolescents treated with ECT for severe mood disorder. Am J Psychiatry 157(3):460–462, 2000 10698827

Cohen LS, Altshuler LL, Harlow BL, et al: Relapse of major depression during pregnancy in women who maintain or discontinue antidepressant treatment. JAMA 295(5):499–507, 2006 16449615

Cole EJ, Stimpson KH, Bentzley BS, et al: Stanford Accelerated Intelligent Neuromodulation Therapy for treatment-resistant depression. Am J Psychiatry 177(8):716–726, 2020 32252538

Cole EJ, Phillips AL, Bentzley BS, et al: Stanford Neuromodulation Therapy (SNT): a double-blind randomized controlled trial. Am J Psychiatry 179(2):132–141, 2022 34711062

Coleman EA, Sackeim HA, Prudic J, et al: Subjective memory complaints prior to and following electroconvulsive therapy. Biol Psychiatry 39(5):346–356, 1996 8704066

Colenda CC, McCall WV: A statistical model predicting the seizure threshold for right unilateral ECT in 106 patients. Convuls Ther 12(1):3–12, 1996 8777650

Conklin M, Nussbaum AM: Electroconvulsive therapy for depression in patient with implanted spinal cord stimulator. J ECT 37(2):e22–e23, 2021 34029307

Connell J, Oldham M, Pandharipande P, et al: Malignant catatonia: a review for the intensivist. J Intensive Care Med 38(2):137–150, 2023 35861966

Consensus Conference: Electroconvulsive therapy. JAMA 254(15):2103–2108, 1985 4046138

Consoli A, Benmiloud M, Wachtel L, et al: Electroconvulsive therapy in adolescents with the catatonia syndrome: efficacy and ethics. J ECT 26(4):259–265, 2010 21099377

Conway CR, Nelson LA: The combined use of bupropion, lithium, and venlafaxine during ECT: a case of prolonged seizure activity. J ECT 17(3):216–218, 2001 11528316

Conway CR, Udaiyar A, Schachter SC: Neurostimulation for depression in epilepsy. Epilepsy Behav 88S:25–32, 2018 30558717

Cook D, Simons DJ: Neuromuscular Blockade. Treasure Island, FL, StatPearls Publishing, 2021

Cooper JJ, Wachtel A, Redleaf M: Electroconvulsive therapy in the presence of an auditory osseointegrated implant. J ECT 35(2):e9, 2019 30095556

Copersino ML, Long MP, Bolton P, et al: First acute-course electroconvulsive therapy for moderate-to-severe depression benefits patients with or without accompanying baseline cognitive impairment. J ECT 38(2):74–80, 2022 34966040

Coryell W, Zimmerman M: Outcome following ECT for primary unipolar depression: a test of newly proposed response predictors. Am J Psychiatry 141(7):862–867, 1984 6731634

Coryell W, Pfohl B, Zimmerman M: Outcome following electroconvulsive therapy: a comparison of primary and secondary depression. Convuls Ther 1(1):10–14, 1985 11940800

Coshal S, Jones K, Coverdale J, et al: An overview of reviews on the safety of electroconvulsive therapy administered during pregnancy. J Psychiatr Pract 25(1):2–6, 2019 30633726

Craighead WE, Evans DD: Factor analysis of the Montgomery-Asberg Depression Rating Scale. Depression 4(1):31–33, 1996 9160651

Crismon ML, Trivedi M, Pigott TA, et al: The Texas Medication Algorithm Project: report of the Texas Consensus Conference Panel on Medication Treatment of Major Depressive Disorder. J Clin Psychiatry 60(3):142–156, 1999 10192589

Cristancho MA, Alici Y, Augoustides JG, et al: Uncommon but serious complications associated with electroconvulsive therapy: recognition and management for the clinician. Curr Psychiatry Rep 10(6):474–480, 2008 18980730

Cristancho MA, Helmer A, Connolly R, et al: Transcranial magnetic stimulation maintenance as a substitute for maintenance electroconvulsive therapy: a case series. J ECT 29(2):106–108, 2013 23519219

Cronemeyer M, Schönfeldt-Lecuona C, Gahr M, et al: Malignant catatonia: severity, treatment and outcome—a systematic case series analysis. World J Biol Psychiatry 23(1):78–86, 2022 33949287

Cronholm B, Ottosson J-O: The experience of memory function after electroconvulsive therapy. Br J Psychiatry 109:251–258, 1963 14023959

Crow S, Meller W, Christenson G, et al: Use of ECT after brain injury. Convuls Ther 12(2):113–116, 1996 8744172

Crowe RR: Current concepts: electroconvulsive therapy—a current perspective. N Engl J Med 311(3):163–167, 1984 6377069

Crowe S, Collins L: Suxamethonium and donepezil: a cause of prolonged paralysis. Anesthesiology 98(2):574–575, 2003 12552219

Crowell AL, Riva-Posse P, Holtzheimer PE, et al: Long-term outcomes of subcallosal cingulate deep brain stimulation for treatment-resistant depression. Am J Psychiatry 176(11):949–956, 2019 31581800

Crozier TA, Flamm C, Speer CP, et al: Effects of etomidate on the adrenocortical and metabolic adaptation of the neonate. Br J Anaesth 70(1):47–53, 1993 8431333

Cui Y, Fang H, Bao C, et al: Efficacy of transcranial magnetic stimulation for reducing suicidal ideation in depression: a meta-analysis. Front Psychiatry 12:764183, 2022 35115959

Culver CM, Ferrell RB, Green RM: ECT and special problems of informed consent. Am J Psychiatry 137(5):586–591, 1980 7369404

Cumper SK, Ahle GM, Liebman LS, et al: Electroconvulsive therapy (ECT) in Parkinson's disease: ECS and dopamine enhancement. J ECT 30(2):122–124, 2014 24810775

Cunningham SJ, Anderson DN: Delusional depression, hyperparathyroidism, and ECT. Convuls Ther 11(2):129–133, 1995 7552053

Currier GE, Cullinan C, Rothschild D: Results of treatment of schizophrenia in a state hospital; changing trends since advent of electroshock therapy. AMA Arch Neurol Psychiatry 67(1):80–88, 1952 14877356

Cusin C, Franco FB, Fernandez-Robles C, et al: Rapid improvement of depression and psychotic symptoms in Huntington's disease: a retrospective chart review of seven patients treated with electroconvulsive therapy. Gen Hosp Psychiatry 35(6):678.e3–678.e5, 2013 23541803

Dalmau J, Gleichman AJ, Hughes EG, et al: Anti-NMDA-receptor encephalitis: case series and analysis of the effects of antibodies. Lancet Neurol 7(12):1091–1098, 2008 18851928

Damkier P, Kaplan YC, Shechtman S, et al: Ondansetron in pregnancy revisited: assessment and pregnancy labelling by the European Medicines Agency (EMA) & Pharmacovigilance Risk Assessment Committee (PRAC). Basic Clin Pharmacol Toxicol 128(4):579–582, 2021 33275828

d'Andrea G, Mancusi G, Santovito MC, et al: Investigating the role of maintenance TMS protocols for major depression: systematic review and future perspectives for personalized interventions. J Pers Med 13(4):697, 2023 37109083

Daniel WF, Crovitz HF: Recovery of orientation after electroconvulsive therapy. Acta Psychiatr Scand 66(6):421–428, 1982 7180562

Daniel WF, Crovitz HF: Acute memory impairment following electroconvulsive therapy. 2. Effects of electrode placement. Acta Psychiatr Scand 67(2):57–68, 1983 6846039

Daniel WF, Crovitz HF: Disorientation during electroconvulsive therapy: technical, theoretical, and neuropsychological issues. Ann N Y Acad Sci 462:293–306, 1986 3458410

Danziger L, Kindwall JA: Prediction of the immediate outcome of shock therapy in dementia praecox. Dis Nerv Syst 7:299–303, 1946 20999123

Daskalakis ZJ, Dimitrova J, McClintock SM, et al: Magnetic seizure therapy (MST) for major depressive disorder. Neuropsychopharmacology 45(2):276–282, 2020 31486777

Davidson J: Seizures and bupropion: a review. J Clin Psychiatry 50(7):256–261, 1989 2500425

Davidson J, McLeod M, Law-Yone B, et al: A comparison of electroconvulsive therapy and combined phenelzine-amitriptyline in refractory depression. Arch Gen Psychiatry 35(5):639–642, 1978 727903

Davis JM, Janicak PG, Sakkas P, et al: Electroconvulsive therapy in the treatment of the neuroleptic malignant syndrome. Convuls Ther 7(2):111–120, 1991 11941110

Dazzi F, Shafer A, Lauriola M: Meta-analysis of the Brief Psychiatric Rating Scale–Expanded (BPRS-E) structure and arguments for a new version. J Psychiatr Res 81:140–151, 2016 27451107

Dean J, Coconcea C: Electroconvulsive therapy in a patient with pulmonary embolism: a case report. J ECT 32(3):e12, 2016 26934276

de A Simoes Moreira D, Gauer LE, Teixeira G, et al: Efficacy and adverse effects of ketamine versus electroconvulsive therapy for major depressive disorder: a systematic review and meta-analysis. J Affect Disord 330:227–238, 2023 36907464

DeBattista C, Mueller K: Sumatriptan prophylaxis for postelectroconvulsive therapy headaches. Headache 35(8):502–503, 1995 7591748

Decina P, Malitz S, Sackeim HA, et al: Cardiac arrest during ECT modified by beta-adrenergic blockade. Am J Psychiatry 141(2):298–300, 1984 6691502

Decina P, Guthrie EB, Sackeim HA, et al: Continuation ECT in the management of relapses of major affective episodes. Acta Psychiatr Scand 75(6):559–562, 1987 3618276

Delamarre L, Galvao F, Gohier B, et al: How much do benzodiazepines matter for electroconvulsive therapy in patients with major depression? J ECT 35(3):184–188, 2019 30720551

de la Serna E, Flamarique I, Castro-Fornieles J, et al: Two-year follow-up of cognitive functions in schizophrenia spectrum disorders of adolescent patients treated with electroconvulsive therapy. J Child Adolesc Psychopharmacol 21(6):611–619, 2011 22136098 d'Elia G: Unilateral electroconvulsive therapy. Acta Psychiatr Scand Suppl 215:1–98, 1970 5271208

d'Elia G: Electrode placement and antidepressant efficacy. Convuls Ther 8(4):294–296, 1992 11941182

Delis DC, Kramer JH, Kaplan E, et al: California Verbal Learning Test-Third Edition (CVLT-3). Bloomington, MN, NCS Pearson, 2017

Deng ZD, Lisanby SH, Peterchev AV: Electric field strength and focality in electroconvulsive therapy and magnetic seizure therapy: a finite element simulation study. J Neural Eng 8(1):016007, 2011 21248385

Deng ZD, Liston C, Gunning FM, et al: Electric field modeling for transcranial magnetic stimulation and electroconvulsive therapy, in Brain and Human Body Modeling: Computational Human Modeling at EMBC 2018. Edited by Makarov SN, Horner M, Noetscher GM. Cham, Switzerland, Springer Nature, 2019, pp 75–84

Denysenko L, Sica N, Penders TM, et al: Catatonia in the medically ill: etiology, diagnosis, and treatment. Ann Clin Psychiatry 30(2):140–155, 2018 29697715

Deocleciano de Araujo C, Schlittler LXC, Sguario RM, et al: Life-threatening catatonia associated with coronavirus disease 2019. J Acad Consult Liaison Psychiatry 62(2):256–257, 2021 33223217

Derikx RL, van Waarde JA, Verwey B, et al: Effects on intracranial pressure of electroconvulsive therapy. J ECT 28(2):e23–e24, 2012 22622301

Dersch R, Zwernemann S, Voderholzer U: Partial status epilepticus after electroconvulsive therapy and medical treatment with bupropion. Pharmacopsychiatry 44(7):344–346, 2011 21979924

DeToledo JC, Minagar A, Lowe MR: Lidocaine-induced seizures in patients with history of epilepsy: effect of antiepileptic drugs. Anesthesiology 97(3):737–739, 2002 12218544

Detweiler MB, Mehra A, Rowell T, et al: Delirious mania and malignant catatonia: a report of 3 cases and review. Psychiatr Q 80(1):23–40, 2009 19199033

Devanand DP, Sackeim HA: Seizure elicitation blocked by pretreatment with lidocaine. Convuls Ther 4(3):225–229, 1988 11940969

Devanand DP, Sackeim HA: Use of increased anesthetic dose prior to electroconvulsive therapy to prevent postictal excitement. Gen Hosp Psychiatry 14(5):345–349, 1992 1521790

Devanand DP, Decina P, Sackeim HA, et al: Status epilepticus following ECT in a patient receiving theophylline. J Clin Psychopharmacol 8(2):153, 1988a 3372714

Devanand DP, Sackeim HA, Decina P, et al: The development of mania and organic euphoria during ECT. J Clin Psychiatry 49(2):69–71, 1988b 3338979

Devanand DP, Briscoe KM, Sackeim HA: Clinical features and predictors of postictal excitement. Convuls Ther 5(2):140–146, 1989 11941004

Devanand DP, Verma AK, Tirumalasetti F, et al: Absence of cognitive impairment after more than 100 lifetime ECT treatments. Am J Psychiatry 148(7):929–932, 1991 2053635

Devanand DP, Prudic J, Sackeim HA: Electroconvulsive therapy–induced hypomania is uncommon. Convuls Ther 8(4):296–298, 1992 11941183

Devanand DP, Dwork AJ, Hutchinson ER, et al: Does ECT alter brain structure? Am J Psychiatry 151(7):957–970, 1994 8010381

Devanand DP, Fitzsimons L, Prudic J, et al: Subjective side effects during electroconvulsive therapy. Convuls Ther 11(4):232–240, 1995 8919573

Devanand DP, Sano M, Tang MX, et al: Depressed mood and the incidence of Alzheimer's disease in the elderly living in the community. Arch Gen Psychiatry 53(2):175–182, 1996 8629893

Devanand DP, Lisanby SH, Nobler MS, et al: The relative efficiency of altering pulse frequency or train duration when determining seizure threshold. J ECT 14(4):227–235, 1998 9871842

Devanand DP, Polanco P, Cruz R, et al: The efficacy of ECT in mixed affective states. J ECT 16(1):32–37, 2000 10735329

Devinsky O, Duchowny MS: Seizures after convulsive therapy: a retrospective case survey. Neurology 33(7):921–925, 1983 6683376

de Vreede IM, Burger H, van Vliet IM: Prediction of response to ECT with routinely collected data in major depression. J Affect Disord 86(2-3):323–327, 2005 15935255

De Wet JST: Evaluation of a common method of convulsion therapy in Bantu schizophrenics. J Ment Sci 103(433):739–757, 1957 13481585

Dhossche DM, Withane N: Electroconvulsive therapy for catatonia in children and adolescents. Child Adolesc Psychiatr Clin N Am 28(1):111–120, 2019 30389071

Dhossche DM, Shettar SM, Kumar T, et al: Electroconvulsive therapy for malignant catatonia in adolescence. South Med J 102(11):1170–1172, 2009 19864990

Diener HC: The risks or lack thereof of migraine treatments in vascular disease. Headache 60(3):649–653, 2020 31967337

Dierckx B, Heijnen WT, van den Broek WW, et al: Efficacy of electroconvulsive therapy in bipolar versus unipolar major depression: a meta-analysis. Bipolar Disord 14(2):146–150, 2012 22420590

Dighe-Deo D, Shah A: Electroconvulsive therapy in patients with long bone fractures. J ECT 14(2):115–119, 1998 9641808

Dillon AE, Wagner CL, Wiest D, et al: Drug therapy in the nursing mother. Obstet Gynecol Clin North Am 24(3):675–696, 1997 9266586

Dillon P: Electroconvulsive therapy patient/family education. Convuls Ther 11(3):188–191, 1995 8528662

Dinan TG, Barry S: A comparison of electroconvulsive therapy with a combined lithium and tricyclic combination among depressed tricyclic nonresponders. Acta Psychiatr Scand 80(1):97–100, 1989 2504034

Dinur-Klein L, Dannon P, Hadar A, et al: Smoking cessation induced by deep repetitive transcranial magnetic stimulation of the prefrontal and insular cortices: a prospective, randomized controlled trial. Biol Psychiatry 76(9):742–749, 2014 25038985

Dinwiddie SH, Spitz D: Resident education in electroconvulsive therapy. J ECT 26(4):310–316, 2010 20357669

Dinwiddie SH, Drevets WC, Smith DR: Treatment of phencyclidine-associated psychosis with ECT. Convuls Ther 4(3):230–235, 1988 11940970

Dinwiddie SH, Huo D, Gottlieb O: The course of myalgia and headache after electroconvulsive therapy. J ECT 26(2):116–120, 2010 19710619

Dodick DW, Shewale AS, Lipton RB, et al: Migraine patients with cardiovascular disease and contraindications: an analysis of real-world claims data. J Prim Care Community Health 11:2150132720963680, 2020 33095099

Dodwell D, Goldberg D: A study of factors associated with response to electroconvulsive therapy in patients with schizophrenic symptoms. Br J Psychiatry 154:635–639, 1989 2597856

Doering EB, Ball WA: Flumazenil before electroconvulsive therapy: outstanding issues. Anesthesiology 83(3):642–643, 1995 7661372

Dolenc TJ, Rasmussen KG: The safety of electroconvulsive therapy and lithium in combination: a case series and review of the literature. J ECT 21(3):165–170, 2005 16127306

Dolenc TJ, Barnes RD, Hayes DL, et al: Electroconvulsive therapy in patients with cardiac pacemakers and implantable cardioverter defibrillators. Pacing Clin Electrophysiol 27(9):1257–1263, 2004a 15461716

Dolenc TJ, Habl SS, Barnes RD, et al: Electroconvulsive therapy in patients taking monoamine oxidase inhibitors. J ECT 20(4):258–261, 2004b 15591861

Dolinski SY, Zvara DA: Anesthetic considerations of cardiovascular risk during electroconvulsive therapy. Convuls Ther 13(3):157–164, 1997 9342131

Dombrovski AY, Mulsant BH, Haskett RF, et al: Predictors of remission after electroconvulsive therapy in unipolar major depression. J Clin Psychiatry 66(8):1043–1049, 2005 16086621

Dominiak M, Antosik-Wójcińska AZ, Goetz Z, et al: Efficacy, safety and tolerability of formula-based unilateral vs bilateral electroconvulsive therapy in the treatment of major depression: a randomized open label controlled trial. J Psychiatr Res 133:52–59, 2021a 33310500

Dominiak M, Antosik-Wójcińska AZ, Wojnar M, et al: Electroconvulsive therapy and age: effectiveness, safety and tolerability in the treatment of major depression among patients under and over 65 years of age. Pharmaceuticals (Basel) 14(6):14, 2021b 34207157

Donahue AB: Electroconvulsive therapy and memory loss: a personal journey. J ECT 16(2):133–143, 2000 10868323

Donders J: The incremental value of neuropsychological assessment: a critical review. Clin Neuropsychol 34(1):56–87, 2020 31014166

Doongaji DR, Jeste DV, Saoji NJ, et al: Unilateral versus bilateral ECT in schizophrenia. Br J Psychiatry 123(572):73–79, 1973 4729877

Døssing E, Pagsberg AK: Electroconvulsive therapy in children and adolescents: a systematic review of current literature and guidelines. J ECT 37(3):158–170, 2021 34424874

Dougherty DD, Rezai AR, Carpenter LL, et al: A randomized sham-controlled trial of deep brain stimulation of the ventral capsule/ventral striatum for chronic treatment-resistant depression. Biol Psychiatry 78(4):240–248, 2015 25726497

Drop LJ, Welch CA: Anesthesia for electroconvulsive therapy in patients with major cardiovascular risk factors. Convuls Ther 5(1):88–101, 1989 11940998

D'Souza RS, Porter BR, Johnson RL: Nondepolarizing Paralytics. Treasure Island, FL, StatPearls Publishing, 2022

Dubin WR, Jaffe R, Roemer R, et al: The efficacy and safety of maintenance ECT in geriatric patients. J Am Geriatr Soc 40(7):706–709, 1992 1607587

Dubuc M, Li G, Tourjman SV: Electroconvulsive therapy after cataract surgery: a review of the literature and a report of 2 cases. J ECT 38(4):256–257, 2022 35462383

Dudley WH Jr, Williams JG: Electroconvulsive therapy in delirium tremens. Compr Psychiatry 13(4):357–360, 1972 5035611

Duffy FF, Chung H, Trivedi M, et al: Systematic use of patient-rated depression severity monitoring: is it helpful and feasible in clinical psychiatry? Psychiatr Serv 59(10):1148–1154, 2008 18832500

Duffy WJ Jr, Conradt H: Electroconvulsive therapy: the perioperative process. AORN J 50(4):806–812, 1989 2636866

Dukakis K, Tye L: Shock: The Healing Power of ECT. New York, Avery-Penguin, 2007

Duma A, Pal S, Johnston J, et al: High-sensitivity cardiac troponin elevation after electroconvulsive therapy: a prospective, observational cohort study. Anesthesiology 126(4):643–652, 2017 28166110

Duma A, Maleczek M, Panjikaran B, et al: Major adverse cardiac events and mortality associated with electroconvulsive therapy: a systematic review and meta-analysis. Anesthesiology 130(1):83–91, 2019 30557212

Dunne RA, McLoughlin DM: Systematic review and meta-analysis of bifrontal electroconvulsive therapy versus bilateral and unilateral electroconvulsive therapy in depression. World J Biol Psychiatry 13(4):248–258, 2012 22098115

Dutt A, Grover S, Chakrabarti S, et al: Phenomenology and treatment of catatonia: a descriptive study from north India. Indian J Psychiatry 53(1):36–40, 2011 21431006

Dwersteg JF, Avery DH: Atracurium as a muscle relaxant for electroconvulsive therapy in a burned patient. Convuls Ther 3(1):49–53, 1987 11940890

Dwork AJ, Arango V, Underwood M, et al: Absence of histological lesions in primate models of ECT and magnetic seizure therapy. Am J Psychiatry 161(3):576–578, 2004 14992989

Dwork AJ, Christensen JR, Larsen KB, et al: Unaltered neuronal and glial counts in animal models of magnetic seizure therapy and electroconvulsive therapy. Neuroscience 164(4):1557–1564, 2009 19782728

Dybedal GS, Tanum L, Sundet K, et al: The role of baseline cognitive function in the neurocognitive effects of electroconvulsive therapy in depressed elderly patients. Clin Neuropsychol 29(4):487–508, 2015 26029851

Ebrahim ZY, O'Hara J Jr, Borden L, et al: Monoamine oxidase inhibitors and elective surgery. Cleve Clin J Med 60(2):129–130, 1993 8443947

Edwards M, Koopowitz LF, Harvey EJ: A naturalistic study of the measurement of seizure adequacy in electroconvulsive therapy. Aust N Z J Psychiatry 37(3):312–318, 2003 12780470

Edwards RM, Stoudemire A, Vela MA, et al: Intraocular pressure changes in nonglaucomatous patients undergoing electroconvulsive therapy. Convuls Ther 6(3):209–213, 1990 11941069

Eggleston K, Porter R: Cognitive screening in electroconvulsive therapy: don't forget subjective cognition. Aust N Z J Psychiatry 55(12):1125–1126, 2021 33637012

Ekstrand J, Fattah C, Persson M, et al: Racemic ketamine as an alternative to electroconvulsive therapy for unipolar depression: a randomized, open-label, non-inferiority trial (KetECT). Int J Neuropsychopharmacol 25(5):339–349, 2022 35020871

Elderkin-Thompson V, Moody T, Knowlton B, et al: Explicit and implicit memory in late-life depression. Am J Geriatr Psychiatry 19(4):249–255, 2011 20808121

el-Ganzouri AR, Ivankovich AD, Braverman B, et al: Monoamine oxidase inhibitors: should they be discontinued preoperatively? Anesth Analg 64(6):592–596, 1985 4003777

Elias A, Phutane VH, Clarke S, et al: Electroconvulsive therapy in the continuation and maintenance treatment of depression: Systematic review and meta-analyses. Aust N Z J Psychiatry 52(5):415–424, 2018 29256252

Elias A, Thomas N, Sackeim HA: Electroconvulsive therapy in mania: a review of 80 years of clinical experience. Am J Psychiatry 178(3):229–239, 2021 33167675

el-Islam MF, Ahmed SA, Erfan ME: The effect of unilateral E.C.T. on schizophrenic delusions and hallucinations. Br J Psychiatry 117(539):447–448, 1970 5481209

Ellison EA, Hamilton DM: The hospital treatment of dementia praecox. Am J Psychiatry 106(6):454–461, 1949 15393324 el-Mallakh RS: Complications of concurrent lithium and electroconvulsive therapy: a review of clinical material and theoretical considerations. Biol Psychiatry 23(6):595–601, 1988 3281716

England ML, Ongür D, Konopaske GT, et al: Catatonia in psychotic patients: clinical features and treatment response. J Neuropsychiatry Clin Neurosci 23(2):223–226, 2011 21677256

Enns M, Karvelas L: Electrical dose titration for electroconvulsive therapy: a comparison with dose prediction methods. Convuls Ther 11(2):86–93, 1995 7552059

Enns M, Peeling J, Sutherland GR: Hippocampal neurons are damaged by caffeine-augmented electroshock seizures. Biol Psychiatry 40(7):642–647, 1996 8886298

Eranti SV, Mogg AJ, Pluck GC, et al: Methohexitone, propofol and etomidate in electroconvulsive therapy for depression: a naturalistic comparison study. J Affect Disord 113(1-2):165–171, 2009 18439686

Erman MK, Welch CA, Mandel MR: A comparison of two unilateral ECT electrode placements: efficacy and electrical energy considerations. Am J Psychiatry 136(10):1317–1319, 1979 484729

Escande M, Nordman S, Loustalan JM, et al: Value of electroconvulsive therapy as maintenance treatment for recurrent depression unresponsive to pharmacologic therapy. Annales de Psychiatrie 7:161–164, 1992

Esener Z, Sarihasan B, Güven H, et al: Thiopentone and etomidate concentrations in maternal and umbilical plasma, and in colostrum. Br J Anaesth 69(6):586–588, 1992 1467101

Esmaeilpour Z, Kronberg G, Reato D, et al: Temporal interference stimulation targets deep brain regions by modulating neural oscillations. Brain Stimul 14(1):55–65, 2021 33186778

Espi Forcen F, Respino M, Eloge J, et al: Catatonia in the medically ill: Differences and parallels in etiology, phenomenology and management. Int J Psychiatry Med 57(1):80–88, 2022 33567935

Espinoza RT, Kellner CH: Electroconvulsive therapy. N Engl J Med 386(7):667–672, 2022 35172057

Espinoza RT, Kellner CH, McCall WV: Electroconvulsive therapy during COVID-19: an essential medical procedure–maintaining service viability and accessibility. J ECT 36(2):78–79, 2020 32433118

Essa H, Hill AM, Lip GYH: Atrial fibrillation and stroke. Card Electrophysiol Clin 13(1):243–255, 2021 33516402

Estime SR, Berg SM, Henry ME: Clozapine-associated aspiration during electroconvulsive therapy. J ECT 35(2):133–134, 2019 30308569

Everman PD Jr, Kellner CH, Beale MD, et al: Modified electrode placement in patients with neurosurgical skull defects. J ECT 15(3):237–239, 1999 10492864

Exner JE Jr, Murillo LG: Effectiveness of regressive ECT with process schizophrenia. Dis Nerv Syst 34(1):44–48, 1973 4709191

Exner JE Jr, Murillo LG: A long term follow-up of schizophrenics treated with regressive ECT. Dis Nerv Syst 38(3):162–168, 1977 402256

Ezion T, Levy A, Levin Y, et al: Should electroconvulsive therapy be used as an ambulatory preventive treatment? Isr J Psychiatry Relat Sci 27(3):168–174, 1990 2125033

Fabbri F, Henry ME, Renshaw PF, et al: Bilateral near-infrared monitoring of the cerebral concentration and oxygen-saturation of hemoglobin during right unilateral electro-convulsive therapy. Brain Res 992(2):193–204, 2003 14625058

Faber R, Trimble MR: Electroconvulsive therapy in Parkinson's disease and other movement disorders. Mov Disord 6(4):293–303, 1991 1758447

Fahy P, Imlah N, Harrington J: A controlled comparison of electroconvulsive therapy, imipramine, and thiopentone sleep in depression. J Neuropsychiatry 4:310–314, 1963 14047828

Fantz RM, Markowitz JS, Kellner CH: Sumatriptan for post-ECT headache. J ECT 14(4):272–274, 1998 9871850

Farah A, McCall WV: Electroconvulsive therapy stimulus dosing: a survey of contemporary practices. Convuls Ther 9(2):90–94, 1993 11941196

Farah A, McCall WV: ECT administration to a hyperthyroid patient. Convuls Ther 11(2):126–128, 1995 7552052

Farah A, McCall WV, Amundson RH: ECT after cerebral aneurysm repair. Convuls Ther 12(3):165–170, 1996 8872405

Farahani A, Correll CU: Are antipsychotics or antidepressants needed for psychotic depression? A systematic review and meta-analysis of trials comparing antidepressant or antipsychotic monotherapy with combination treatment. J Clin Psychiatry 73(4):486–496, 2012 22579147

Fava M, Freeman MP, Flynn M, et al: Double-blind, proof-of-concept (POC) trial of low-field magnetic stimulation (LFMS) augmentation of antidepressant therapy in treatment-resistant depression (TRD). Brain Stimul 11(1):75–84, 2018 29030111

Federici S, Bracalenti M, Meloni F, et al: World Health Organization disability assessment schedule 2.0: an international systematic review. Disabil Rehabil 39(23):2347–2380, 2017 27820966

Feenstra TC, Blake Y, Hoogendoorn AW, et al: Pharmacological prevention of postictal agitation after electroconvulsive therapy: a systematic review and meta-analysis. Front Psychiatry 14:1170931, 2023 37151968

Fenoy AJ, Schulz PE, Sanches M, et al: Deep brain stimulation of the "medial forebrain bundle": sustained efficacy of antidepressant effect over years. Mol Psychiatry 27(5):2546–2553, 2022 35288633

Ferrando SJ, Nims C: HIV-associated mania treated with electroconvulsive therapy and highly-active antiretroviral therapy. Psychosomatics 47(2):170–174, 2006 16508032

Ferreira-Garcia R, da Rocha Freire RC, Appolinário JC, et al: Tranylcypromine plus amitriptyline for electroconvulsive therapy-resistant depression: a long-term study. J Clin Psychopharmacol 38(5):502–504, 2018 30106881

Ferrier IN, Waite J (eds): The ECT Handbook, Fourth Edition. New York, Cambridge University Press, 2019

Feske U, Mulsant BH, Pilkonis PA, et al: Clinical outcome of ECT in patients with major depression and comorbid borderline personality disorder. Am J Psychiatry 161(11):2073–2080, 2004 15514409

Ffytche DH, Pereira JB, Ballard C, et al: Risk factors for early psychosis in PD: insights from the Parkinson's Progression Markers Initiative. J Neurol Neurosurg Psychiatry 88(4):325–331, 2017 28315846

Figiel GS, Coffey CE, Djang WT, et al: Brain magnetic resonance imaging findings in ECT-induced delirium. J Neuropsychiatry Clin Neurosci 2(1):53–58, 1990 2136061

Figiel GS, Hassen MA, Zorumski C, et al: ECT-induced delirium in depressed patients with Parkinson's disease. J Neuropsychiatry Clin Neurosci 3(4):405–411, 1991 1821261

Finestone DH, Weiner RD: Effects of ECT on diabetes mellitus. An attempt to account for conflicting data. Acta Psychiatr Scand 70(4):321–326, 1984 6496156

Fink M: Convulsive Therapy: Theory and Practice. New York, Raven Press, 1979

Fink M: New technology in convulsive therapy: a challenge in training. Am J Psychiatry 144(9):1195–1198, 1987 3631317

Fink M: Is catatonia a primary indication for ECT? Convuls Ther 6(1):1–4, 1990 11941041

Fink M: Delirious mania. Bipolar Disord 1(1):54–60, 1999 11256658

Fink M: Electroconvulsive Therapy: A Guide for Professionals and their Patients. New York, Oxford University Press, 2009

Fink M: Rediscovering catatonia: the biography of a treatable syndrome. Acta Psychiatr Scand Suppl (441):1–47, 2013 23215963

Fink M: What was learned: studies by the consortium for research in ECT (CORE) 1997–2011. Acta Psychiatr Scand 129(6):417–426, 2014 24571807

Fink M: Electroshock therapy and catatonia: a productive synergism. J ECT 35(4):219–221, 2019 31764441

Fink M, Kellner CH: Certification in ECT. J ECT 14(1):1–4, 1998 9661087

Fink M, Kellner CH: Belling the cat: ECT practice standards in the United States. J ECT 23(1):3–5, 2007 17435562

Fink M, Sackeim HA: Convulsive therapy in schizophrenia? Schizophr Bull 22(1):27–39, 1996 8685661

Fink M, Sackeim HA: Theophylline and ECT. J ECT 14:286–290, 1998 9871854

Fink M, Abrams R, Bailine S, et al: Ambulatory electroconvulsive therapy: report of a task force of the association for convulsive therapy. Convuls Ther 12(1):42–55, 1996 8777654

Fink M, Kellner CH, Sackeim HA: Intractable seizures, status epilepticus, and ECT. J ECT 15(4):282–284, 1999 10614038

Fink M, Rush AJ, Knapp R, et al: DSM melancholic features are unreliable predictors of ECT response: a CORE publication. J ECT 23(3):139–146, 2007 17804986

Fink M, Kellner CH, McCall WV: Optimizing ECT technique in treating catatonia. J ECT 32(3):149–150, 2016 27428478

Finlayson AJ, Vieweg WV, Wilkey WD, et al: Hyponatremic seizure following ECT. Can J Psychiatry 34(5):463–464, 1989 2504479

Finnegan M, Ryan K, Shanahan E, et al: Ketamine for depression relapse prevention following electroconvulsive therapy: protocol for a randomised pilot trial (the KEEP-WELL trial). Pilot Feasibility Stud 2:38, 2016 27965856

Finnegan M, Galligan T, Ryan K, et al: Ketamine versus midazolam for depression relapse prevention following successful electroconvulsive therapy: a randomized controlled pilot trial. J ECT 35(2):115–121, 2019 30531397

Fischer C, Schweizer TA, Atkins JH, et al: Neurocognitive profiles in older adults with and without major depression. Int J Geriatr Psychiatry 23(8):851–856, 2008 18311855

Fitzgerald PB, Daskalakis ZJ: rTMS Treatment for Depression: A Practical Guide, 2nd Edition. New York, Springer, 2023

Fitzsimons MG, Welch CA, Haspel KL, et al: The safety and efficacy of ECT and anesthesia in the setting of multiple sclerosis. J Psychiatr Pract 13(3):195–198, 2007 17522564

Fleisher LA, Fleischmann KE, Auerbach AD, et al: 2014 ACC/AHA guideline on perioperative cardiovascular evaluation and management of patients undergoing noncardiac surgery: executive summary: a report of the American College of Cardiology/American Heart Association Task Force on Practice Guidelines. Circulation 130(24):2215–2245, 2014 25085962

Fleminger JJ, de Horne DJ, Nair NPV, et al: Differential effect of unilateral and bilateral ECT. Am J Psychiatry 127(4):430–436, 1970 4918113

Flexman AM, Abcejo AS, Avitsian R, et al: Neuroanesthesia practice during the COVID-19 pandemic: recommendations from Society for Neuroscience in Anesthesiology and Critical Care (SNACC). J Neurosurg Anesthesiol 32(3):202–209, 2020 32301764

Flint AJ, Rifat SL: Two-year outcome of psychotic depression in late life. Am J Psychiatry 155(2):178–183, 1998 9464195

Focht A, Kellner CH: Electroconvulsive therapy (ECT) in the treatment of postpartum psychosis. J ECT 28(1):31–33, 2012 22330704

Fogg-Waberski JH, Szarek BL, Knauft RF: Electroconvulsive therapy for treatment of refractory depression in a patient with cystic fibrosis. J ECT 22(1):72–73, 2006 16633213

Folkerts H: Electroconvulsive therapy in neurologic diseases [in German]. Nervenarzt 66(4):241–251, 1995 7783810

Folkerts H: The ictal electroencephalogram as a marker for the efficacy of electroconvulsive therapy. Eur Arch Psychiatry Clin Neurosci 246(3):155–164, 1996 8739401

Folkerts HW, Michael N, Tölle R, et al: Electroconvulsive therapy vs. paroxetine in treatment-resistant depression—a randomized study. Acta Psychiatr Scand 96(5):334–342, 1997 9395150

Folstein M, Folstein S, McHugh PR: Clinical predictors of improvement after electroconvulsive therapy of patients with schizophrenia, neurotic reactions, and affective disorders. Biol Psychiatry 7(2):147–152, 1973 4748846

Folstein MF, Folstein SE, McHugh PR: "Mini-mental state": a practical method for grading the cognitive state of patients for the clinician. J Psychiatr Res 12(3):189–198, 1975 1202204

Folstein MF, Folstein SE, Messer MA, et al: Mini-Mental State Examination, 2nd Edition. Lutz, FL, Psychological Assessment Resources, 2010

Fomenko A, Neudorfer C, Dallapiazza RF, et al: Low-intensity ultrasound neuromodulation: an overview of mechanisms and emerging human applications. Brain Stimul 11(6):1209–1217, 2018 30166265

Forkmann T, Scherer A, Boecker M, et al: The Clinical Global Impression Scale and the influence of patient or staff perspective on outcome. BMC Psychiatry 11:83, 2011 21569566

Fornaro M, Carvalho AF, Fusco A, et al: The concept and management of acute episodes of treatment-resistant bipolar disorder: a systematic review and exploratory meta-analysis of randomized controlled trials. J Affect Disord 276:970–983, 2020 32750614

Forray A, Ostroff RB: The use of electroconvulsive therapy in postpartum affective disorders. J ECT 23(3):188–193, 2007 17804998

Fortney JC, Unützer J, Wrenn G, et al: A tipping point for measurement-based care. Psychiatr Serv 68(2):179–188, 2017 27582237

Fountoulakis KN, Yatham LN, Grunze H, et al: The CINP guidelines on the definition and evidence-based interventions for treatment-resistant bipolar disorder. Int J Neuropsychopharmacol 23(4):230–256, 2020 31802122

Frajo-Apor B, Edinger M, Schmidinger S, et al: Successful electroconvulsive therapy in a clozapine-refractory schizophrenia patient with meningioma. Clin Schizophr Relat Psychoses 10(4):225–226, 2017 24846879

Francis A, Fochtmann L: Caffeine augmentation of electroconvulsive seizures. Psychopharmacology (Berl) 115(3):320–324, 1994 7871071

Francis-Taylor R, Ophel G, Martin D, et al: The ictal EEG in ECT: a systematic review of the relationships between ictal features, ECT technique, seizure threshold and outcomes. Brain Stimul 13(6):1644–1654, 2020 32998055

Francois D, Snow C, Kotbi N, et al: Electroconvulsive therapy in the presence of cranial metallic objects. J ECT 30(4):e51, 2014 25181020

Frankenburg FR, Suppes T, McLean PE: Combined clozapine and electroconvulsive therapy. Convuls Ther 9(3):176–180, 1993 11941210

Fraser LM, O'Carroll RE, Ebmeier KP: The effect of electroconvulsive therapy on autobiographical memory: a systematic review. J ECT 24(1):10–17, 2008 18379329

Freeman CP, Kendell RE: ECT: I. Patients' experiences and attitudes. Br J Psychiatry 137:8–16, 1980 7459545

Freeman CP, Basson JV, Crighton A: Double-blind controlled trial of electroconvulsive therapy (E.C.T.) and simulated E.C.T. in depressive illness. Lancet 1(8067):738–740, 1978 76748

Freeman CP, Weeks D, Kendell RE: ECT: II: patients who complain. Br J Psychiatry 137:17–25, 1980 7459536

Freeman SA: The effect of lamotrigine on electroconvulsive therapy outcomes. J ECT 23(1):38, author reply 38–39, 2007 17435576

Freese KJ: Can patients safely undergo electroconvulsive therapy while receiving monoamine oxidase inhibitors? Convuls Ther 1(3):190–194, 1985 11940823

Fregni F, El-Hagrassy MM, Pacheco-Barrios K, et al: Evidence-based guidelines and secondary meta-analysis for the use of transcranial direct current stimulation in neurological and psychiatric disorders. Int J Neuropsychopharmacol 24(4):256–313, 2021 32710772

Fricchione G, Mann SC, Caroff SN: Catatonia, lethal catatonia, and neuroleptic malignant syndrome. Psychiatr Ann 30(5):347–355, 2000

Fricchione GL, Kaufman LD, Gruber BL, et al: Electroconvulsive therapy and cyclophosphamide in combination for severe neuropsychiatric lupus with catatonia. Am J Med 88(4):442–443, 1990 2327432

Fried D, Mann JJ: Electroconvulsive treatment of a patient with known intracranial tumor. Biol Psychiatry 23(2):176–180, 1988 3334886

Fried EI, Epskamp S, Nesse RM, et al: What are "good" depression symptoms? Comparing the centrality of DSM and non-DSM symptoms of depression in a network analysis. J Affect Disord 189:314–320, 2016a 26458184

Fried EI, van Borkulo CD, Epskamp S, et al: Measuring depression over time...or not? Lack of unidimensionality and longitudinal measurement invariance in four common rating scales of depression. Psychol Assess 28(11):1354–1367, 2016b 26821198

Friedlander R, Francois D: Efficacious use of electroconvulsive therapy in the setting of previous retinal detachment. J ECT 36(4):e51–e52, 2020 32558762

Friedman J, Gordon N: Electroconvulsive therapy in Parkinson's disease: a report on five cases. Convuls Ther 8(3):204–210, 1992 11941171

Friedman JM: Teratogen update: anesthetic agents. Teratology 37(1):69–77, 1988 3279563

Frith CD, Stevens M, Johnstone EC, et al: Effects of ECT and depression on various aspects of memory. Br J Psychiatry 142:610–617, 1983 6882984

Froimson L, Creed P, Mathew L: State of the art: nursing knowledge and electroconvulsive therapy. Convuls Ther 11(3):205–211, 1995 8528665

Fromholt P, Christensen AL, Strömgren LS: The effects of unilateral and bilateral electroconvulsive therapy on memory. Acta Psychiatr Scand 49(4):466–478, 1973 4746012

Fruitman K, Francois D: Role of electroconvulsive therapy in managing major depressive episodes in patients with dementia with Lewy bodies. J ECT 38(2):e21–e22, 2022 34966041

Fryml L, Fox J, Manett AJ, et al: Neurogenic pulmonary edema complicating ECT. J ECT 34(2):78, 2018 29166318

Fuenmayor AJ, el Fakih Y, Moreno J, et al: Effects of electroconvulsive therapy on cardiac function in patients without heart disease. Cardiology 88(3):254–257, 1997 9129846

Gahr M, Connemann BJ, Freudenmann RW, et al: Safety of electroconvulsive therapy in the presence of cranial metallic objects. J ECT 30(1):62–68, 2014 24553318

Gaitz CM, Pokorny AD, Mills M Jr: Death following electroconvulsive therapy: report of three cases. AMA Arch Neurol Psychiatry 75(5):493–499, 1956 13312731

Gálvez V, Loo CK, Alonzo A, et al: Do benzodiazepines moderate the effectiveness of bitemporal electroconvulsive therapy in major depression? J Affect Disord 150(2):686–690, 2013 23668903

Gálvez V, Hadzi-Pavlovic D, Smith D, et al: Predictors of seizure threshold in right unilateral ultrabrief electroconvulsive therapy: role of concomitant medications and anaesthesia used. Brain Stimul 8(3):486–492, 2015 25683317

Ganesh R, Kebede E, Mueller M, et al: Perioperative cardiac risk reduction in noncardiac surgery. Mayo Clin Proc 96(8):2260–2276, 2021 34226028

Gangadhar BN (ed): Proceedings of the National Workshop on ECT: Priorities for Research and Practice in India. Bangalore, India, National Institute of Mental Health and Neurologic Sciences, 1992

Gangadhar BN, Kapur RL, Kalyanasundaram S: Comparison of electroconvulsive therapy with imipramine in endogenous depression: a double blind study. Br J Psychiatry 141:367–371, 1982 6756530

Gangadhar BN, Janakiramaiah N, Subbakrishna DK, et al: Twice versus thrice weekly ECT in melancholia: a double-blind prospective comparison. J Affect Disord 27(4):273–278, 1993 8509527

Gangadhar BN, Girish K, Janakiramiah N, et al: Formula method for stimulus setting in bilateral electroconvulsive therapy: relevance of age. J ECT 14(4):259–265, 1998 9871848

García-López B, Gómez-Menéndez AI, Vázquez-Sánchez F, et al: Electroconvulsive therapy in super refractory status epilepticus: case series with a defined protocol. Int J Environ Res Public Health 17(11):4023, 2020 32516983

Gardno AG, Simpson CJ: Electroconvulsive therapy in Paget's disease and hydrocephalus. Convuls Ther 7(1):48–51, 1991 11941097

Garg R, Chavan BS, Arun P: Quality of life after electroconvulsive therapy in persons with treatment resistant schizophrenia. Indian J Med Res 133(6):641–644, 2011 21727663

Garrett MD: Use of ECT in a depressed hypothyroid patient. J Clin Psychiatry 46(2):64–66, 1985 3968048

Gass JP: The knowledge and attitudes of mental health nurses to electro-convulsive therapy. J Adv Nurs 27(1):83–90, 1998 9515612

Gazdag G, Iványi Z: Hemodynamic effects of etomidate and propofol. J ECT 23(3):206, 2007 17805003

Gazdag G, Barna I, Iványi Z, et al: The impact of neuroleptic medication on seizure threshold and duration in electroconvulsive therapy. Ideggyogy Sz 57(11-12):385–390, 2004a 15662766

Gazdag G, Kocsis N, Tolna J, et al: Etomidate versus propofol for electroconvulsive therapy in patients with schizophrenia. J ECT 20(4):225–229, 2004b 15591855

Gbyl K, Videbech P: Electroconvulsive therapy increases brain volume in major depression: a systematic review and meta-analysis. Acta Psychiatr Scand 138(3):180–195, 2018 29707778

Geoghegan JJ, Stevenson GH: Prophylactic electroshock. Am J Psychiatry 105(7):494–496, 1949 18121767

George MS, Rush AJ, Marangell LB, et al: A one-year comparison of vagus nerve stimulation with treatment as usual for treatment-resistant depression. Biol Psychiatry 58(5):364–373, 2005 16139582

Geretsegger C, Nickel M, Judendorfer B, et al: Propofol and methohexital as anesthetic agents for electroconvulsive therapy: a randomized, double-blind comparison of electroconvulsive therapy seizure quality, therapeutic efficacy, and cognitive performance. J ECT 23(4):239–243, 2007 18090696

Gershon RC, Lai JS, Bode R, et al: Neuro-QOL: quality of life item banks for adults with neurological disorders: item development and calibrations based upon clinical and general population testing. Qual Life Res 21(3):475–486, 2012 21874314

Ghaemi SN, Miller CJ, Berv DA, et al: Sensitivity and specificity of a new bipolar spectrum diagnostic scale. J Affect Disord 84(2-3):273–277, 2005 15708426

Ghanshani S, Chen C, Lin B, et al: Risk of acute myocardial infarction, heart failure, and death in migraine patients treated with triptans. Headache 60(10):2166–2175, 2020 33017476

Ghasemi M, Kazemi MH, Yoosefi A, et al: Rapid antidepressant effects of repeated doses of ketamine compared with electroconvulsive therapy in hospitalized patients with major depressive disorder. Psychiatry Res 215(2):355–361, 2014 24374115

Ghaziuddin N, Walter G: Electroconvulsive Therapy in Children and Adolescents. New York, Oxford University Press, 2013

Ghaziuddin N, Kaza M, Ghazi N, et al: Electroconvulsive therapy for minors: experiences and attitudes of child psychiatrists and psychologists. J ECT 17(2):109–117, 2001 11417921

Ghaziuddin N, Kutcher SP, Knapp P, et al: Practice parameter for use of electroconvulsive therapy with adolescents. J Am Acad Child Adolesc Psychiatry 43(12):1521–1539, 2004 15564821

Ghaziuddin N, Dumas S, Hodges E: Use of continuation or maintenance electroconvulsive therapy in adolescents with severe treatment-resistant depression. J ECT 27(2):168–174, 2011 21233763

Ghaziuddin N, Hendriks M, Patel P, et al: Neuroleptic malignant syndrome/malignant catatonia in child psychiatry: literature review and a case series. J Child Adolesc Psychopharmacol 27(4):359–365, 2017 28398818

Ghaziuddin N, Shamseddeen W, Gettys G, et al: Electroconvulsive therapy for the treatment of severe mood disorders during adolescence: a retrospective chart review. J Child Adolesc Psychopharmacol 30(4):235–243, 2020 32125885

Ghaziuddin N, Yaqub T, Shamseddeen W, et al: Maintenance electroconvulsive therapy is an essential medical treatment for patients with catatonia: a COVID-19 related experience. Front Psychiatry 12:670476, 2021 34335326

Ghignone E, Rosenthal L, Lloyd RB, et al: Electroconvulsive therapy in a patient with moyamoya syndrome. J ECT 31(1):e14–e16, 2015 24901428

Ghio L, Gotelli S, Marcenaro M, et al: Duration of untreated illness and outcomes in unipolar depression: a systematic review and meta-analysis. J Affect Disord 152-154:45–51, 2014 24183486

Giacobbe P, Rakita U, Penner-Goeke K, et al: Improvements in health-related quality of life with electroconvulsive therapy: a meta-analysis. J ECT 34(2):87–94, 2018 29461332

Gill SP, Kellner CH: Clinical practice recommendations for continuation and maintenance electroconvulsive therapy for depression: outcomes from a review of the evidence and a consensus workshop held in Australia in May 2017. J ECT 35(1):14–20, 2019 29419559

Gillman PK: Monoamine oxidase inhibitors, opioid analgesics and serotonin toxicity. Br J Anaesth 95(4):434–441, 2005 16051647

Gillman PK: A reassessment of the safety profile of monoamine oxidase inhibitors: elucidating tired old tyramine myths. J Neural Transm (Vienna) 125(11):1707–1717, 2018 30255284

Giltay EJ, Kho KH, Keijzer LT, et al: Electroconvulsive therapy (ECT) in a patient with a dual-chamber sensing, VDDR pacemaker. J ECT 21(1):35–38, 2005 15793358

Giné-Servén E, Serra-Mestres J, Martinez-Ramirez M, et al: Anti-NMDA receptor encephalitis in older adults: a systematic review of case reports. Gen Hosp Psychiatry 74:71–77, 2022 34929551

Girish K, Jayaprakash MS, Gangadhar BN, et al: Etophylline as a proconvulsant. Convuls Ther 12(3):196–198, 1996 8872408

Glaub T, Telek B, Boda Z, et al: Successful electroconvulsive treatment of a schizophrenic patient suffering from severe haemophilia A. Thromb Haemost 75(6):978, 1996 8822600

Glauser T, Shinnar S, Gloss D, et al: Evidence-based guideline: treatment of convulsive status epilepticus in children and adults: report of the guideline committee of the American Epilepsy Society. Epilepsy Curr 16(1):48–61, 2016 26900382

Glezer A, Murray E, Price B, et al: Effective use of electroconvulsive therapy after craniofacial reconstructive surgery. J ECT 25(3):208–209, 2009 19145209

Godemann F, Hellweg R: 20 years unsuccessful prevention of bipolar affective psychosis recurrence [in German]. Nervenarzt 68(7):582–585, 1997 9333720

Goetz KL, Price TRP: Electroconvulsive therapy in Creutzfeldt-Jakob disease. Convuls Ther 9(1):58–62, 1993 11941194

Gold L, Chiarello CJ: Prognostic value of clinical findings in cases treated with electroshock. J Nerv Ment Dis 100:577–583, 1944

Gold MI, Duarte I, Muravchick S: Arterial oxygenation in conscious patients after 5 minutes and after 30 seconds of oxygen breathing. Anesth Analg 60(5):313–315, 1981 7194597

Goldberg E, Barnett J: The Goldberg-Barnett Remote Memory Questionnaire. New York, Albert Einstein Medical College, 1985

Goldberg RJ, Badger JM: Major depressive disorder in patients with the implantable cardioverter defibrillator: two cases treated with ECT. Psychosomatics 34(3):273–277, 1993 8493312

Goldfarb W, Kiene HE: The treatment of the psychotic-like regressions of the combat soldier. Psychiatr Q 19:555–565, 1945 21006527

Goldman D: Brief stimulus electric shock therapy. J Nerv Ment Dis 110(1):36–45, 1949 18132845

Gomez J: Subjective side-effects of ECT. Br J Psychiatry 127:609–611, 1975 1201457

Gómez-Arnau J, de Arriba-Arnau A, Correas-Lauffer J, et al: Hyperventilation and electroconvulsive therapy: a literature review. Gen Hosp Psychiatry 50:54–62, 2018 29054017

Gonzales N, Quinn DK, Rayburn W: Perinatal catatonia: a case report and literature review. Psychosomatics 55(6):708–714, 2014 25262045

Gonzalez-Arriaza HL, Mueller PS, Rummans TA: Successful electroconvulsive therapy in an elderly man with severe thrombocytopenia: case report and literature review. J ECT 17(3):198–200, 2001 11528312

Gonzalez-Pinto A, Gutierrez M, Gonzalez N, et al: Efficacy and safety of venlafaxine-ECT combination in treatment-resistant depression. J Neuropsychiatry Clin Neurosci 14(2):206–209, 2002 11983797

Good MS, Dolenc TJ, Rasmussen KG: Electroconvulsive therapy in a patient with glaucoma. J ECT 20(1):48–49, 2004 15087998

Goodman T, McCall WV: Electroconvulsive therapy malpractice: verdict for the defense. J ECT 31(3):155–158, 2015 25373562

Goodwin GM, Haddad PM, Ferrier IN, et al: Evidence-based guidelines for treating bipolar disorder: revised third edition recommendations from the British Association for Psychopharmacology. J Psychopharmacol 30(6):495–553, 2016 26979387

Goswami U, Dutta S, Kuruvilla K, et al: Electroconvulsive therapy in neuroleptic-induced parkinsonism. Biol Psychiatry 26(3):234–238, 1989 2568133

Gottlieb JS, Huston PE: Treatment of schizophrenia; a comparison of three methods: brief psychotherapy, insulin coma and electric shock. J Nerv Ment Dis 113(3):237–246, 1951 14824956

Gournellis R, Tournikioti K, Touloumi G, et al: Psychotic (delusional) depression and completed suicide: a systematic review and meta-analysis. Ann Gen Psychiatry 17:39, 2018 30258483

Grassi L, Caruso R, Da Ronch C, et al: Quality of life, level of functioning, and its relationship with mental and physical disorders in the elderly: results from the MentDis_ICF65+ study. Health Qual Life Outcomes 18(1):61, 2020 32143635

Graveland PE, Wierdsma AI, van den Broek WW, et al: A retrospective comparison of the effects of propofol and etomidate on stimulus variables and efficacy of electroconvulsive therapy in depressed inpatients. Prog Neuropsychopharmacol Biol Psychiatry 45:230–235, 2013 23774194

Green A, Nutt D, Cowen P: Increased seizure threshold following convulsion, in Psychopharmacology of Anticonvulsants. Edited by Sandler M. Oxford, UK, Oxford University Press, 1982, pp 16–26

Greenan J, Dewar M, Jones CJ: Intravenous glycopyrrolate and atropine at induction of anaesthesia: a comparison. J R Soc Med 76(5):369–371, 1983 6864702

Greenberg LB, Mofson R, Fink M: Prospective electroconvulsive therapy in a delusional depressed patient with a frontal meningioma: a case report. Br J Psychiatry 153:105–107, 1988 3224230

Greenberg RM, Pettinati HM: Benzodiazepines and electroconvulsive therapy. Convuls Ther 9(4):262–273, 1993 11941222

Greenblatt M, Grosser GH, Wechsler H: A comparative study of selected antidepressant medications and EST. Am J Psychiatry 119:144–153, 1962 13901499

Greenblatt M, Grosser GH, Wechsler H: Differential response of hospitalized depressed patients in somatic therapy. Am J Psychiatry 120:935–943, 1964 14138843

Greene YM, McDonald WM, Duggan J, et al: Ventricular ectopy associated with low-dose intravenous haloperidol and electroconvulsive therapy. J ECT 16(3):309–311, 2000 11005056

Greer RA, Stewart RB: Hyponatremia and ECT. Am J Psychiatry 150(8):1272, 1993 8328581

Gregory S, Shawcross CR, Gill D: The Nottingham ECT Study: a double-blind comparison of bilateral, unilateral and simulated ECT in depressive illness. Br J Psychiatry 146:520–524, 1985 3893601

Gressier F, Rotenberg S, Cazas O, et al: Postpartum electroconvulsive therapy: a systematic review and case report. Gen Hosp Psychiatry 37(4):310–314, 2015 25929986

Griesemer DA, Kellner CH, Beale MD, et al: Electroconvulsive therapy for treatment of intractable seizures. Initial findings in two children. Neurology 49(5):1389–1392, 1997 9371927

Grisso T, Appelbaum PS: Comparison of standards for assessing patients' capacities to make treatment decisions. Am J Psychiatry 152(7):1033–1037, 1995 7793439

Grisso T, Appelbaum PS, Hill-Fotouhi C: The MacCAT-T: a clinical tool to assess patients' capacities to make treatment decisions. Psychiatr Serv 48(11):1415–1419, 1997 9355168

Grossman N, Bono D, Dedic N, et al: Noninvasive deep brain stimulation via temporally interfering electric fields. Cell 169(6):1029.e16–1041.e16, 2017 28575667

Grover S, Hazari N, Kate N: Combined use of clozapine and ECT: a review. Acta Neuropsychiatr 27(3):131–142, 2015 25697225

Grover S, Chakrabarti S, Hazari N, Avasthi A: Effectiveness of electroconvulsive therapy in patients with treatment resistant schizophrenia: a retrospective study. Psychiatry Res 249:349–353, 2017 28152470

Grover S, Somani A, Sahni N, et al: Effectiveness of electroconvulsive therapy (ECT) in parkinsonian symptoms: a case series. Innov Clin Neurosci 15(1-2):23–27, 2018 29497576

Grover S, Sahoo S, Rabha A, et al: ECT in schizophrenia: a review of the evidence. Acta Neuropsychiatr 31(3):115–127, 2019 30501675

Gruber NP, Dilsaver SC, Shoaib AM, et al: ECT in mixed affective states: a case series. J ECT 16(2):183–188, 2000 10868328

Grunhaus L, Dilsaver S, Greden JF, et al: Depressive pseudodementia: a suggested diagnostic profile. Biol Psychiatry 18(2):215–225, 1983 6830931

Grunhaus L, Pande AC, Haskett RF: Full and abbreviated courses of maintenance electroconvulsive therapy. Convuls Ther 6(2):130–138, 1990 11941054

Grunhaus L, Dolberg O, Lustig M: Relapse and recurrence following a course of ECT: reasons for concern and strategies for further investigation. J Psychiatr Res 29(3):165–172, 1995 7473293

Grützner TM, Sharma A, Listunova L, et al: Neurocognitive performance in patients with depression compared to healthy controls: association of clinical variables and remission state. Psychiatry Res 271:343–350, 2019 30529317

Guay J, Grenier Y, Varin F: Clinical pharmacokinetics of neuromuscular relaxants in pregnancy. Clin Pharmacokinet 34(6):483–496, 1998 9646009

Gunderson-Falcone G: Developing an outpatient electroconvulsive therapy program: a nursing perspective. Convuls Ther 11(3):202–204, 1995 8528664

Güney P, Ekman CJ, Hammar Å, et al: Electroconvulsive therapy in depression: improvement in quality of life depending on age and sex. J ECT 36(4):242–246, 2020 32108666

Guo T, Xiang Y-T, Xiao L, et al: Measurement-based care versus standard care for major depression: a randomized controlled trial with blind raters. Am J Psychiatry 172(10):1004–1013, 2015 26315978

Gutheil TG, Bursztajn H: Clinicians' guidelines for assessing and presenting subtle forms of patient incompetence in legal settings. Am J Psychiatry 143(8):1020–1023, 1986 3728716

Gutierrez-Esteinou R, Pope HG Jr: Does fluoxetine prolong electrically induced seizures? Convuls Ther 5(4):344–348, 1989 11941033

Guttmann E, Mayer-Gross W, Slater ET: Short-distance prognosis of schizophrenia. J Neurol Psychiatry 2(1):25–34, 1939 21610940

Guy W (ed): ECDEU Assessment Manual for Psychopharmacology. Rockville, MD, U.S. Department of Health, Education, and Welfare, 1976

Guze BH, Baxter LR Jr, Liston EH, et al: Attorneys' perceptions of electroconvulsive therapy: impact of instruction with an ECT videotape demonstration. Compr Psychiatry 29(5):520–522, 1988 3180762

Haddad PM, Benbow SM: Electroconvulsive therapy–related psychiatric knowledge among British anesthetists. Convuls Ther 9(2):101–107, 1993 11941198

Haeck M, Gillmann B, Janouschek H, et al: Electroconvulsive therapy can benefit from controlled hyperventilation using a laryngeal mask. Eur Arch Psychiatry Clin Neurosci 261(Suppl 2):S172–S176, 2011 21901267

Hafeiz HB: Psychiatric manifestations of enteric fever. Acta Psychiatr Scand 75(1):69–73, 1987 3577842

Haghighi M, Bajoghli H, Bigdelou G, et al: Assessment of cognitive impairments and seizure characteristics in electroconvulsive therapy with and without sodium valproate in manic patients. Neuropsychobiology 67(1):14–24, 2013 23221898

Hamilton M: The assessment of anxiety states by rating. Br J Med Psychol 32(1):50–55, 1959 13638508

Hamilton M: A rating scale for depression. J Neurol Neurosurg Psychiatry 23(1):56–62, 1960 14399272

Hamilton M, White JM: Factors related to the outcome of depression treated with E.C.T. J Ment Sci 106:1031–1041, 1960 13711022

Hamilton RW, Walter-Ryan WG: ECT and thrombocythemia. Am J Psychiatry 143(2):258, 1986 3946669

Hanmer J, Jensen RE, Rothrock N: A reporting checklist for HealthMeasures' patient-reported outcomes: ASCQ-Me, Neuro-QoL, NIH Toolbox, and PROMIS. J Patient Rep Outcomes 4(1):21, 2020 32215788

Hannay HJ, Levin HS: Selective reminding test: an examination of the equivalence of four forms. J Clin Exp Neuropsychol 7(3):251–263, 1985 3998090

Hanretta AT, Malek-Ahmadi P: Use of ECT in a patient with a Harrington rod implant. Convuls Ther 11(4):266–270, 1995 8919579

Hannigan K: Nursing care of the patient receiving ECT and the roles of the ECT nurse, in The ECT Handbook. Edited by Ferrier IN, Waite J. Cambridge, UK, Cambridge University Press, 2019, pp 173–182

Haq AU, Sitzmann AF, Goldman ML, et al: Response of depression to electroconvulsive therapy: a meta-analysis of clinical predictors. J Clin Psychiatry 76(10):1374–1384, 2015 26528644

Harmandayan M, Romanowicz M, Sola C: Successful use of ECT in post-stroke depression. Gen Hosp Psychiatry 34(1):102.e5–102.e6, 2012 21937120

Harris M, Merz ZC: High elevation rates of the Structured Inventory of Malingered Symptomatology (SIMS) in neuropsychological patients. Appl Neuropsychol Adult 4:1–8, 2021 33662216

Harsch HH: Atrial fibrillation, cardioversion, and electroconvulsive therapy. Convuls Ther 7(2):139–142, 1991 11941115

Harsch HH, Haddox JD: Electroconvulsive therapy and fluoxetine. Convuls Ther 6(3):250–251, 1990 11941076

Hartmann SJ, Saldivia A: ECT in an elderly patient with skull defects and shrapnel. Convuls Ther 6(2):165–171, 1990 11941059

Hassani V, Amniati S, Kashaninasab F, et al: Electroconvulsive therapy for a patient with suicide by drinking bleach during treatment of COVID-19: a case report. Anesth Pain Med 10(6):e107513, 2020 34150573

Hasselbalch BJ, Knorr U, Kessing LV: Cognitive impairment in the remitted state of unipolar depressive disorder: a systematic review. J Affect Disord 134(1-3):20–31, 2011 21163534

Hasselbalch BJ, Knorr U, Hasselbalch SG, et al: Cognitive deficits in the remitted state of unipolar depressive disorder. Neuropsychology 26(5):642–651, 2012 22823136

Hatta K, Kitajima A, Ito M, et al: Pulmonary edema after electroconvulsive therapy in a patient treated for long-standing asthma with a beta2 stimulant. J ECT 23(1):26–27, 2007 17435570

Hausner L, Damian M, Sartorius A, et al: Efficacy and cognitive side effects of electroconvulsive therapy (ECT) in depressed elderly inpatients with coexisting mild cognitive impairment or dementia. J Clin Psychiatry 72(1):91–97, 2011 21208587

Hawken ER, Delva NJ, Lawson JS: Successful use of propranolol in migraine associated with electroconvulsive therapy. Headache 41(1):92–96, 2001 11168610

Hawkins J, Khanna S, Argalious M: Sugammadex for reversal of neuromuscular blockade: Uses and limitations. Curr Pharm Des 25(19):2140–2148, 2019 31272347

Haxton C, Kelly S, Young D, et al: The efficacy of electroconvulsive therapy in a perinatal population: a comparative pilot study. J ECT 32(2):113–115, 2016 26479488

Heath ES, Adams A, Wakeling PL: Short courses of ECT and simulated ECT in chronic schizophrenia. Br J Psychiatry 110:800–807, 1964 14211696

Heijnen WT, Birkenhäger TK, Wierdsma AI, et al: Antidepressant pharmacotherapy failure and response to subsequent electroconvulsive therapy: a meta-analysis. J Clin Psychopharmacol 30(5):616–619, 2010 20814336

Heijnen WT, Pluijms EM, Birkenhager TK: Refractory major depression successfully treated with electroconvulsive therapy in a patient with Addison disease. J ECT 29(2):137–138, 2013 23377750

Heijnen WTCJ, Kamperman AM, Tjokrodipo LD, et al: Influence of age on ECT efficacy in depression and the mediating role of psychomotor retardation and psychotic features. J Psychiatr Res 109:41–47, 2019 30472527

Heinonen OP, Slone D, Shapiro S: Birth Defects and Drugs in Pregnancy. Littleton, MA, Publishing Sciences Group, 1977

Henssler J, Bschor T, Baethge C: Combining antidepressants in acute treatment of depression: a meta-analysis of 38 studies including 4511 patients. Can J Psychiatry 61(1):29–43, 2016 27582451

Henstra MJ, Jansma EP, van der Velde N, et al: Acetylcholinesterase inhibitors for electroconvulsive therapy-induced cognitive side effects: a systematic review. Int J Geriatr Psychiatry 32(5):522–531, 2017 28295591

Hermida AP, Janjua AU, Tang Y, et al: Use of orally disintegrating olanzapine during electroconvulsive therapy for prevention of postictal agitation. J Psychiatr Pract 22(6):459–462, 2016 27824778

Hermida AP, Goldstein FC, Loring DW, et al: ElectroConvulsive therapy Cognitive Assessment (ECCA) tool: a new instrument to monitor cognitive function in patients undergoing ECT. J Affect Disord 269:36–42, 2020a 32217341

Hermida AP, Tang YL, Glass O, et al: Efficacy and safety of ECT for behavioral and psychological symptoms of dementia (BPSD): a retrospective chart review. Am J Geriatr Psychiatry 28(2):157–163, 2020b 31668364

Hermida AP, Mohsin M, Marques Pinheiro AP, et al: The cardiovascular side effects of electroconvulsive therapy and their management. J ECT 38(1):2–9, 2022 34699395

Hersh JK: Struck by Living: From Depression to Hope. Dallas, TX, Brown Books, 2010

Hersh JK: Electroconvulsive therapy (ECT) from the patient's perspective. J Med Ethics 39(3):171–172, 2013 23197793

Herzberg F: Prognostic variables for electro-shock therapy. J Gen Psychol 50:79–86, 1954

Herzig SJ, LaSalvia MT, Naidus E, et al: Antipsychotics and the risk of aspiration pneumonia in individuals hospitalized for nonpsychiatric conditions: a cohort study. J Am Geriatr Soc 65(12):2580–2586, 2017 29095482

Herzog A, Detre T: Psychotic reactions associated with childbirth. Dis Nerv Syst 37(4):229–235, 1976 767081

Heshe J, Roeder E: Electroconvulsive therapy in Denmark. Br J Psychiatry 128:241–245, 1976 1252687

Hickey DR, O'Connor JP, Donati F: Comparison of atracurium and succinylcholine for electroconvulsive therapy in a patient with atypical plasma cholinesterase. Can J Anaesth 34(3 (Pt 1)):280–283, 1987 3581397

Hickie I, Parsonage B, Parker G: Prediction of response to electroconvulsive therapy. preliminary validation of a sign-based typology of depression. Br J Psychiatry 157:65–71, 1990 1975760

Hickie I, Mason C, Parker G, et al: Prediction of ECT response: validation of a refined sign-based (CORE) system for defining melancholia. Br J Psychiatry 169(1):68–74, 1996 8818371

Hicks FG: ECT modified by atracurium. Convuls Ther 3(1):54–59, 1987 11940891

Higgins ES, George MS: Brain Stimulation Therapies for Clinicians, Revised Edition. Washington, DC, American Psychiatric Publishing, 2019

Hillow MA, Kwobah EK, Gakinya B, et al: Sudden death after electroconvulsive therapy in the context of coronavirus disease 2019. J ECT 37(3):209–210, 2021 33907074

Hinkle PE, Coffey CE, Weiner RD, et al: Use of caffeine to lengthen seizures in ECT. Am J Psychiatry 144(9):1143–1148, 1987 3631312

Hiremani RM, Thirthalli J, Tharayil BS, et al: Double-blind randomized controlled study comparing short-term efficacy of bifrontal and bitemporal electroconvulsive therapy in acute mania. Bipolar Disord 10(6):701–707, 2008 18837864

Hirschfeld RM, Williams JB, Spitzer RL, et al: Development and validation of a screening instrument for bipolar spectrum disorder: the Mood Disorder Questionnaire. Am J Psychiatry 157(11):1873–1875, 2000 11058490

Hitti FL, Cristancho MA, Yang AI, et al: Deep brain stimulation of the ventral capsule/ventral striatum for treatment-resistant depression: a decade of clinical follow-up. J Clin Psychiatry 82(6):21m13973, 2021 34670026

Hjerrild S, Kahlert J, Buchholtz PE, et al: Long-term risk of developing dementia after electroconvulsive therapy for affective disorders. J ECT 37(4):250–255, 2021 33907075

Hobo M, Uezato A, Nishiyama M, et al: A case of malignant catatonia with idiopathic pulmonary arterial hypertension treated by electroconvulsive therapy. BMC Psychiatry 16:130, 2016 27153810

Hobson RF: Prognostic factors in ECT. J Neurol Neurosurg Psychiatry 16:275–281, 1953 13109543

Hodgson RE, Dawson P, Hold AR, et al: Anaesthesia for electroconvulsive therapy: a comparison of sevoflurane with propofol. Anaesth Intensive Care 32(2):241–245, 2004 15957723

Höflich G, Kasper S, Burghof KW, et al: Maintenance ECT for treatment of therapy-resistant paranoid schizophrenia and Parkinson's disease. Biol Psychiatry 37(12):892–894, 1995 7548464

Holdcroft A, Robinson MJ, Gordon H, et al: Comparison of effect of two induction doses of methohexitone on infants delivered by elective caesarean section. BMJ 2(5917):472–475, 1974 4834097

Holmberg C, Gremyr A, Torgerson J, et al: Clinical validity of the 12-item WHODAS-2.0 in a naturalistic sample of outpatients with psychotic disorders. BMC Psychiatry 21(1):147, 2021 33691655

Holtzheimer PE, Husain MM, Lisanby SH, et al: Subcallosal cingulate deep brain stimulation for treatment-resistant depression: a multisite, randomised, sham-controlled trial. Lancet Psychiatry 4(11):839–849, 2017 28988904

Honing G, Martini CH, Bom A, et al: Safety of sugammadex for reversal of neuromuscular block. Expert Opin Drug Saf 18(10):883–891, 2019 31359807

Hood DD, Mecca RS: Failure to initiate electroconvulsive seizures in a patient pretreated with lidocaine. Anesthesiology 58(4):379–381, 1983 6837980

Hooten WM, Rasmussen KG Jr: Effects of general anesthetic agents in adults receiving electroconvulsive therapy: a systematic review. J ECT 24(3):208–223, 2008 18628717

Hořínková J, Barteček R, Fedorová S: Electroconvulsive therapy in the treatment of patient with depressive disorder after traumatic brain injury, intracranial bleeding, and polytrauma. J ECT 33(3):e22–e24, 2017 28445184

Hoshi H, Kadoi Y, Kamiyama J, et al: Use of rocuronium-sugammadex, an alternative to succinylcholine, as a muscle relaxant during electroconvulsive therapy. J Anesth 25(2):286–290, 2011 21293886

Hovorka EJ, Schumsky DA, Work MS: Electroconvulsive thresholds as related to stimulus parameters of unidirectional ECS. J Comp Physiol Psychol 53:412–414, 1960 14403427

Howes OD, McCutcheon R, Agid O, et al: Treatment-resistant schizophrenia: treatment response and resistance in psychosis (TRRIP) working group consensus guidelines on diagnosis and terminology. Am J Psychiatry 174(3):216–229, 2017 27919182

Howland M, Tatsuoka C, Smyth KA, et al: Evaluating PROMIS® applied cognition items in a sample of older adults at risk for cognitive decline. Psychiatry Res 247:39–42, 2017 27863317

Hoyer C, Kranaster L, Janke C, et al: Impact of the anesthetic agents ketamine, etomidate, thiopental, and propofol on seizure parameters and seizure quality in electroconvulsive therapy: a retrospective study. Eur Arch Psychiatry Clin Neurosci 264(3):255–261, 2014 23835527

Hsiao JK, Evans DL: ECT in a depressed patient after craniotomy. Am J Psychiatry 141(3):442–444, 1984 6703116

Hsiao JK, Messenheimer JA, Evans DL: ECT and neurological disorders. Convuls Ther 3(2):121–136, 1987 11940905

Hsieh KY, Tsai KY, Chou FH, et al: Reduced risk of stroke among psychiatric patients receiving ECT: a population-based cohort study in Taiwan. Psychiatry Res 276:107–111, 2019 31048180

Huang CJ, Lin CH, Wu JI, et al: The relationship between depression symptoms and anxiety symptoms during acute ECT for patients with major depressive disorder. Int J Neuropsychopharmacol 22(10):609–615, 2019 31282929

Hudcova J, Schumann R: Electroconvulsive therapy complicated by life-threatening hyperkalemia in a catatonic patient. Gen Hosp Psychiatry 28(5):440–442, 2006 16950383

Huffman JC, Niazi SK, Rundell JR, et al: Essential articles on collaborative care models for the treatment of psychiatric disorders in medical settings: a publication by the academy of psychosomatic medicine research and evidence-based practice committee. Psychosomatics 55(2):109–122, 2014 24370112

Hung CI, Liu CY, Yang CH: Untreated duration predicted the severity of depression at the two-year follow-up point. PLoS One 12(9):e0185119, 2017 28934289

Husain MM, Meyer DE, Muttakin MH, et al: Maintenance ECT for treatment of recurrent mania. Am J Psychiatry 150(6):985, 1993 8494084

Husain MM, Rush AJ, Fink M, et al: Speed of response and remission in major depressive disorder with acute electroconvulsive therapy (ECT): a Consortium for Research in ECT (CORE) report. J Clin Psychiatry 65(4):485–491, 2004 15119910

Hutchinson JT, Smedberg D: Treatment of depression: a comparative study of E.C.T. and six drugs. Br J Psychiatry 109:536–538, 1963 13955929

Hutson MM, Blaha JD: Patients' recall of preoperative instruction for informed consent for an operation. J Bone Joint Surg Am 73(2):160–162, 1991 1993710

Huuhka MJ, Seinelä L, Reinikainen P, et al: Cardiac arrhythmias induced by ECT in elderly psychiatric patients: experience with 48-hour Holter monitoring. J ECT 19(1):22–25, 2003 12621273

Huybrechts KF, Hernández-Díaz S, Straub L, et al: Association of maternal first-trimester ondansetron use with cardiac malformations and oral clefts in offspring. JAMA 320(23):2429–2437, 2018 30561479

Hyrman V, Palmer LH, Cernik J, et al: ECT: the search for the perfect stimulus. Biol Psychiatry 20(6):634–645, 1985 3995110

Ibrahim L, Diazgranados N, Luckenbaugh DA, et al: Rapid decrease in depressive symptoms with an N-methyl-D-aspartate antagonist in ECT-resistant major depression. Prog Neuropsychopharmacol Biol Psychiatry 35(4):1155–1159, 2011 21466832

Imashuku Y, Kanemoto K, Senda M, et al: Relationship between blood levels of propofol and recovery of memory in electroconvulsive therapy. Psychiatry Clin Neurosci 68(4):270–274, 2014 24313665

Imlah NW, Ryan E, Harrington JA: The influence of antidepressant drugs on the response to electroconvulsive therapy and on subsequent relapse rates. Neuropsychopharmacology 4:438–442, 1965

Impastato D, Almansi N: A study of over 2000 cases of electrofit treated patients. N Z Med J 43:2057–2065, 1943

Ingram A, Saling MM, Schweitzer I: Cognitive side effects of brief pulse electroconvulsive therapy: a review. J ECT 24(1):3–9, 2008 18379328

Iodice AJ, McCall WV: ECT resistance and early relapse: two cases of subsequent response to venlafaxine. J ECT 19(4):238–241, 2003 14657779

Iosifescu DV, Norton RJ, Tural U, et al: Very low-level transcranial photobiomodulation for major depressive disorder: the ELATED-3 multicenter, randomized, sham-controlled trial. J Clin Psychiatry 83(5):21m14226, 2022 35950904

Irving AD, Drayson AM: Bladder rupture during ECT. Br J Psychiatry 144:670, 1984 6743939

Isenberg KE, Dinwiddie S, Heath AC, et al: Effect of electrical parameters on ECT convulsive threshold and duration. Ann Clin Psychiatry 28(2):105–116, 2016 27285391

Isserles M, Daskalakis ZJ, Kumar S, et al: Clinical effectiveness and tolerability of electroconvulsive therapy in patients with neuropsychiatric symptoms of dementia. J Alzheimers Dis 57(1):45–51, 2017 28222513

Ithal D, Arumugham SS, Kumar CN, et al: Comparison of cognitive adverse effects and efficacy of 2 pulse widths (0.5 ms and 1.5 ms) of brief pulse bilateral electroconvulsive therapy in patients with schizophrenia: a randomized single blind controlled trial. Schizophr Res 216:520–522, 2020 31839555

Ithman M, O'Connell C, Ogunleye A, et al: Pre- and post-clerkship knowledge, perceptions, and acceptability of electroconvulsive therapy (ECT) in 3rd year medical students. Psychiatr Q 89(4):869–880, 2018 29804233

Ittasakul P, Likitnukul A, Pitidhrammabhorn U, et al: Stimulus intensity determined by dose-titration versus age-based methods in electroconvulsive therapy in Thai patients. Neuropsychiatr Dis Treat 15:429–434, 2019 30799921

Izquierdo-Guerra KI, Montoya-Arenas D, Franco JG, et al: Relationship between depressive symptomatology and cognitive performance in older people. Int J Psychol Res (Medellin) 11(2):35–45, 2018 32612777

Jacobowski NL, Heckers S, Bobo WV: Delirious mania: detection, diagnosis, and clinical management in the acute setting. J Psychiatr Pract 19(1):15–28, 2013 23334676

Jacobs DG, Brewer ML: Application of the APA practice guidelines on suicide to clinical practice. CNS Spectr 11(6):447–454, 2006 16816784

Jacobsma B: A balancing act: continuing education for staff nurses. J Psychosoc Nurs Ment Health Serv 29(2):15–21, 1991 2005591

Jadhav T, Sriganesh K, Thirthalli J, et al: Effect of atropine premedication on cardiac autonomic function during electroconvulsive therapy: a randomized crossover study. J ECT 33(3):176–180, 2017 28471773

Jaffe R: ECT training: can the case be made for certification? J ECT 21(2):73–74, 2005 15905746

Jaffe R, Brubaker G, Dubin WR, et al: Caffeine-associated cardiac dysrhythmia during ECT: report of three cases. Convuls Ther 6(4):308–313, 1990a 11941084

Jaffe R, Dubin W, Shoyer B, et al: Outpatient electroconvulsive therapy: efficacy and safety. Convuls Ther 6(3):231–238, 1990b 11941073

Jaffe RL, Rives W, Dubin WR, et al: Problems in maintenance ECT in bipolar disorder: replacement by lithium and anticonvulsants. Convuls Ther 7(4):288–294, 1991 11941135

Jagadisha, Gangadhar B, Janakiramiah N, et al: Post-seizure EEG fractal dimension and spectral power predict antidepressant response to unilateral ECT. Indian J Psychiatry 45(1):16–20, 2003 21206807

Jahangard L, Haghighi M, Bigdelou G, et al: Comparing efficacy of ECT with and without concurrent sodium valproate therapy in manic patients. J ECT 28(2):118–123, 2012 22531205

Jaimes-Albornoz W, Ruiz de Pellon-Santamaria A, Nizama-Vía A, et al: Catatonia in older adults: a systematic review. World J Psychiatry 12(2):348–367, 2022 35317341

Janakiramaiah N, Motreja S, Gangadhar BN, et al: Once vs. three times weekly ECT in melancholia: a randomized controlled trial. Acta Psychiatr Scand 98(4):316–320, 1998 9821454

Janicak PG, Davis JM, Gibbons RD, et al: Efficacy of ECT: a meta-analysis. Am J Psychiatry 142(3):297–302, 1985 3882006

Janicak PG, Sharma RP, Israni TH, et al: Effects of unilateral-nondominant vs. bilateral ECT on memory and depression: a preliminary report. Psychopharmacol Bull 27(3):353–357, 1991 1775610

Janis K, Hess J, Fabian JA, Gillis M: Substitution of mivacurium for succinylcholine for ECT in elderly patients. Can J Anaesth 42(7):612–613, 1995 7553998

Jarde A, Morais M, Kingston D, et al: Neonatal outcomes in women with untreated antenatal depression compared with women without depression: a systematic review and meta-analysis. JAMA Psychiatry 73(8):826–837, 2016 27276520

Jarvis MR, Goewert AJ, Zorumski CF: Novel antidepressants and maintenance electroconvulsive therapy: a review. Ann Clin Psychiatry 4:275–284, 1992

Jeanneau A: Electroconvulsive therapy in the treatment of Parkinson disease [in French]. Encephale 19(5):573–578, 1993 8306926

Jelovac A, Kolshus E, McLoughlin DM: Relapse following successful electro-convulsive therapy for major depression: a meta-analysis. Neuropsycho-pharmacology 38(12):2467–2474, 2013 23774532

Jelovac A, O'Connor S, McCarron S, et al: Autobiographical memory specificity in major depression treated with electroconvulsive therapy. J ECT 32(1):38–43, 2016 26252557

Jensen FS, Mogensen JV: Plasma cholinesterase and abnormal reaction to suxamethonium injection: 20-year experience with the Danish Cholinesterase Registry [in Danish]. Ugeskr Laeger 158(13):1835–1839, 1996 8650760

Jewell M, Delva NJ, Graf P, et al: A national survey on nursing in Canadian ECT departments. Arch Psychiatr Nurs 31(3):302–305, 2017 28499572

Jha A, Stein G: Decreased efficacy of combined benzodiazepines and unilateral ECT in treatment of depression. Acta Psychiatr Scand 94(2):101–104, 1996 8883570

Jha AK, Stein GS, Fenwick P: Negative interaction between lithium and electro-convulsive therapy: a case-control study. Br J Psychiatry 168(2):241–243, 1996 8837918

Jiam NT, Li D, Kramer K, et al: Preserved cochlear implant function after multiple electroconvulsive therapy treatments. Laryngoscope 131(5):E1695–E1698, 2021 33252138

Johnson SY: Regulatory pressures hamper the effectiveness of electroconvulsive therapy. Law Psychol Rev 17:155–170, 1993 11659924

Johnstone EC, Deakin JF, Lawler P, et al: The Northwick Park electroconvulsive therapy trial. Lancet 2(8208–8209):1317–1320, 1980 6109147

Joo SW, Joo YH, Kim CY, et al: Effects of stimulus parameters on motor seizure duration in electroconvulsive therapy. Neuropsychiatr Dis Treat 13:1427–1434, 2017 28603421

Joo SW, Kim H, Jo YT, et al: One-year clinical outcomes following electrocon-vulsive therapy for patients with schizophrenia: a nationwide health insurance data-based study. Neuropsychiatr Dis Treat 18:1645–1652, 2022 35968513

Julian LJ: Measures of anxiety: State-Trait Anxiety Inventory (STAI), Beck Anxiety Inventory (BAI), and Hospital Anxiety and Depression Scale—Anxiety (HADS-A). Arthritis Care Res (Hoboken) 63 Suppl(0 11):S467–S472, 2011 22588767

Jurica PJ, Leitten CL, Mattis S: DRS-2 Dementia Rating Scale-2: Professional Manual. Lutz, FL, Psychological Assessment Resources, 1988

Kales H, Raz J, Tandon R, et al: Relationship of seizure duration to antidepres-sant efficacy in electroconvulsive therapy. Psychol Med 27(6):1373–1380, 1997 9403909

Kalinowsky LB: Electric convulsion therapy with emphasis on importance of adequate treatment. AMA Archives of Neurology and Psychiatry (Chica-go) 50:652–660, 1943

Kalinowsky LB, Hoch PH: Shock Treatments and Other Somatic Procedures in Psychiatry. New York, Grune & Stratton, 1946

Kalinowsky LB, Kennedy F: Observation in electroshock therapy applied to problems in epilepsy. J Nerv Ment Dis 98:56–67, 1943

Kalinowsky LB, Worthing H: Results with electric convulsive therapy in 200 cases of schizophrenia. Psychiatr Q 17:144–153, 1943

Kamigaichi R, Kubo S, Ishikawa K, et al: Effective control of catatonia in Parkinson's disease by electroconvulsive therapy: a case report. Eur J Neurol 16(2):e6, 2009 19146631

Kane JM: Tools to assess negative symptoms in schizophrenia. J Clin Psychiatry 74(6):e12, 2013 23842020

Kang N, Passmore MJ: Successful ECT in a patient with an orbital cavernous hemangioma. J ECT 20(4):267–271, 2004 15591864

Kant R, Bogyi AM, Carosella NW, et al: ECT as a therapeutic option in severe brain injury. Convuls Ther 11(1):45–50, 1995 7796068

Kant R, Coffey CE, Bogyi AM: Safety and efficacy of ECT in patients with head injury: a case series. J Neuropsychiatry Clin Neurosci 11(1):32–37, 1999 9990553

Kaplan YC, Richardson JL, Keskin-Arslan E, et al: Use of ondansetron during pregnancy and the risk of major congenital malformations: a systematic review and meta-analysis. Reprod Toxicol 86:1–13, 2019 30849498

Kardener SH: EST in a patient with idiopathic thrombocytopenic purpura. Dis Nerv Syst 29(7):465–466, 1968 5692089

Karimi M, Brazier J: Health, health-related quality of life, and quality of life: what is the difference? PharmacoEconomics 34(7):645–649, 2016 26892973

Karmacharya R, England ML, Ongür D: Delirious mania: clinical features and treatment response. J Affect Disord 109(3):312–316, 2008 18191210

Karthik N, Jolly AJ, Selvaraj S, et al: Electroconvulsive therapy in a patient with mania and ventriculoperitoneal shunt: a case report. J ECT 38(3):e41–e42, 2022 35462390

Kashaninasab F, Panahi Dashdebi R, Ghalehbandi MF: Comorbidity of Coronavirus disease (COVID-19) and the first episode of bipolar disorder and its treatment challenges: a case report. Med J Islam Repub Iran 34:103, 2020 33315969

Kaster TS, Goldbloom DS, Daskalakis ZJ, et al: Electroconvulsive therapy for depression with comorbid borderline personality disorder or post-traumatic stress disorder: a matched retrospective cohort study. Brain Stimul 11(1):204–212, 2018 29111076

Kaster TS, Vigod SN, Gomes T, et al: Risk of serious medical events in patients with depression treated with electroconvulsive therapy: a propensity score-matched, retrospective cohort study. Lancet Psychiatry 8(8):686–695, 2021 34265274

Kaster TS, Blumberger DM, Gomes T, et al: Risk of suicide death following electroconvulsive therapy treatment for depression: a propensity score-weighted, retrospective cohort study in Canada. Lancet Psychiatry 9(6):435–446, 2022 35487236

Katona CL: Puerperal mental illness: comparisons with non-puerperal controls. Br J Psychiatry 141:447–452, 1982 7150880

Katz G: Electroconvulsive therapy from a social work perspective. Soc Work Health Care 16(4):55–68, 1992 1529408

Katz RB, Toprak M, Ostroff R: A successful course of electroconvulsive therapy in a patient with epilepsy and a posterior fossa titanium plate. J ECT 33(2):e17–e18, 2017 28009626

Katzell L, Beydler EM, Holbert R, et al: Electroconvulsive therapy use for refractory status epilepticus in an implantable vagus nerve stimulation patient: a case report. Front Psychiatry 14:1126956, 2023 36816412

Kaur G, Khavarian Z, Basith SA, et al: New-onset catatonia and delirium in a COVID-positive patient. Cureus 13(10):e18422, 2021 34729258

Kavanagh A, McLoughlin DM: Electroconvulsive therapy and nursing care. Br J Nurs 18(22):1370–1377, 1372, 1374–1377, 2009 20081692

Kay DW, Fahy T, Garside RF: A seven-month double-blind trial of amitriptyline and diazepam in ECT-treated depressed patients. Br J Psychiatry 117(541):667–671, 1970 4923720

Kay SR, Fiszbein A, Opler LA: The positive and negative syndrome scale (PANSS) for schizophrenia. Schizophr Bull 13(2):261–276, 1987 3616518

Keilp JG, Madden SP, Gorlyn M, et al: The lack of meaningful association between depression severity measures and neurocognitive performance. J Affect Disord 241:164–172, 2018 30121449

Kellner C, Batterson JR, Monroe R: ECT as an alternative to lithium for preventive treatment of bipolar disorder. Am J Psychiatry 147(7):953, 1990 2356888

Kellner C, Lisanby SH; Consortium for Research on ECT (CORE) Investigator Group: Flexible dosing schedules for continuation electroconvulsive therapy. J ECT 24(3):177–178, 2008 18772701

Kellner CH: ECT education. J ECT 17(3):157, 2001 11528303

Kellner CH: Handbook of ECT: A Guide to Electroconvulsive Therapy for Practitioners. New York, Cambridge University Press, 2019

Kellner CH, Bruno RM: Fluoxetine and ECT (letter). Convuls Ther 5(4):367–368, 1989 11941039

Kellner CH, Farber KG: The role of bilateral ECT when right unilateral ECT is inferior. Am J Psychiatry 173(7):731, 2016 27363553

Kellner CH, Rames L: Dexamethasone pretreatment for ECT in a patient with meningioma. Clin Gerontol 10:67–72, 1990

Kellner CH, Monroe RR, Burns C, et al: Electroconvulsive therapy in a patient with a heart transplant. N Engl J Med 325(9):663, 1991a 1861707

Kellner CH, Tolhurst JE, Burns CM: ECT in the presence of severe cervical spine disease (case report). Convuls Ther 7(1):52–55, 1991b 11941098

Kellner CH, Monroe RR Jr, Pritchett J, et al: Weekly ECT in geriatric depression. Convuls Ther 8(4):245–252, 1992a 11941174

Kellner CH, Rubey RN, Burns C, et al: Safe administration of ECT in a patient taking selegiline. Convuls Ther 8(2):144–145, 1992b 11941163

Kellner CH, Beale MD, Pritchett JT, et al: Electroconvulsive therapy and Parkinson's disease: the case for further study. Psychopharmacol Bull 30(3):495–500, 1994a 7878188

Kellner CH, Pritchett JT, Jackson CW: Bupropion coadministration with electroconvulsive therapy: two case reports. J Clin Psychopharmacol 14(3):215–216, 1994b 8027425

Kellner CH, Knapp RG, Petrides G, et al: Continuation electroconvulsive therapy vs pharmacotherapy for relapse prevention in major depression: a multisite study from the Consortium for Research in Electroconvulsive Therapy (CORE). Arch Gen Psychiatry 63(12):1337–1344, 2006 17146008

Kellner CH, Knapp R, Husain MM, et al: Bifrontal, bitemporal and right unilateral electrode placement in ECT: randomised trial. Br J Psychiatry 196(3):226–234, 2010 20194546

Kellner CH, Kaicher DC, Banerjee H, et al: Depression severity in electroconvulsive therapy (ECT) versus pharmacotherapy trials. J ECT 31(1):31–33, 2015 24839981

Kellner CH, Husain MM, Knapp RG, et al: Right unilateral ultrabrief pulse ECT in geriatric depression: phase 1 of the PRIDE study. Am J Psychiatry 173(11):1101–1109, 2016b 27418379

Kellner CH, Husain MM, Knapp RG, et al: A novel strategy for continuation ECT in geriatric depression: phase 2 of the PRIDE study. Am J Psychiatry 173(11):1110–1118, 2016a 27418381

Kellner CH, Farber KG, Chen XR, et al: A systematic review of left unilateral electroconvulsive therapy. Acta Psychiatr Scand 136(2):166–176, 2017 28422271

Kellner CH, McCall WV, Spaans HP, et al: The FDA final order on ECT devices, finally. J ECT 35(2):69–70, 2019 31022040

Kellner CH, Obbels J, Sienaert P: When to consider electroconvulsive therapy (ECT). Acta Psychiatr Scand 141(4):304–315, 2020 31774547

Kelway B, Simpson KH, Smith RJ, et al: Effects of atropine and glycopyrrolate on cognitive function following anaesthesia and electroconvulsive therapy (ECT). Int Clin Psychopharmacol 1(4):296–302, 1986 3549875

Kennedy CJ, Anchel D: Regressive electric-shock in schizophrenics refractory to other shock therapies. Psychiatr Q 22(2):317–320, 1948 18874318

Kennedy R, Mittal D, O'Jile J: Electroconvulsive therapy in movement disorders: an update. J Neuropsychiatry Clin Neurosci 15(4):407–421, 2003 14627767

Kerman EF: Electroshock therapy: with special reference to relapses and an effort to prevent them. J Nerv Ment Dis 102:231–242, 1945

Kerner N, Prudic J: Current electroconvulsive therapy practice and research in the geriatric population. Neuropsychiatry (London) 4(1):33–54, 2014 24778709

Kessing L, LaBianca JH, Bolwig TG: HIV-induced stupor treated with ECT. Convuls Ther 10(3):232–235, 1994 7834262

Keyloun KR, Hansen RN, Hepp Z, et al: Adherence and persistence across antidepressant therapeutic classes: a retrospective claims analysis among insured US patients with major depressive disorder (MDD). CNS Drugs 31(5):421–432, 2017 28378157

Kho KH, van Vreeswijk MF, Simpson S, et al: A meta-analysis of electroconvulsive therapy efficacy in depression. J ECT 19(3):139–147, 2003 12972983

Kho KH, Zwinderman AH, Blansjaar BA: Predictors for the efficacy of electroconvulsive therapy: chart review of a naturalistic study. J Clin Psychiatry 66(7):894–899, 2005 16013905

Kibret B, Premaratne M, Sullivan C, et al: Electroconvulsive therapy (ECT) during pregnancy: quantifying and assessing the electric field strength inside the foetal brain. Sci Rep 8(1):4128, 2018 29515221

Kikuchi A, Yasui-Furukori N, Fujii A, et al: Identification of predictors of post-ictal delirium after electroconvulsive therapy. Psychiatry Clin Neurosci 63(2):180–185, 2009 19335388

Kiloh LG, Child JP, Latner G: A controlled trial of iproniazid in the treatment of endogenous depression. J Ment Sci 106:1139–1144, 1960 13755968

Kiloh LG, Smith JS, Johnson GF: Physical Treatments in Psychiatry. Melbourne, Australia, Blackwell Scientific, 1988

King PD: Phenelzine and ECT in the treatment of depressions. Am J Psychiatry 116(1):64–65, 1959 13661451

King PD: Chlorpromazine and electroconvulsive therapy in the treatment of newly hospitalized schizophrenics. J Clin Exp Psychopathol Q Rev Psychiatry Neurol 21:101–105, 1960 14409198

Kino FF, Thorpe FT: Electrical convulsion therapy in 500 selected psychotics. J Ment Sci 92:138–145, 1946 20984299

Kivler CA: Will I Ever Be the Same Again? Transforming the Face of Depression and Anxiety. Lawrence, NJ, Three Gem Publishing/Kivler Communications, 2018

Klapheke MM: Electroconvulsive therapy consultation: an update. Convuls Ther 13(4):227–241, 1997 9437567

Koch M, Chandragiri S, Rizvi S, et al: Catatonic signs in neuroleptic malignant syndrome. Compr Psychiatry 41(1):73–75, 2000 10646623

Koenig HG, Kuchibhatla M: Use of health services by hospitalized medically ill depressed elderly patients. Am J Psychiatry 155(7):871–877, 1998 9659849

Koester J: Voltage-gated channels and the generation of the action potential, in Principles of Neural Science. Edited by Kandel ER, Schwartz JH. New York, Elsevier, 1985, pp 75–86

Kohler CG, Burock M: ECT for psychotic depression associated with a brain tumor. Am J Psychiatry 158(12):2089, 2001 11729041

Kolano JE, Chhibber A, Calalang CC: Use of esmolol to control bleeding and heart rate during electroconvulsive therapy in a patient with an intracranial aneurysm. J Clin Anesth 9(6):493–495, 1997 9278838

Kolshus E, Jelovac A, McLoughlin DM: Bitemporal v. high-dose right unilateral electroconvulsive therapy for depression: a systematic review and meta-analysis of randomized controlled trials. Psychol Med 47(3):518–530, 2017 27780482

Koong FJ, Chen WC: Maintaining electroconvulsive therapy for refractory epilepsy combined with psychotic symptoms. BMJ Case Rep 2010:bcr1120092506, 2010 22802485

Koopowitz LF, Chur-Hansen A, Reid S, et al: The subjective experience of patients who received electroconvulsive therapy. Aust N Z J Psychiatry 37(1):49–54, 2003 12534656

Kopelman MD: Anomalies of autobiographical memory. J Int Neuropsychol Soc 25(10):1061–1075, 2019 31474234

Koren G, Zemlickis DM: Outcome of pregnancy after first trimester exposure to H2 receptor antagonists. Am J Perinatol 8(1):37–38, 1991 1670987

Koyama Y, Tsuzaki K, Suzuki T, et al: Prevention of oxygen desaturation in morbidly obese patients during electroconvulsive therapy: a narrative review. J ECT 36(3):161–167, 2020 32040021

Kramer BA: Use of ECT in California, 1977–1983. Am J Psychiatry 142(10):1190–1192, 1985 3898873

Kramer BA: Maintenance ECT: a survey of practice (1986). Convuls Ther 3(4):260–268, 1987 11940927

Kramer BA: Maintenance electroconvulsive therapy in clinical practice. Convuls Ther 6(4):279–286, 1990 11941081

Kramer BA: A naturalistic view of maintenance ECT at a university setting. J ECT 15(4):262–269, 1999 10614033

Kramer BA, Afrasiabi A: Atypical cholinesterase and prolonged apnea during electroconvulsive therapy. Convuls Ther 7(2):129–132, 1991 11941113

Kramer BA, Allen RE, Friedman B: Atropine and glycopyrrolate as ECT preanesthesia. J Clin Psychiatry 47(4):199–200, 1986 3957880

Kramp P, Bolwig TG: Electroconvulsive therapy in acute delirious states. Compr Psychiatry 22(4):368–371, 1981 7261577

Kranaster L, Janke C, Mindt S, et al: Protein S-100 and neuron-specific enolase serum levels remain unaffected by electroconvulsive therapy in patients with depression. J Neural Transm (Vienna) 121(11):1411–1415, 2014 24801966

Kraus C, Kadriu B, Lanzenberger R, et al: Prognosis and improved outcomes in major depression: a review. Transl Psychiatry 9(1):127, 2019 30944309

Kristiansen ES: A comparison of treatment of endogenous depression with electroshock and with imipramine (tofranil). Acta Psychiatr Scand Suppl 162:179–188, 1961 14459717

Kriston L, von Wolff A, Westphal A, et al: Efficacy and acceptability of acute treatments for persistent depressive disorder: a network meta-analysis. Depress Anxiety 31(8):621–630, 2014 24448972

Kroenke K, Spitzer RL, Williams JBW: The PHQ-9: validity of a brief depression severity measure. J Gen Intern Med 16(9):606–613, 2001 11556941

Kroessler D: Relative efficacy rates for therapies of delusional depression. Convuls Ther 1(3):173–182, 1985 11940821

Kronsell A, Nordenskjöld A, Bell M, et al: The effect of anaesthetic dose on response and remission in electroconvulsive therapy for major depressive disorder: nationwide register-based cohort study. BJPsych Open 7(2):e71, 2021 33752777

Krueger RB, Sackeim HA: Electroconvulsive therapy and schizophrenia, in Schizophrenia. Edited by Hirsch SR, Weinberger D. Oxford, UK, Blackwell Scientific, 1995, pp 503–545

Krueger RB, Fama JM, Devanand DP, et al: Does ECT permanently alter seizure threshold? Biol Psychiatry 33(4):272–276, 1993 8471681

Krystal AD, Coffey CE: Neuropsychiatric considerations in the use of electroconvulsive therapy. J Neuropsychiatry Clin Neurosci 9(2):283–292, 1997 9144111

Krystal AD, Weiner RD: Low-frequency ictal EEG activity and ECT therapeutic impact. Convuls Ther 9(3):220–224, 1993 11941217

Krystal AD, Weiner RD: ECT seizure duration: reliability of manual and computer-automated determinations. Convuls Ther 11(3):158–169, 1995 8528657

Krystal AD, Weiner RD, McCall WV, et al: The effects of ECT stimulus dose and electrode placement on the ictal electroencephalogram: an intraindividual crossover study. Biol Psychiatry 34(11):759–767, 1993 8292679

Krystal AD, Weiner RD, Coffey CE: The ictal EEG as a marker of adequate stimulus intensity with unilateral ECT. J Neuropsychiatry Clin Neurosci 7(3):295–303, 1995 7580187

Krystal AD, Weiner RD, Coffey CE, et al: Effect of ECT treatment number on the ictal EEG. Psychiatry Res 62(2):179–189, 1996 8771615

Krystal AD, Coffey CE, Weiner RD, et al: Changes in seizure threshold over the course of electroconvulsive therapy affect therapeutic response and are detected by ictal EEG ratings. J Neuropsychiatry Clin Neurosci 10(2):178–186, 1998a 9608406

Krystal AD, Watts BV, Weiner RD, et al: The use of flumazenil in the anxious and benzodiazepine-dependent ECT patient. J ECT 14(1):5–14, 1998b 9661088

Krystal AD, Dean MD, Weiner RD, et al: ECT stimulus intensity: are present ECT devices too limited? Am J Psychiatry 157(6):963–967, 2000a 10831477

Krystal AD, Holsinger T, Weiner RD, et al: Prediction of the utility of a switch from unilateral to bilateral ECT in the elderly using treatment 2 ictal EEG indices. J ECT 16(4):327–337, 2000b 11314870

Krystal AD, Weiner RD, Lindahl V, et al: The development and retrospective testing of an electroencephalographic seizure quality-based stimulus dosing paradigm with ECT. J ECT 16(4):338–349, 2000c 11314871

Krystal AD, Weiner RD, Dean MD, et al: Comparison of seizure duration, ictal EEG, and cognitive effects of ketamine and methohexital anesthesia with ECT. J Neuropsychiatry Clin Neurosci 15(1):27–34, 2003 12556568

Kucuker MU, Almorsy AG, Sonmez AI, et al: A systematic review of neuromodulation treatment effects on suicidality. Front Hum Neurosci 15:660926, 2021 34248523

Kufner M, Nothdurfter C, Steffling D, et al: Electroconvulsive therapy in a patient with hypertrophic cardiomyopathy: a case report. Clin Case Rep 10(9):e6286, 2022 36093461

Kukopulos A, Reginaldi D, Tondo L, et al: Spontaneous length of depression and response to ECT. Psychol Med 7(4):625–629, 1977 594243

Kumar A, Bunker MT, Aaronson ST, et al: Durability of symptomatic responses obtained with adjunctive vagus nerve stimulation in treatment-resistant depression. Neuropsychiatr Dis Treat 15:457–468, 2019 30858703

Kumar S, Mulsant BH, Liu AY, et al: Systematic review of cognitive effects of electroconvulsive therapy in late-life depression. Am J Geriatr Psychiatry 24(7):547–565, 2016 27067067

Kupchik M, Spivak B, Mester R, et al: Combined electroconvulsive-clozapine therapy. Clin Neuropharmacol 23(1):14–16, 2000 10682225

Kurnutala LN, Kamath S, Koyfman S, et al: Aspiration during electroconvulsive therapy under general anesthesia. J ECT 29(4):e68, 2013 24263279

Kurup V, Ostroff R: When cardiac patients need ECT—challenges for the anesthesiologist. Int Anesthesiol Clin 50(2):128–140, 2012 22481560

Labadie RF, Clark NK, Cobb CM, et al: Electroconvulsive therapy in a cochlear implant patient. Otol Neurotol 31(1):64–66, 2010 19816223

Labbate LA, Miller JP: Midazolam for treatment of agitation after ECT. Am J Psychiatry 152(3):472–473, 1995 7864283

Ladenheim J, Looman JE, Lewis SK: Informed consent: is it a myth? Neurosurgery 31(2):380–381, 1992 1513448

LaGrone D: ECT in secondary mania, pregnancy, and sickle cell anemia. Convuls Ther 6(2):176–180, 1990 11941061

Lalla FR, Milroy T: The current status of seizure duration in the practice of electroconvulsive therapy. Can J Psychiatry 41(5):299–304, 1996 8793149

Lally J, Tully J, Robertson D, et al: Augmentation of clozapine with electroconvulsive therapy in treatment resistant schizophrenia: a systematic review and meta-analysis. Schizophr Res 171(1-3):215–224, 2016 26827129

Lambourn J, Gill D: A controlled comparison of simulated and real ECT. Br J Psychiatry 133:514–519, 1978 367479

Lambrecq V, Villéga F, Marchal C, et al: Refractory status epilepticus: electroconvulsive therapy as a possible therapeutic strategy. Seizure 21(9):661–664, 2012 22877995

Lambrichts S, Vansteelandt K, Crauwels B, et al: Relapse after abrupt discontinuation of maintenance electroconvulsive therapy during the COVID-19 pandemic. Acta Psychiatr Scand 144(3):230–237, 2021 34086984

Landmark J, Joseph L, Merskey H: Characteristics of schizophrenic patients and the outcome of fluphenazine and of electroconvulsive treatments. Can J Psychiatry 32(6):425–428, 1987 3690470

Landry M, Lafrenière S, Patry S, et al: The clinical relevance of dose titration in electroconvulsive therapy: a systematic review of the literature. Psychiatry Res 294:113497, 2020 33039882

Lang B, Zhang L, Yang C, et al: Pretreatment with lidocaine reduces both incidence and severity of etomidate-induced myoclonus: a meta-analysis of randomized controlled trials. Drug Des Devel Ther 12:3311–3319, 2018 30323563

Langsley DG, Enterline JD, Hickerson GX Jr: A comparison of chlorpromazine and EST in treatment of acute schizophrenic and manic reactions. AMA Arch Neurol Psychiatry 81(3):384–391, 1959 13626291

Lapid MI, Rummans TA, Poole KL, et al: Decisional capacity of severely depressed patients requiring electroconvulsive therapy. J ECT 19(2):67–72, 2003 12792453

Lapid MI, Rummans TA, Pankratz VS, et al: Decisional capacity of depressed elderly to consent to electroconvulsive therapy. J Geriatr Psychiatry Neurol 17(1):42–46, 2004 15018698

Lapid MI, Seiner S, Heintz H, et al: Electroconvulsive therapy practice changes in older individuals due to COVID-19: expert consensus statement. Am J Geriatr Psychiatry 28(11):1133–1145, 2020 32863137

Lapidus KA, Kellner CH: When to switch from unilateral to bilateral electroconvulsive therapy. J ECT 27(3):244–246, 2011 21681108

Lauritzen L, Odgaard K, Clemmesen L, et al: Relapse prevention by means of paroxetine in ECT-treated patients with major depression: a comparison with imipramine and placebo in medium-term continuation therapy. Acta Psychiatr Scand 94(4):241–251, 1996 8911559

Lawson JS, Inglis J, Delva NJ, et al: Electrode placement in ECT: cognitive effects. Psychol Med 20(2):335–344, 1990 2356258

Le A, Patel S: Extravasation of noncytotoxic drugs: a review of the literature. Ann Pharmacother 48(7):870–886, 2014 24714850

Lee AJ, Landau R: Aortocaval compression syndrome: time to revisit certain dogmas. Anesth Analg 125(6):1975–1985, 2017 28759487

Lee HB, Jayaram G, Teitelbaum ML: Electroconvulsive therapy for depression in a cardiac transplant patient. Psychosomatics 42(4):362–364, 2001 11496030

Lee JH, Kung S, Rasmussen KG, et al: Effectiveness of electroconvulsive therapy in patients with major depressive disorder and comorbid borderline personality disorder. J ECT 35(1):44–47, 2019 30113988

Lee JJ, Rubin AP: Breast feeding and anaesthesia. Anaesthesia 48(7):616–625, 1993 8346780

Lee LA, Athanassoglou V, Pandit JJ: Neuromuscular blockade in the elderly patient. J Pain Res 9:437–444, 2016 27382330

Lee WH, Lisanby SH, Laine AF, et al: Comparison of electric field strength and spatial distribution of electroconvulsive therapy and magnetic seizure therapy in a realistic human head model. Eur Psychiatry 36:55–64, 2016 27318858

Lee WH, Lisanby SH, Laine AF, et al: Minimum electric field exposure for seizure induction with electroconvulsive therapy and magnetic seizure therapy. Neuropsychopharmacology 42(6):1192–1200, 2017 27934961

Leentjens AF, van den Broek WW, Kusuma A, et al: Facilitation of ECT by intravenous administration of theophylline. Convuls Ther 12(4):232–237, 1996 9034698

Legon W, Sato TF, Opitz A, et al: Transcranial focused ultrasound modulates the activity of primary somatosensory cortex in humans. Nat Neurosci 17(2):322–329, 2014 24413698

Leiknes KA, Jarosh-von Schweder L, Høie B: Contemporary use and practice of electroconvulsive therapy worldwide. Brain Behav 2(3):283–344, 2012 22741102

Lerer B, Shapira B, Calev A, et al: Antidepressant and cognitive effects of twice- versus three-times-weekly ECT. Am J Psychiatry 152(4):564–570, 1995 7694905

Letemendia FJ, Delva NJ, Rodenburg M, et al: Therapeutic advantage of bifrontal electrode placement in ECT. Psychol Med 23(2):349–360, 1993 8332652

Leucht S, Fennema H, Engel RR, et al: Translating the HAM-D into the MADRS and vice versa with equipercentile linking. J Affect Disord 226:326–331, 2018 29031182

Leuchter AF, Cook IA, Feifel D, et al: Efficacy and safety of low-field synchronized transcranial magnetic stimulation (sTMS) for treatment of major depression. Brain Stimul 8(4):787–794, 2015 26143022

Leung M, Hollander Y, Brown GR: Pretreatment with ibuprofen to prevent electroconvulsive therapy–induced headache. J Clin Psychiatry 64(5):551–553, 2003 12755658

Levine SB, Blank K, Schwartz HI, et al: Informed consent in the electroconvulsive treatment of geriatric patients. Bull Am Acad Psychiatry Law 19(4):395–403, 1991 1786419

Levkovitz Y, Isserles M, Padberg F, et al: Efficacy and safety of deep transcranial magnetic stimulation for major depression: a prospective multicenter randomized controlled trial. World Psychiatry 14(1):64–73, 2015 25655160

Levy E, Reinoso P, Shoaib H, et al: Adolescents and young adults with anti-N-methyl-D-aspartate receptor encephalitis with excited catatonia: literature review and 2 illustrative cases. J Acad Consult Liaison Psychiatry 64(2):177–182, 2023 35948253

Levy SD: "Cuff" monitoring, osteoporosis, and fracture. Convuls Ther 4(3):248–249, 1988 11940974

Lew JK, Eastley RJ, Hanning CD: Oxygenation during electroconvulsive therapy: a comparison of two anaesthetic techniques. Anaesthesia 41(11):1092–1097, 1986 3789366

Lezak MD: Neuropsychological Assessment, 3rd Edition. New York, Oxford University Press, 1995

Li D, Hall SE, Tong LD, et al: The electroconvulsive therapy and anesthesia exercise (ECTAE): the creation of an interdisciplinary learning activity for medical students. J ECT 29(3):214–218, 2013 23377747

Li JM, Zhang Y, Su WJ, et al: Cognitive behavioral therapy for treatment-resistant depression: a systematic review and meta-analysis. Psychiatry Res 268:243–250, 2018 30071387

Liberson WT: Time factors in electric convulsive therapy. Yale J Biol Med 17(4):571–578, 1945 21434229

Liberson WT: Some technical observations concerning brief stimulus therapy. Dig Neurol Psychiatr 15:72–78, 1947

Liberson WT: Brief stimulus therapy; psysiological and clinical observations. Am J Psychiatry 105(1):28–39, 1948 18874254

Lieberman P, Nicklas RA, Randolph C, et al: Anaphylaxis—a practice parameter update 2015. Ann Allergy Asthma Immunol 115(5):341–384, 2015 26505932

Lim J, Oh IK, Han C, et al: Sensitivity of cognitive tests in four cognitive domains in discriminating MDD patients from healthy controls: a meta-analysis. Int Psychogeriatr 25(9):1543–1557, 2013 23725644

Limoncelli J, Marino T, Smetana R, et al: General anesthesia recommendations for electroconvulsive therapy during the coronavirus disease 2019 pandemic. J ECT 36(3):152–155, 2020 32483035

Lin CH, Huang CJ, Chen CC: ECT has greater efficacy than fluoxetine in alleviating the burden of illness for patients with major depressive disorder: a Taiwanese pooled analysis. Int J Neuropsychopharmacol 21(1):63–72, 2018 29228200

Lin HT, Liu SK, Hsieh MH, et al: Impacts of electroconvulsive therapy on 1-year outcomes in patients with schizophrenia: a controlled, population-based mirror-image study. Schizophr Bull 44(4):798–806, 2018 29036711

Ling T III, Manepalli J, Grossberg G: Electroconvulsive therapy in the presence of a metallic skull plate after meningioma resection. J ECT 26(2):136–138, 2010 19935094

Link MS, Berkow LC, Kudenchuk PJ, et al: Part 7: adult advanced cardiovascular life support: 2015 American Heart Association guidelines update for cardiopulmonary resuscitation and emergency cardiovascular care. Circulation 132(18)(Suppl 2):S444–S464, 2015 26472995

Lippi G, Plebani M: False myths and legends in laboratory diagnostics. Clin Chem Lab Med 51(11):2087–2097, 2013 23525875

Lippman S, Manshadi M, Wehry M, et al: 1,250 electroconvulsive treatments without evidence of brain injury. Br J Psychiatry 147:203–204, 1985 4041696

Lippmann SB, Tao CA: Electroconvulsive therapy and lithium: safe and effective treatment. Convuls Ther 9(1):54–57, 1993 11941193

Lisanby SH: Electroconvulsive therapy for depression. N Engl J Med 357(19):1939–1945, 2007 17989386

Lisanby SH, Devanand DP, Nobler MS, et al: Exceptionally high seizure threshold: ECT device limitations. Convuls Ther 12(3):156–164, 1996 8872404

Lisanby S, Luber B, Osman M, et al: The effect of pulse width on seizure threshold during electroconvulsive shock (ECS). Convuls Ther 13:56, 1997

Lisanby SH, Maddox JH, Prudic J, et al: The effects of electroconvulsive therapy on memory of autobiographical and public events. Arch Gen Psychiatry 57(6):581–590, 2000 10839336

Lisanby SH, Bazil CW, Resor SR, et al: ECT in the treatment of status epilepticus. J ECT 17(3):210–215, 2001a 11528315

Lisanby SH, Schlaepfer TE, Fisch HU, et al: Magnetic seizure therapy of major depression. Arch Gen Psychiatry 58(3):303–305, 2001b 11231838

Lisanby SH, Sampson S, Husain MM, et al: Toward individualized post-electroconvulsive therapy care: piloting the Symptom-Titrated, Algorithm-Based Longitudinal ECT (STABLE) intervention. J ECT 24(3):179–182, 2008 18708943

Lisanby SH, McClintock SM, Alexopoulos G, et al: Neurocognitive effects of combined electroconvulsive therapy (ECT) and venlafaxine in geriatric depression: phase 1 of the PRIDE study. Am J Geriatr Psychiatry 28(3):304–316, 2020 31706638

Lisanby SH, McClintock SM, McCall WV, et al: Longitudinal neurocognitive effects of combined electroconvulsive therapy (ECT) and pharmacotherapy in major depressive disorder in older adults: phase 2 of the PRIDE study. Am J Geriatr Psychiatry 30(1):15–28, 2022 34074611

Livingston R, Wu C, Mu K, et al: Regulation of electroconvulsive therapy: systematic review of US state laws. J ECT 34(1):60–68, 2018 28991068

LoBiondo-Wood G, Haber J: Nursing Research: Methods and Critical Appraisal for Evidence-Based Practice, 9th Edition. St. Louis, MO, Elsevier, 2018

Locala JA, Irefin SA, Malone D, et al: The comparative hemodynamic effects of methohexital and remifentanil in electroconvulsive therapy. J ECT 21(1):12–15, 2005 15791171

Logan CJ, Stewart JT: Treatment of post-electroconvulsive therapy delirium and agitation with donepezil. J ECT 23(1):28–29, 2007 17435571

Lohr WD, Figiel GS, Hudziak JJ, et al: Maintenance electroconvulsive therapy in schizophrenia. J Clin Psychiatry 55(5):217–218, 1994 8071275

Longcope JC, Fink M: Guidelines for long-term use of electroconvulsive therapy. JAMA 264:1174, 1990

Loo C, Simpson B, MacPherson R: Augmentation strategies in electroconvulsive therapy. J ECT 26(3):202–207, 2010 20562640

Loo CK, Sainsbury K, Sheehan P, et al: A comparison of RUL ultrabrief pulse (0.3 ms) ECT and standard RUL ECT. Int J Neuropsychopharmacol 11(7):883–890, 2008 18752719

Loo CK, Katalinic N, Garfield JB, et al: Neuropsychological and mood effects of ketamine in electroconvulsive therapy: a randomised controlled trial. J Affect Disord 142(1-3):233–240, 2012 22858219

Loo CK, Garfield JB, Katalinic N, et al: Speed of response in ultrabrief and brief pulse width right unilateral ECT. Int J Neuropsychopharmacol 16(4):755–761, 2013 22963997

Loo CK, Katalinic N, Smith DJ, et al: A randomized controlled trial of brief and ultrabrief pulse right unilateral electroconvulsive therapy. Int J Neuropsychopharmacol 18(1):18, 2014 25522389

Loo CK, Husain MM, McDonald WM, et al: International randomized-controlled trial of transcranial direct current stimulation in depression. Brain Stimul 11(1):125–133, 2018 29111077

Lôo H, de Carvalho W, Galinowski A: Towards the rehabilitation of maintenance electroconvulsive therapy? [in French]. Ann Med Psychol (Paris) 148(1):1–15, 1990 2191618

Luber B, Nobler MS, Moeller JR, et al: Quantitative EEG during seizures induced by electroconvulsive therapy: relations to treatment modality and clinical features II: topographic analyses. J ECT 16(3):229–243, 2000 11005044

Luccarelli J, Fernandez-Robles C, Fernandez-Robles C, et al: Modified anesthesia protocol for electroconvulsive therapy permits reduction in aerosol-generating bag-mask ventilation during the COVID-19 pandemic. Psychother Psychosom 89(5):314–319, 2020a 32554959

Luccarelli J, Henry ME, McCoy TH Jr: Demographics of patients receiving electroconvulsive therapy based on state-mandated reporting data. J ECT 36(4):229–233, 2020b 32453188

Luccarelli J, Henry ME, McCoy TH Jr: Quantification of fracture rate during electroconvulsive therapy (ECT) using state-mandated reporting data. Brain Stimul 13(3):523–524, 2020c 32289667

Luccarelli J, McCoy TH Jr, Horvath RJ, et al: The effects of anesthetic change on electrographic seizure duration during electroconvulsive therapy. Brain Stimul 14(5):1084–1086, 2021a 34293513

Luccarelli J, McCoy TH Jr, Seiner SJ, et al: Total charge required to induce a seizure in a retrospective cohort of patients undergoing dose titration of right unilateral ultrabrief pulse electroconvulsive therapy. J ECT 37(1):40–45, 2021b 32826707

Luccarelli J, McCoy TH, Uchida M, et al: The efficacy and cognitive effects of acute course electroconvulsive therapy are equal in adolescents, transitional age youth, and young adults. J Child Adolesc Psychopharmacol 31(8):538–544, 2021c 34619038

Luccarelli J, Forester BP, Dooley M, et al: The effects of baseline impaired global cognitive function on the efficacy and cognitive effects of electroconvulsive therapy in geriatric patients: a retrospective cohort study. Am J Geriatr Psychiatry 30(7):790–798, 2022 34996701

Luchini F, Medda P, Mariani MG, et al: Electroconvulsive therapy in catatonic patients: efficacy and predictors of response. World J Psychiatry 5(2):182–192, 2015 26110120

Lui PW, Ma JY, Chan KK: Modification of tonic-clonic convulsions by atracurium in multiple-monitored electroconvulsive therapy. J Clin Anesth 5(1):16–21, 1993 8442962

Lukoff D, Liberman RP, Nuechterlein KH: Symptom monitoring in the rehabilitation of schizophrenic patients. Schizophr Bull 12(4):578–602, 1986 3810065

Lunde ME, Lee EK, Rasmussen KG: Electroconvulsive therapy in patients with epilepsy. Epilepsy Behav 9(2):355–359, 2006 16876485

Lupke K, Warren N, Teodorczuk A, et al: A systematic review of modified electroconvulsive therapy (ECT) to treat delirium. Acta Psychiatr Scand 147(5):403–419, 2023 35996219

Lykouras E, Malliaras D, Christodoulou GN, et al: Delusional depression: phenomenology and response to treatment: a prospective study. Acta Psychiatr Scand 73(3):324–329, 1986 2872774

Mackenzie TB, Thurston J, Rogers L, et al: Placement of an implantable venous access device for use in maintenance ECT. Convuls Ther 12(2):122–124, 1996 8744174

MacKinnon AL: Electric shock therapy in a private psychiatric hospital. Can Med Assoc J 58(5):478–483, 1948 18862237

MacPherson RD, Loo CK, Barrett N: Electroconvulsive therapy in patients with cardiac pacemakers. Anaesth Intensive Care 34(4):470–474, 2006 16913344

Madan S, Anderson K: ECT for a patient with a metallic skull plate. J ECT 17(4):289–291, 2001 11731732

Magee LA, Inocencion G, Kamboj L, et al: Safety of first trimester exposure to histamine H2 blockers: a prospective cohort study. Dig Dis Sci 41(6):1145–1149, 1996 8654145

Magen JG, D'Mello D: Acute lymphocytic leukemia and psychosis: treatment with electroconvulsive therapy. Ann Clin Psychiatry 7(3):133–137, 1995 8646273

Magid M, Lapid MI, Sampson SM, et al: Use of electroconvulsive therapy in a patient 10 days after myocardial infarction. J ECT 21(3):182–185, 2005 16127311

Magni G, Fisman M, Helmes E: Clinical correlates of ECT-resistant depression in the elderly. J Clin Psychiatry 49(10):405–407, 1988 3170492

Mahler H, Co BT Jr, Dinwiddie S: Studies in involuntary civil commitment and involuntary electroconvulsive therapy. J Nerv Ment Dis 174(2):97–106, 1986 3944600

Maixner DF, Weiner R, Reti IM, et al: Electroconvulsive therapy is an essential procedure. Am J Psychiatry 178(5):381–382, 2021 33979536

Malaty G, Godbe K, Elmouchtari M, et al: Electroconvulsive therapy in a renal transplantation patient: a rare combination of disease and treatment. Case Rep Psychiatry 2020:8889883, 2020 33178474

Malek-Ahmadi P, Hanretta AT: Successful ECT in a patient with intracranial venous angioma. J ECT 18(2):99–102, 2002 12195139

Malek-Ahmadi P, Hanretta AT: Cochlear implant and ECT. J ECT 19(1):51, 2003 12621280

Malek-Ahmadi P, Sedler RR: Electroconvulsive therapy and asymptomatic meningioma. Convuls Ther 5(2):168–170, 1989 11941009

Maletzky BM: Multiple-Monitored Electroconvulsive Therapy. Boca Raton, FL, CRC Press, 1981

Malhi GS, Bell E, Bassett D, et al: The 2020 Royal Australian and New Zealand College of Psychiatrists clinical practice guidelines for mood disorders. Aust N Z J Psychiatry 55(1):7–117, 2021 33353391

Malik M, Batchvarov VN: Measurement, interpretation and clinical potential of QT dispersion. J Am Coll Cardiol 36(6):1749–1766, 2000 11092641

Maltbie AA, Wingfield MS, Volow MR, et al: Electroconvulsive therapy in the presence of brain tumor. Case reports and an evaluation of risk. J Nerv Ment Dis 168(7):400–405, 1980 7400788

Malur C, Pasol E, Francis A: ECT for prolonged catatonia. J ECT 17(1):55–59, 2001 11281518

Mamah D, Lammle M, Isenberg KE: Pulmonary embolism after ECT. J ECT 21(1):39–40, 2005 15791176

Mandel MR, Welch CA, Mieske M, et al: Prediction of response to ECT in tricyclic-intolerant or tricyclic-resistant depressed patients. McLean Hospital Journal 4:203–209, 1977

Manjunatha N, Ram Kumar GS, Vidyendaran R, et al: Delayed onset, protracted delirium and aspiration pneumonitis associated with a combination of clozapine and electroconvulsive therapy. Indian J Psychol Med 33(1):80–82, 2011 22021960

Mankad M, Beyer J, Weiner RE, et al: Clinical Manual of Electroconvulsive Therapy. Washington, DC, American Psychiatric Publishing, 2010

Manne JR, Kasirye Y, Epperla N, et al: Non-cardiogenic pulmonary edema complicating electroconvulsive therapy: short review of the pathophysiology and diagnostic approach. Clin Med Res 10(3):131–136, 2012 22031475

Mann-Wrobel MC, Carreno JT, Dickinson D: Meta-analysis of neuropsychological functioning in euthymic bipolar disorder: an update and investigation of moderator variables. Bipolar Disord 13(4):334–342, 2011 21843273

Mansoor D, Trevino C, Ganzini L, et al: Negative pressure pulmonary edema after electroconvulsive therapy. J ECT 32(2):e2–e3, 2016 26579637

Marangell LB, Rush AJ, George MS, et al: Vagus nerve stimulation (VNS) for major depressive episodes: one year outcomes. Biol Psychiatry 51(4):280–287, 2002 11958778

Marazziti D, Consoli G, Picchetti M, et al: Cognitive impairment in major depression. Eur J Pharmacol 626(1):83–86, 2010 19835870

Marcus SM: Depression during pregnancy: rates, risks and consequences—Motherisk update 2008. Can J Clin Pharmacol 16(1):e15–e22, 2009 19164843

Markowitz JS, Kellner CH, DeVane CL, et al: Intranasal sumatriptan in post-ECT headache: results of an open-label trial. J ECT 17(4):280–283, 2001 11731730

Marques Macedo I, Gama Marques J: Catatonia secondary to anti-N-methyl-D-aspartate receptor (NMDAr) encephalitis: a review. CNS Spectr 25(4):475–492, 2020 31663486

Mårtensson B, Bartfai A, Hallén B, et al: A comparison of propofol and methohexital as anesthetic agents for ECT: effects on seizure duration, therapeutic outcome, and memory. Biol Psychiatry 35(3):179–189, 1994 8173018

Martin BA, Bean GJ: Competence to consent to electroconvulsive therapy. Convuls Ther 8(2):92–102, 1992 11659635

Martin BA, Glancy GD: Consent to electroconvulsive therapy: investigation of the validity of a competency questionnaire. Convuls Ther 10(4):279–286, 1994 7850398

Martin DM, Katalinic N, Ingram A, et al: A new early cognitive screening measure to detect cognitive side-effects of electroconvulsive therapy? J Psychiatr Res 47(12):1967–1974, 2013 24074514

Martin DM, Gálvez V, Loo CK: Predicting retrograde autobiographical memory changes following electroconvulsive therapy: relationships between individual, treatment, and early clinical factors. Int J Neuropsychopharmacol 18(12):pyv067, 2015 26091817

Martin DM, Wong A, Kumar DR, et al: Validation of the 10-item Orientation Questionnaire: a new tool for monitoring post-electroconvulsive therapy disorientation. J ECT 34(1):21–25, 2018 28976441

Martin DM, McClintock SM, Loo CK: Brief cognitive screening instruments for electroconvulsive therapy: which one should I use? Aust N Z J Psychiatry 54(9):867–873, 2020a 32436734

Martin DM, Wollny-Huttarsch D, Nikolin S, et al: Neurocognitive subgroups in major depressive disorder. Neuropsychology 34(6):726–734, 2020b

Martin M, Figiel G, Mattingly G, et al: ECT-induced interictal delirium in patients with a history of a CVA. J Geriatr Psychiatry Neurol 5(3):149–155, 1992 1497792

Martinez MW, Rasmussen KG, Mueller PS, et al: Troponin elevations after electroconvulsive therapy: the need for caution. Am J Med 124(3):229–234, 2011 21396506

Martínez-Amorós E, Real Barrero E, Fuste Fusares C, et al: Bilateral posterior vitreous detachment after electroconvulsive therapy. Gen Hosp Psychiatry 31(4):385–387, 2009 19555802

Martino C, Krysko M, Petrides G, et al: Cognitive tolerability of electroconvulsive therapy in a patient with a history of traumatic brain injury. J ECT 24(1):92–95, 2008 18379342

Martyn JA, Richtsfeld M: Succinylcholine-induced hyperkalemia in acquired pathologic states: etiologic factors and molecular mechanisms. Anesthesiology 104(1):158–169, 2006 16394702

Mashimo K, Kanaya M, Yamauchi T: Electroconvulsive therapy for a schizophrenic patient in catatonic stupor with joint contracture. Convuls Ther 11(3):216–219, 1995 8528667

Mashimo K, Sato Y, Yamauchi T: Effective electroconvulsive therapy for stupor in the high risk patient: a report of two cases. Psychiatry Clin Neurosci 50(3):129–131, 1996 9201758

Mashimo K, Yamauchi T, Harada T: Electroconvulsive therapy for a schizophrenic patient with burns in the critical care centre. Burns 23(1):85–86, 1997 9115620

Masoudzadeh A, Khalilian AR: Comparative study of clozapine, electroshock and the combination of ECT with clozapine in treatment-resistant schizophrenic patients. Pak J Biol Sci 10(23):4287–4290, 2007 19086588

Matsuda Y, Sakuma K, Kishi T, et al: Repetitive transcranial magnetic stimulation for preventing relapse in antidepressant treatment-resistant depression: a systematic review and meta-analysis of randomized controlled trials. Brain Stimul 16(2):458–461, 2023 36736857

Mattes JA, Pettinati HM, Stephens S, et al: A placebo-controlled evaluation of vasopressin for ECT-induced memory impairment. Biol Psychiatry 27(3):289–303, 1990 2405915

Matthews JD, Blais M, Park L, et al: The impact of galantamine on cognition and mood during electroconvulsive therapy: a pilot study. J Psychiatr Res 42(7):526–531, 2008 17681545

Matthews JD, Siefert CJ, Blais MA, et al: A double-blind, placebo-controlled study of the impact of galantamine on anterograde memory impairment during electroconvulsive therapy. J ECT 29(3):170–178, 2013 23519225

Mattingly G, Baker K, Zorumski CF, et al: Multiple sclerosis and ECT: possible value of gadolinium-enhanced magnetic resonance scans for identifying high-risk patients. J Neuropsychiatry Clin Neurosci 4(2):145–151, 1992 1627975

Matz O, Schwerz S, Dafotakis M, et al: Cardiac stress after electroconvulsive therapy and spontaneous generalized convulsive seizures: a prospective echocardiographic and blood biomarker study. Epilepsy Behav 101(Pt A):106565, 2019 31675603

Matzen TA, Martin RL, Watt TJ, et al: The use of maintenance electroconvulsive therapy for relapsing depression. Jefferson J Psychiatry 6:52–58, 1988

May PR, Tuma AH: Treatment of schizophrenia: an experimental study of five treatment methods. Br J Psychiatry 111:503–510, 1965

May PR, Tuma AH, Yale C, et al: Schizophrenia—a follow-up study of results of treatment. Arch Gen Psychiatry 33(4):481–486, 1976 938185

May PR, Tuma AH, Dixon WJ, et al: Schizophrenia: a follow-up study of the results of five forms of treatment. Arch Gen Psychiatry 38(7):776–784, 1981 6113821

Mayur P, Bray A, Fernandes J, et al: Impact of hyperventilation on stimulus efficiency during the early phase of an electroconvulsive therapy course: a randomized double-blind study. J ECT 26(2):91–94, 2010 20514695

Mayur P, Byth K, Harris A: Acute antidepressant effects of right unilateral ultrabrief ECT: a double-blind randomised controlled trial. J Affect Disord 149(1-3):426–429, 2013 23287525

Mayur PM, Shree RS, Gangadhar BN, et al: Atropine premedication and the cardiovascular response to electroconvulsive therapy. Br J Anaesth 81(3):466–467, 1998 9861141

Mayur PM, Gangadhar BN, Janakiramaiah N, et al: Motor seizure monitoring during electroconvulsive therapy. Br J Psychiatry 174:270–272, 1999 10448455

McAllister DA, Perri MG, Jordan RC, et al: Effects of ECT given two vs. three times weekly. Psychiatry Res 21(1):63–69, 1987 3602221

McAllister TW, Price TR: Severe depressive pseudodementia with and without dementia. Am J Psychiatry 139(5):626–629, 1982 7072850

McCall WV: Asystole in electroconvulsive therapy: report of four cases. J Clin Psychiatry 57(5):199–203, 1996 8626350

McCall WV, Coffey CE, Maltbie AA: Successful electroconvulsive therapy in a depressed patient with pseudohypoparathyroidism. Convuls Ther 5:114–117, 1989

McCall WV, Weiner RD, Shelp FE, et al: ECT in a state hospital setting. Convuls Ther 8(1):12–18, 1992 11941144

McCall WV, Reid S, Rosenquist P, et al: A reappraisal of the role of caffeine in ECT. Am J Psychiatry 150(10):1543–1545, 1993 8379563

McCall WV, Reid S, Ford M: Electrocardiographic and cardiovascular effects of subconvulsive stimulation during titrated right unilateral ECT. Convuls Ther 10(1):25–33, 1994 8055289

McCall WV, Farah BA, Reboussin D, et al: Comparison of the efficacy of titrated, moderate dose and fixed, high-dose right unilateral ECT in elderly patients. Am J Geriatr Psychiatry 3(4):317–324, 1995 28531065

McCall WV, Colenda CC, Farah BA: Ictal EEG regularity declines during a course of RUL ECT. Convuls Ther 12(4):213–216, 1996a 9034695

McCall WV, Robinette GD, Hardesty D: Relationship of seizure morphology to the convulsive threshold. Convuls Ther 12(3):147–151, 1996b 8872402

McCall WV, Reboussin DM, Weiner RD, et al: Titrated moderately suprathreshold vs fixed high-dose right unilateral electroconvulsive therapy: acute antidepressant and cognitive effects. Arch Gen Psychiatry 57:438–444, 2000 10807483

McCall WV, Arias L, Onafuye R, et al: What the electroconvulsive therapy practitioner needs to know about obstructive sleep apnea. J ECT 25(1):50–53, 2009 18580817

McCall WV, Reboussin D, Prudic J, et al: Poor health-related quality of life prior to ECT in depressed patients normalizes with sustained remission after ECT. J Affect Disord 147(1-3):107–111, 2013 23158959

McCall WV, Lisanby SH, Rosenquist PB, et al: Effects of a right unilateral ultrabrief pulse electroconvulsive therapy course on health related quality of life in elderly depressed patients. J Affect Disord 209:39–45, 2017 27886569

McCall WV, Lisanby SH, Rosenquist PB, et al: Effects of continuation electroconvulsive therapy on quality of life in elderly depressed patients: a randomized clinical trial. J Psychiatr Res 97:65–69, 2018 29195125

McCarron RH, Rathee R, Yang S, et al: ECT in two elderly patients with COVID-19: weighing up unknown risks in unprecedented times. Clin Neuropsychiatry 17(5):295–299, 2020 34909007

McClellan J, Kowatch R, Findling RL: Practice parameter for the assessment and treatment of children and adolescents with bipolar disorder. J Am Acad Child Adolesc Psychiatry 46(1):107–125, 2007 17195735

McClellan J, Stock S; American Academy of Child and Adolescent Psychiatry (AACAP) Committee on Quality Issues (CQI): Practice parameter for the assessment and treatment of children and adolescents with schizophrenia. J Am Acad Child Adolesc Psychiatry 52(9):976–990, 2013 23972700

McClintock SM, Husain MM, Greer TL, et al: Association between depression severity and neurocognitive function in major depressive disorder: a review and synthesis. Neuropsychology 24(1):9–34, 2010 20063944

McClintock SM, Brandon AR, Husain MM, et al: A systematic review of the combined use of electroconvulsive therapy and psychotherapy for depression. J ECT 27(3):236–243, 2011a 21206376

McClintock SM, Haley C, Bernstein IH: Psychometric considerations of depression symptom rating scales. Neuropsychiatry (London) 1(6):611–623, 2011b

McClintock SM, Husain MM, Bernstein IH, et al: Assessing anxious features in depressed outpatients. Int J Methods Psychiatr Res 20(4):e69–e82, 2011c 22057975

McClintock SM, Tirmizi O, Chansard M, et al: A systematic review of the neurocognitive effects of magnetic seizure therapy. Int Rev Psychiatry 23(5):413–423, 2011d 22200131

McClintock SM, Choi J, Deng ZD, et al: Multifactorial determinants of the neurocognitive effects of electroconvulsive therapy. J ECT 30(2):165–176, 2014 24820942

McClintock SM, Reti IM, Carpenter LL, et al: Consensus recommendations for the clinical application of repetitive transcranial magnetic stimulation (rTMS) in the treatment of depression. J Clin Psychiatry 79(1):16cs10905, 2018 28541649

McClintock SM, Minto L, Denney DA, et al: Clinical neuropsychological evaluation in older adults with major depressive disorder. Curr Psychiatry Rep 23(9):55, 2021 34255167

McCormick AS, Saunders DA: Oxygen saturation of patients recovering from electroconvulsive therapy. Anaesthesia 51(7):702–704, 1996 8758171

McCutchen TM, Gligorovic PV, Tighe NTG, et al: Alfentanil pretreatment for electroconvulsive therapy-associated hemodynamic lability: a prospective randomized crossover trial. J ECT 39(2):84–90, 2023 36215414

McDonald IM, Perkins M, Marjerrison G, et al: A controlled comparison of amitriptyline and electroconvulsive therapy in the treatment of depression. Am J Psychiatry 122(12):1427–1431, 1966 5326021

McDonald WM: Neuromodulation treatments for geriatric mood and cognitive disorders. Am J Geriatr Psychiatry 24(12):1130–1141, 2016 27889282

McElhiney MC, Moody BJ, Steif BL, et al: Autobiographical memory and mood: effects of electroconvulsive therapy. Neuropsychology 9:501–517, 1995

McGarvey KA, Zis AP, Brown EE, et al: ECS-induced dopamine release: effects of electrode placement, anticonvulsant treatment, and stimulus intensity. Biol Psychiatry 34(3):152–157, 1993 8399807

McGrane IR, Munjal RC, Skauge SL, et al: Successful electroconvulsive therapy after failed pharmacotherapies in an older female on hemodialysis with bipolar mania. Bipolar Disord 24(5):556–558, 2022 35165989

McHorney CA, Ware JE Jr, Raczek AE: The MOS 36-Item Short-Form Health Survey (SF-36): II. Psychometric and clinical tests of validity in measuring physical and mental health constructs. Med Care 31(3):247–263, 1993 8450681

McKinney P, Kellner C: Multiple ECT late in the course of neuroleptic malignant syndrome. Convuls Ther 13(4):269–273, 1997 9437570

McKinney PA, Beale MD, Kellner CH: Electroconvulsive therapy in a patient with a cerebellar meningioma. J ECT 14(1):49–52, 1998 9661094

McParlin C, O'Donnell A, Robson SC, et al: Treatments for hyperemesis gravidarum and nausea and vomiting in pregnancy: a systematic review. JAMA 316(13):1392–1401, 2016 27701665

McRackan TR, Rivas A, Hedley-Williams A, et al: Impedance testing on cochlear implants after electroconvulsive therapy. J ECT 30(4):303–308, 2014 24755726

Medda P, Perugi G, Zanello S, et al: Comparative response to electroconvulsive therapy in medication-resistant bipolar I patients with depression and mixed state. J ECT 26(2):82–86, 2010 19710623

Medda P, Toni C, Perugi G: The mood-stabilizing effects of electroconvulsive therapy. J ECT 30(4):275–282, 2014 25010031

Mehdi SMA, Devanand DP: Electroconvulsive therapy in elderly patients with cerebral aneurysms: a systematic review with clinical recommendations. J Geriatr Psychiatry Neurol 34(6):504–512, 2021 34402339

Mehta S, Downar J, Mulsant BH, et al: Effect of high frequency versus theta-burst repetitive transcranial magnetic stimulation on suicidality in patients with treatment-resistant depression. Acta Psychiatr Scand 145(5):529–538, 2022 35188677

Mehta V, Mueller PS, Gonzalez-Arriaza HL, et al: Safety of electroconvulsive therapy in patients receiving long-term warfarin therapy. Mayo Clin Proc 79(11):1396–1401, 2004 15544018

Meisel A, Roth LH: Toward an informed discussion of informed consent: a review and critique of the empirical studies. Ariz Law Rev 25(2):265–346, 1983 11658677

Meister R, von Wolff A, Mohr H, et al: Comparative safety of pharmacologic treatments for persistent depressive disorder: a systematic review and network meta-analysis. PLoS One 11(5):e0153380, 2016 27187783

Mendels J: Electroconvulsive therapy and depression, I: the prognostic significance of clinical factors. Br J Psychiatry 111:675–681, 1965a 14337414

Mendels J: Electroconvulsive therapy and depression, III: a method for prognosis. Br J Psychiatry 111:687–690, 1965b 14337416

Mendels J: The prediction of response to electroconvulsive therapy. Am J Psychiatry 124(2):153–159, 1967 4951568

Menon V, Varadharajan N, Faheem A, et al: Ketamine vs electroconvulsive therapy for major depressive episode: a systematic review and meta-analysis. JAMA Psychiatry 80(6):639–642, 2023 37043224

Messer GJ, Stoudemire A, Knos G, et al: Electroconvulsive therapy and the chronic use of pseudocholinesterase-inhibitor (echothiophate iodide) eye drops for glaucoma: a case report. Gen Hosp Psychiatry 14(1):56–60, 1992 1730402

Messina AG, Paranicas M, Katz B, et al: Effect of electroconvulsive therapy on the electrocardiogram and echocardiogram. Anesth Analg 75(4):511–514, 1992 1530163

Methfessel I, Besse M, Belz M, et al: Effectiveness of maintenance electroconvulsive therapy: evidence from modifications due to the COVID-19 pandemic. Acta Psychiatr Scand 144(3):238–245, 2021 33960406

Meyer JP, Swetter SK, Kellner CH: Electroconvulsive therapy in geriatric psychiatry: a selective review. Clin Geriatr Med 36(2):265–279, 2020 32222301

Meyers BS: Geriatric delusional depression. Clin Geriatr Med 8(2):299–308, 1992 1600480

Milev RV, Giacobbe P, Kennedy SH, et al: Canadian Network for Mood and Anxiety Treatments (CANMAT) 2016 clinical guidelines for the management of adults with major depressive disorder: section 4: neurostimulation treatments. Can J Psychiatry 61(9):561–575, 2016 27486154

Miller AL, Faber RA, Hatch JP, et al: Factors affecting amnesia, seizure duration, and efficacy in ECT. Am J Psychiatry 142(6):692–696, 1985 4003587

Miller DH, Clancy J, Cumming E: A comparison between unidirectional current nonconvulsive electrical stimulation given with Reiter's machine, standard alternating current electro-shock (Cerletti method), and pentothal in chronic schizophrenia. Am J Psychiatry 109(8):617–620, 1953 13030821

Miller J, Jones T, Upston J, et al: Ictal theta power as an electroconvulsive therapy safety biomarker: a pilot study. J ECT 38(2):88–94, 2022 35613008

Miller ME, Siris SG, Gabriel AN: Treatment delays in the course of electroconvulsive therapy. Hosp Community Psychiatry 37(8):825–827, 1986 3733014

Miller ML, Luu H, Gaasedelen O, et al: Long-term cognitive and psychological functioning in post-electroconvulsive therapy patients. J ECT 35(1):27–34, 2019 29727307

Mills MJ, Avery D: The legal regulation of electroconvulsive therapy, in Mood Disorders: The World's Major Public Health Problem. Edited by Ayd FJ. Baltimore, MD, Frank Ayd Communications, 1978, pp 154–183

Milstein V, Small JG, Klapper MH, et al: Uni- versus bilateral ECT in the treatment of mania. Convuls Ther 3(1):1–9, 1987 11940883

Milstein V, Small IF, French RN: ECT in a patient with Harrington rods. Convuls Ther 8(2):137–140, 1992 11941160

Minelli A, Abate M, Zampieri E, et al: Seizure adequacy markers and the prediction of electroconvulsive therapy response. J ECT 32(2):88–92, 2016 26397151

Mingo K, Kominsky A: Electroconvulsive therapy for depression in a patient with an Inspire hypoglossal nerve stimulator device for obstructive sleep apnea: a case report. Am J Otolaryngol 39(4):462–463, 2018 29703415

Minichino A, Bersani FS, Capra E, et al: ECT, rTMS, and deepTMS in pharmacoresistant drug-free patients with unipolar depression: a comparative review. Neuropsychiatr Dis Treat 8:55–64, 2012 22347797

Minnai GP, Salis PG, Oppo R, et al: Effectiveness of maintenance electroconvulsive therapy in rapid-cycling bipolar disorder. J ECT 27(2):123–126, 2011 20559148

Minneman SA: A history of oral protection for the ECT patient: past, present, and future. Convuls Ther 11(2):94–103, 1995 7552060

Mirzakhani H, Guchelaar HJ, Welch CA, et al: Minimum effective doses of succinylcholine and rocuronium during electroconvulsive therapy: a prospective, randomized, crossover trial. Anesth Analg 123(3):587–596, 2016 26967896

Mischel NA, Mooneyham GC, Lau C, et al: Non-N-methyl-D-aspartate autoimmune encephalopathy and catatonia treated with electroconvulsive therapy: a pediatric case series and treatment guidelines. Psychosomatics 61(6):834–839, 2020 31980211

Mishra BR, Agrawal K, Biswas T, et al: Comparison of acute followed by maintenance ECT vs clozapine on psychopathology and regional cerebral blood flow in treatment-resistant schizophrenia: a randomized controlled trial. Schizophr Bull 48(4):814–825, 2022 35556138

Mitchell S, Hassan E, Ghaziuddin N: A follow-up study of electroconvulsive therapy in children and adolescents. J ECT 34(1):40–44, 2018 28937548

Mizrak A, Koruk S, Ganidagli S, et al: Premedication with dexmedetomidine and midazolam attenuates agitation after electroconvulsive therapy. J Anesth 23(1):6–10, 2009 19234815

Mohan TS, Tharyan P, Alexander J, et al: Effects of stimulus intensity on the efficacy and safety of twice-weekly, bilateral electroconvulsive therapy (ECT) combined with antipsychotics in acute mania: a randomised controlled trial. Bipolar Disord 11(2):126–134, 2009 19267695

Moirand R, Galvao F, Lecompte M, et al: Usefulness of the Montreal Cognitive Assessment (MoCA) to monitor cognitive impairments in depressed patients receiving electroconvulsive therapy. Psychiatry Res 259:476–481, 2018 29149717

Möller H-J: Standardised rating scales in psychiatry: methodological basis, their possibilities and limitations and descriptions of important rating scales. World J Biol Psychiatry 10(1):6–26, 2009 18663668

Monaco JT, Delaplaine P: Tranylcypromine with ECT. Am J Psychiatry 120:1003, 1964 14138828

Monroe RR Jr: Maintenance electroconvulsive therapy. Psychiatr Clin North Am 14(4):947–960, 1991 1771156

Montgomery SA, Åsberg M: A new depression scale designed to be sensitive to change. Br J Psychiatry 134:382–389, 1979 444788

Mooneyham GC, Ferrafiat V, Stolte E, et al: Developing consensus in the assessment and treatment pathways for autoimmune encephalitis in child and adolescent psychiatry. Front Psychiatry 12:638901, 2021 33854451

Moore N: The maintenance treatment of chronic psychotics by electrically induced convulsions. J Ment Sci 89(375):257–269, 1943

Morcos N, Rosinski A, Maixner DF: Electroconvulsive therapy for neuroleptic malignant syndrome: a case series. J ECT 35(4):225–230, 2019 31764444

Morgan DH: ECT given to people with pacemakers. Bulletin of the Royal College of Psychiatrists 11:135–135, 1987

Mormando C, Francis A: Catatonia revived: a unique syndrome updated. Int Rev Psychiatry 32(5-6):403–411, 2020 32067538

Moscarillo FM, Annunziata CM: ECT in a patient with a deep brain-stimulating electrode in place. J ECT 16(3):287–290, 2000 11005051

Mueller PS, Schak KM, Barnes RD, et al: Safety of electroconvulsive therapy in patients with asthma. Neth J Med 64(11):417–421, 2006 17179572

Mueller PS, Barnes RD, Varghese R, et al: The safety of electroconvulsive therapy in patients with severe aortic stenosis. Mayo Clin Proc 82(11):1360–1363, 2007 17976355

Mueller PS, Albin SM, Barnes RD, et al: Safety of electroconvulsive therapy in patients with unrepaired abdominal aortic aneurysm: report of 8 patients. J ECT 25(3):165–169, 2009 19730028

Mukherjee S: Combined ECT and lithium therapy. Convuls Ther 9(4):274–284, 1993 11941223

Mukherjee S, Sackeim HA, Lee C: Unilateral ECT in the treatment of manic episodes. Convuls Ther 4(1):74–80, 1988 11940944

Mukherjee S, Sackeim HA, Schnur DB: Electroconvulsive therapy of acute manic episodes: a review of 50 years' experience. Am J Psychiatry 151(2):169–176, 1994 8296883

Mulder LAC, Grootens KP: The incidence of post-electroconvulsive therapy headache: a systematic review. J ECT 36(3):e22–e28, 2020 32205737

Muller D: 1. Nardil (phenelzine) as a potentiator of electroconvulsive therapy (E.C.T.). 2. A survey of outpatient E.C.T. J Ment Sci 107:994–996, 1961 14477115

Mulsant BH, Rosen J, Thornton JE, et al: A prospective naturalistic study of electroconvulsive therapy in late-life depression. J Geriatr Psychiatry Neurol 4(1):3–13, 1991 2054049

Mulsant BH, Haskett RF, Prudic J, et al: Low use of neuroleptic drugs in the treatment of psychotic major depression. Am J Psychiatry 154(4):559–561, 1997 9090348

Munday J, Deans C, Little J: Effectiveness of a training program for ECT nurses. J Psychosoc Nurs Ment Health Serv 41(11):20–26, 2003 14621443

Munk-Olsen T, Laursen TM, Videbech P, et al: All-cause mortality among recipients of electroconvulsive therapy: register-based cohort study. Br J Psychiatry 190:435–439, 2007 17470959

Muntingh AD, van der Feltz-Cornelis CM, van Marwijk HW, et al: Is the Beck Anxiety Inventory a good tool to assess the severity of anxiety? A primary care study in the Netherlands Study of Depression and Anxiety (NESDA). BMC Fam Pract 12:66, 2011 21726443

Murayama T, Kobayashi S, Matsuoka T, et al: Effectiveness of electroconvulsive therapy in patients with advanced Parkinson disease. J ECT 37(2):88–93, 2021 33337651

Murillo LG, Exner JE Jr: The effect of regressive ECT with process schizophrenics. Am J Psychiatry 130(3):269–273, 1973 4143944

Musgrave N, Madden A, Mehta M, et al: The safety of electroconvulsive therapy in cervical fusion. J ECT 36(4):e43–e44, 2020 32205734

Mutz J, Vipulananthan V, Carter B, et al: Comparative efficacy and acceptability of non-surgical brain stimulation for the acute treatment of major depressive episodes in adults: systematic review and network meta-analysis. BMJ 364:l1079, 2019 30917990

Myers CL, Gopalka A, Glick D, et al: A case of negative-pressure pulmonary edema after electroconvulsive therapy. J ECT 23(4):281–283, 2007 18090704

Nagler J, Geppert M: Predictors of bradycardia during the stimulation phase of electroconvulsive therapy. J ECT 27(3):201–206, 2011 21673585

Naguib M, Koorn R: Interactions between psychotropics, anaesthetics and electroconvulsive therapy: implications for drug choice and patient management. CNS Drugs 16(4):229–247, 2002 11945107

Nahar A, Kondapuram N, Desai G, et al: Catatonia among women with postpartum psychosis in a mother-baby inpatient psychiatry unit. Gen Hosp Psychiatry 45:40–43, 2017 28274337

Nahas Z, Marangell LB, Husain MM, et al: Two-year outcome of vagus nerve stimulation (VNS) for treatment of major depressive episodes. J Clin Psychiatry 66(9):1097–1104, 2005 16187765

Najjar F, Guttmacher LB: ECT in the presence of intracranial aneurysm. J ECT 14(4):266–271, 1998 9871849

Nakatake M, Teraishi T, Ide M, et al: Modified electroconvulsive therapy for recurrent major depressive disorder in a meningioma patient: a case report of clinical experience. Fukuoka Igaku Zasshi 101(9):198–206, 2010 21222352

Narang P, Glowacki A, Lippmann S: Electroconvulsive therapy intervention for Parkinson's disease. Innov Clin Neurosci 12(9-10):25–28, 2015 26634178

Narrow WE, Clarke DE, Kuramoto SJ, et al: DSM-5 field trials in the United States and Canada, part III: development and reliability testing of a cross-cutting symptom assessment for DSM-5. Am J Psychiatry 170(1):71–82, 2013 23111499

Nasr S, Murillo A, Katariwala N, et al: Case report of electroconvulsive therapy in a patient with Parkinson disease concomitant with deep brain stimulation. J ECT 27(1):89–90, 2011 20386114

Nasreddine ZS, Phillips NA, Bédirian V, et al: The Montreal Cognitive Assessment, MoCA: a brief screening tool for mild cognitive impairment. J Am Geriatr Soc 53(4):695–699, 2005 15817019

Nasseri K, Arasteh MT, Maroufi A, et al: Effects of remifentanil on convulsion duration and hemodynamic responses during electroconvulsive therapy: a double-blind, randomized clinical trial. J ECT 25(3):170–173, 2009 19755938

Nath M, Shah YD, Theroux LM, et al: A role for electroconvulsive therapy in the management of new onset refractory status epilepticus (NORSE) in a young child. Neurol India 69(5):1374–1379, 2021 34747817

National Fire Protection Association: NFPA 70: National Electrical Code 2020. Quincy, MA, National Fire Protection Association, 2020

National Fire Protection Association: NFPA 99, Health Care Facilities Code. Quincy, MA, National Fire Protection Association, 2021

National Institutes of Health: Confirmatory Efficacy and Safety Trial of Magnetic Seizure Therapy for Depression (CREST-MST). U.S. National Library of Medicine, January 26, 2022a. Available at: https://clinicaltrials.gov/ct2/show/NCT03191058. Accessed June 26, 2022.

National Institutes of Health: Safety and Feasibility of Individualized Low Amplitude Seizure Therapy (iLAST). U.S. National Library of Medicine, June 24, 2022b. Available at: www.clinicaltrials.gov/ct2/show/NCT03895658. Accessed June 26, 2022.

National Library of Medicine: Drugs and Lactation Database (LactMed): Acetaminophen. Bethesda, MD, National Institute of Child Health and Human Development. October 31, 2018a. Available at: www.ncbi.nlm.nih.gov/books/NBK501194. Accessed May 15, 2022.

National Library of Medicine: Drugs and Lactation Database (LactMed): Ibuprofen. Bethesda, MD, National Institute of Child Health and Human Development, October 31, 2018b. Available at: www.ncbi.nlm.nih.gov/books/NBK500986/. Accessed May 15, 2022.

National Library of Medicine: Drugs and Lactation Database (LactMed): Aspirin. Bethesda, MD, National Institute of Child Health and Human Development, March 16, 2020a. Available at: www.ncbi.nlm.nih.gov/books/NBK501196/. Accessed May 15, 2022.

National Library of Medicine: Drugs and Lactation Database (LactMed): Cimetidine. Bethesda, MD, National Institute of Child Health and Human Development, September 21, 2020b. Available at: www.ncbi.nlm.nih.gov/books/NBK501206/. Accessed May 15, 2022.

National Library of Medicine: Drugs and Lactation Database (LactMed): Famotidine. Bethesda, MD, National Institute of Child Health and Human Development, September 21, 2020c. Available at: www.ncbi.nlm.nih.gov/books/NBK501267/. Accessed May 15, 2022.

Navarro V, Gastó C, Torres X, et al: Continuation/maintenance treatment with nortriptyline versus combined nortriptyline and ECT in late-life psychotic depression: a two-year randomized study. Am J Geriatr Psychiatry 16(6):498–505, 2008 18515694

Nelson JC, Price LH, Jatlow PI: Neuroleptic dose and desipramine concentrations during combined treatment of unipolar delusional depression. Am J Psychiatry 143(9):1151–1154, 1986 3752299

Nelson JC, Baumann P, Delucchi K, et al: A systematic review and meta-analysis of lithium augmentation of tricyclic and second generation antidepressants in major depression. J Affect Disord 168:269–275, 2014 25069082

Nelson JP, Benjamin L: Efficacy and safety of combined ECT and tricyclic antidepressant drugs in the treatment of depressed geriatric patients. Convuls Ther 5(4):321–329, 1989 11941030

Nelson JP, Rosenberg DR: ECT treatment of demented elderly patients with major depression: a retrospective study of efficacy and safety. Convuls Ther 7(3):157–165, 1991 11941118

Nettelbladt P: Factors influencing number of treatments and seizure duration in ECT: drug treatment, social class. Convuls Ther 4(2):160–168, 1988 11940957

Netzel PJ, Mueller PS, Rummans TA, et al: Safety, efficacy, and effects on glycemic control of electroconvulsive therapy in insulin-requiring type 2 diabetic patients. J ECT 18(1):16–21, 2002 11925516

Newport DJ, Carpenter LL, McDonald WM, et al: Ketamine and other NMDA antagonists: early clinical trials and possible mechanisms in depression. Am J Psychiatry 172(10):950–966, 2015 26423481

Nibuya M, Sugiyama H, Shioda K, et al: ECT for the treatment of psychiatric symptoms in Basedow's disease. J ECT 18(1):54–57, 2002 11925523

Nicolini AP, Sienaert P: Borderline personality disorder and outcome of electroconvulsive therapy in patients with depression: a systematic review. J ECT 39(2):74–80, 2023 36821825

Nielsen RM, Olsen KS, Lauritsen AO, et al: Electroconvulsive therapy as a treatment for protracted refractory delirium in the intensive care unit: five cases and a review. J Crit Care 29(5):881.e1–881.e6, 2014 24975569

Niemantsverdriet L, Birkenhäger TK, van den Broek WW: The efficacy of ultrabrief-pulse (0.25 millisecond) versus brief-pulse (0.50 millisecond) bilateral electroconvulsive therapy in major depression. J ECT 27(1):55–58, 2011 21343712

Nikolin S, Moffa A, Razza L, et al: Time-course of the tDCS antidepressant effect: an individual participant data meta-analysis. Prog Neuropsychopharmacol Biol Psychiatry 125:110752, 2023 36931456

Nisijima K, Ishiguro T: Electroconvulsive therapy for the treatment of neuroleptic malignant syndrome with psychotic symptoms: a report of five cases. J ECT 15(2):158–163, 1999 10378156

Nitsun M, Szokol JW, Saleh HJ, et al: Pharmacokinetics of midazolam, propofol, and fentanyl transfer to human breast milk. Clin Pharmacol Ther 79(6):549–557, 2006 16765143

Niu Y, Ye D, You Y, et al: Prophylactic cognitive enhancers for improvement of cognitive function in patients undergoing electroconvulsive therapy: a systematic review and meta-analysis. Medicine (Baltimore) 99(11):e19527, 2020 32176105

Nobler MS, Sackeim HA: Augmentation strategies in electroconvulsive therapy: a synthesis. Convuls Ther 9(4):331–351, 1993 11941229

Nobler MS, Sackeim HA: Electroconvulsive therapy: clinical and biological aspects, in Predictors of Response in Mood Disorders. Edited by Goodnick PJ. Washington, DC, American Psychiatric Press, 1996, pp 177–198

Nobler MS, Sackeim HA, Solomou M, et al: EEG manifestations during ECT: effects of electrode placement and stimulus intensity. Biol Psychiatry 34(5):321–330, 1993 8399832

Nobler MS, Sackeim HA, Moeller JR, et al: Quantifying the speed of symptomatic improvement with electroconvulsive therapy: comparison of alternative statistical methods. Convuls Ther 13(4):208–221, 1997 9437565

Nordenskjöld A, Güney P, Nordenskjöld AM: Major adverse cardiovascular events following electroconvulsive therapy in depression: a register-based nationwide Swedish cohort study with 1-year follow-up. J Affect Disord 296:298–304, 2022 34606801

Norris AS, Clancy J: Hospitalized depressions: drugs or electrotherapy? Arch Gen Psychiatry 5:276–279, 1961 13729593

Northoff G, Koch A, Wenke J, et al: Catatonia as a psychomotor syndrome: a rating scale and extrapyramidal motor symptoms. Mov Disord 14(3):404–416, 1999 10348462

Nothdurfter C, Eser D, Schüle C, et al: The influence of concomitant neuroleptic medication on safety, tolerability and clinical effectiveness of electroconvulsive therapy. World J Biol Psychiatry 7(3):162–170, 2006 16861142

Nuñez NA, Joseph B, Pahwa M, et al: Augmentation strategies for treatment resistant major depression: a systematic review and network meta-analysis. J Affect Disord 302:385–400, 2022 34986373

Nuttall GA, Bowersox MR, Douglass SB, et al: Morbidity and mortality in the use of electroconvulsive therapy. J ECT 20(4):237–241, 2004 15591857

Nykamp MJ, Marks L, Kerby PW, et al: Negative pressure pulmonary edema after electroconvulsive therapy. J ECT 37(4):220–221, 2021 34519683

Nymeyer L, Grossberg GT: Delirium in a 75-year-old woman receiving ECT and levodopa. Convuls Ther 13(2):114–116, 1997 9253532

Nystrom S: On relation between clinical factors and efficacy of ECT in depression. Acta Psychiatr Neurol Scand, Suppl 181:11–135, 1964

Obbels J, Verwijk E, Bouckaert F, et al: ECT-related anxiety: a systematic review. J ECT 33(4):229–236, 2017 28009627

Obbels J, Verwijk E, Vansteelandt K, et al: Long-term neurocognitive functioning after electroconvulsive therapy in patients with late-life depression. Acta Psychiatr Scand 138(3):223–231, 2018 30003550

Obbels J, Vansteelandt K, Verwijk E, et al: MMSE changes during and after ECT in late-life depression: a prospective study. Am J Geriatr Psychiatry 27(9):934–944, 2019 31104967

Obbels J, Vanbrabant K, Verwijk E, et al: Monitoring electroconvulsive therapy-related anxiety: the ECT-Related Anxiety Questionnaire. J ECT 36(3):180–186, 2020a 32118688

Obbels J, Vansteelandt K, Verwijk E, et al: Understanding electroconvulsive therapy-related anxiety: a prospective study. Acta Psychiatr Scand 142(2):132–140, 2020b 32474903

O'Brien PD, Morgan DH: Bladder rupture during ECT. Convuls Ther 7(1):56–59, 1991 11941099

O'Connor DW, Gardner B, Presnell I, et al: The effectiveness of continuation-maintenance ECT in reducing depressed older patients' hospital re-admissions. J Affect Disord 120(1-3):62–66, 2010 19411112

O'Connor MK, Knapp R, Husain M, et al: The influence of age on the response of major depression to electroconvulsive therapy: a C.O.R.E. Report. Am J Geriatr Psychiatry 9(4):382–390, 2001 11739064

Odeberg H, Rodriguez-Silva B, Salander P, et al: Individualized continuation electroconvulsive therapy and medication as a bridge to relapse prevention after an index course of electroconvulsive therapy in severe mood disorders: a naturalistic 3-year cohort study. J ECT 24(3):183–190, 2008 18695624

Ogami S, Yamada M, Kanazawa M, et al: The effectiveness of a mouth guard to protect against strong occlusion caused by modified electroconvulsive therapy. Dent Traumatol 30(5):368–373, 2014 25364808

Ogyu K, Kurose S, Uchida H, et al: Clinical features of catatonic non-convulsive status epilepticus: a systematic review of cases. J Psychosom Res 151:110660, 2021 34768095

Okamoto N, Nakai T, Sakamoto K, et al: Rapid antidepressant effect of ketamine anesthesia during electroconvulsive therapy of treatment-resistant depression: comparing ketamine and propofol anesthesia. J ECT 26(3):223–227, 2010 19935085

Olariu E, Forero CG, Castro-Rodriguez JI, et al: Detection of anxiety disorders in primary care: a meta-analysis of assisted and unassisted diagnoses. Depress Anxiety 32(7):471–484, 2015 25826526

Oldfield RC: The assessment and analysis of handedness: the Edinburgh inventory. Neuropsychologia 9(1):97–113, 1971 5146491

Oldham MA: The probability that catatonia in the hospital has a medical cause and the relative proportions of its causes: a systematic review. Psychosomatics 59(4):333–340, 2018 29776679

Oldham MA, Desan PH: Alcohol and sedative-hypnotic withdrawal catatonia: two case reports, systematic literature review, and suggestion of a potential relationship with alcohol withdrawal delirium. Psychosomatics 57(3):246–255, 2016 26949118

Oliva LR, Santos MFL, Leal GC: Neurogenic pulmonary edema after electroconvulsive therapy in 2 young patients. J ECT 38(2):e20–e21, 2022 35613012

O'Reardon JP, Takieddine N, Datto CJ, et al: Propofol for the management of emergence agitation after electroconvulsive therapy: review of a case series. J ECT 22(4):247–252, 2006 17143155

O'Reardon JP, Solvason HB, Janicak PG, et al: Efficacy and safety of transcranial magnetic stimulation in the acute treatment of major depression: a multisite randomized controlled trial. Biol Psychiatry 62(11):1208–1216, 2007 17573044

O'Shea B, Lynch T, Falvey J, et al: Electroconvulsive therapy and cognitive improvement in a very elderly depressed patient. Br J Psychiatry 150:255–257, 1987 3651685

Osler M, Rozing MP, Jorgensen MB, Jorgensen A: Mortality and acute somatic events following electroconvulsive therapy in patients with pre-existing somatic comorbidity—a register-based nationwide Danish cohort study. World J Biol Psychiatry 23(4):318–326, 2022 34668447

Østergaard SD, Meyers BS, Flint AJ, et al: Measuring treatment response in psychotic depression: the Psychotic Depression Assessment Scale (PDAS) takes both depressive and psychotic symptoms into account. J Affect Disord 160:68–73, 2014 24439830

Østergaard SD, Rothschild AJ, Flint AJ, et al: Rating scales measuring the severity of psychotic depression. Acta Psychiatr Scand 132(5):335–344, 2015 26016647

O'Toole JK, Dyck G: Report of psychogenic fever in catatonia responding to electroconvulsive therapy. Dis Nerv Syst 38(10):852–853, 1977 908250

Ott SM: Review article: bone density in patients with chronic kidney disease stages 4–5. Nephrology (Carlton) 14(4):395–403, 2009 19563381

Otto MW, Bruder GE, Fava M, et al: Norms for depressed patients for the California verbal learning test: associations with depression severity and self-report of cognitive difficulties. Arch Clin Neuropsychol 9(1):81–88, 1994 14589514

Ottosson J-O: Experimental studies of the mode of action of electroconvulsive therapy: introduction. Acta Psychiatr Scand Suppl 35(145):5–6, 1960 14429446

Ottosson J-O: Ethics of electroconvulsive therapy. Convuls Ther 8(4):233–236, 1992 11941173

Overall JE: The brief psychiatric rating scale in psychopharmacology research, in Psychological Measurements in Psychopharmacology: Modern Problems in Psychopharmacology. Edited by Pichot P, Olivier-Martin E. Basel, Switzerland, Karger, 1974, pp 67–78

Overall JE, Gorham DR: The brief psychiatric rating scale. Psychol Rep 10(3):799–812, 1962

Packman PM, Meyer DA, Verdun RM: Hazards of succinylcholine administration during electrotherapy. Arch Gen Psychiatry 35(9):1137–1141, 1978 686974

Pagnin D, de Queiroz V, Pini S, et al: Efficacy of ECT in depression: a meta-analytic review. J ECT 20(1):13–20, 2004 15087991

Palma M, Ferreira B, Borja-Santos N, et al: Efficacy of electroconvulsive therapy in bipolar disorder with mixed features. Depress Res Treat 2016:8306071, 2016 26881069

Palmer DM, Sprang HE, Hans CL: Electroshock therapy in schizophrenia; a statistical survey of 455 cases. J Nerv Ment Dis 114(2):162–171, 1951 14861659

Palmio J, Huuhka M, Laine S, et al: Electroconvulsive therapy and biomarkers of neuronal injury and plasticity: serum levels of neuron-specific enolase and S-100b protein. Psychiatry Res 177(1-2):97–100, 2010 20378182

Panchal AR, Berg KM, Kudenchuk PJ, et al: 2018 American Heart Association focused update on advanced cardiovascular life support use of antiarrhythmic drugs during and immediately after cardiac arrest: an update to the American Heart Association guidelines for cardiopulmonary resuscitation and emergency cardiovascular care. Circulation 138(23):e740–e749, 2018 30571262

Pande AC, Grunhaus LJ: ECT for depression in the presence of myasthenia gravis. Convuls Ther 6(2):172–175, 1990 11941060

Pande AC, Grunhaus LJ, Haskett RF, Greden JF: Electroconvulsive therapy in delusional and non-delusional depressive disorder. J Affect Disord 19(3):215–219, 1990 2145342

Pantuck EJ: Plasma cholinesterase: gene and variations. Anesth Analg 77(2):380–386, 1993 8346840

Pargger H, Kaufmann MA, Schouten R, et al: Hemodynamic responses to electroconvulsive therapy in a patient 5 years after cardiac transplantation. Anesthesiology 83(3):625–627, 1995 7661366

Park LT, Falodun TB, Zarate CA Jr: Ketamine for treatment-resistant mood disorders. Focus Am Psychiatr Publ 17(1):8–12, 2019 31975953

Parker G, Roy K, Hadzi-Pavlovic D, et al: Psychotic (delusional) depression: a meta-analysis of physical treatments. J Affect Disord 24(1):17–24, 1992 1347545

Parker G, Hadzi-Pavlovic D, Tully L: Distinguishing bipolar and unipolar disorders: an isomer model. J Affect Disord 96(1-2):67–73, 2006 16815557

Parker V, Nobler MS, Pedley TA, et al: A unilateral, prolonged, nonconvulsive seizure in a patient treated with bilateral ECT. J ECT 17:141–144, 2001 11417926

Parry J: Legal parameters of informed consent for ECT administered to mentally disabled persons. Psychopharmacol Bull 22:490–494, 1986

Patel AS, Gorst-Unsworth C, Venn RM, et al: Anesthesia and electroconvulsive therapy: a retrospective study comparing etomidate and propofol. J ECT 22(3):179–183, 2006 16957533

Patel RS, Manikkara G, Chopra A: Bipolar disorder and comorbid borderline personality disorder: patient characteristics and outcomes in US hospitals. Medicina (Kaunas) 55(1):55, 2019 30646620

Patel RS, Bachu A, Youssef NA: Combination of lithium and electroconvulsive therapy (ECT) is associated with higher odds of delirium and cognitive problems in a large national sample across the United States. Brain Stimul 13(1):15–19, 2020 31492631

Patkar AA, Hill KP, Weinstein SP, et al: ECT in the presence of brain tumor and increased intracranial pressure: evaluation and reduction of risk. J ECT 16(2):189–197, 2000 10868329

Patry S, Graf P, Delva NJ, et al: Electroconvulsive therapy teaching in Canada: cause for concern. J ECT 29(2):109–112, 2013 23303423

Paul SM, Extein I, Calil HM, et al: Use of ECT with treatment-resistant depressed patients at the National Institute of Mental Health. Am J Psychiatry 138(4):486–489, 1981 6111228

Pawełczyk T, Kołodziej-Kowalska E, Pawełczyk A, et al: Augmentation of antipsychotics with electroconvulsive therapy in treatment-resistant schizophrenia patients with dominant negative symptoms: a pilot study of effectiveness. Neuropsychobiology 70(3):158–164, 2014 25358377

Pearce CJ, Wallin JD: Labetalol and other agents that block both alpha- and beta-adrenergic receptors. Cleve Clin J Med 61(1):59–69, quiz 80–82, 1994 8124849

Pearlman C, Carson W, Metz A: Hemodialysis, chronic renal failure, and ECT. Convuls Ther 4(4):332–333, 1988 11940984

Pearlman CA: Electroconvulsive therapy for patient with cardiac pacemaker. JAMA 255:1501, 1986

Peltzman T, Gottlieb DJ, Shiner B, et al: Electroconvulsive therapy in Veterans Health Administration hospitals: prevalence, patterns of use, and patient characteristics. J ECT 36(2):130–136, 2020 31913928

Pelzer ACM, van der Heijden FMMA, den Boer E: Systematic review of catatonia treatment. Neuropsychiatr Dis Treat 14:317–326, 2018 29398916

Penland HR, Ostroff RB: Combined use of lamotrigine and electroconvulsive therapy in bipolar depression: a case series. J ECT 22(2):142–147, 2006 16801832

Perera TD, Luber B, Nobler MS, et al: Seizure expression during electroconvulsive therapy: relationships with clinical outcome and cognitive side effects. Neuropsychopharmacology 29(4):813–825, 2004 14735129

Pergolizzi JV Jr, Philip BK, Leslie JB, et al: Perspectives on transdermal scopolamine for the treatment of postoperative nausea and vomiting. J Clin Anesth 24(4):334–345, 2012 22608591

Perugi G, Medda P, Zanello S, et al: Episode length and mixed features as predictors of ECT nonresponse in patients with medication-resistant major depression. Brain Stimul 5(1):18–24, 2012 22037132

Perugi G, Medda P, Toni C, et al: The role of electroconvulsive therapy (ECT) in bipolar disorder: effectiveness in 522 patients with bipolar depression, mixed-state, mania and catatonic features. Curr Neuropharmacol 15(3):359–371, 2017 28503107

Perugi G, Medda P, Barbuti M, et al: The role of electroconvulsive therapy in the treatment of severe bipolar mixed state. Psychiatr Clin North Am 43(1):187–197, 2020 32008684

Peterchev AV, Rosa MA, Deng ZD, et al: Electroconvulsive therapy stimulus parameters: rethinking dosage. J ECT 26(3):159–174, 2010 20805726

Peterchev AV, Krystal AD, Rosa MA, et al: Individualized low-amplitude seizure therapy: minimizing current for electroconvulsive therapy and magnetic seizure therapy. Neuropsychopharmacology 40(9):2076–2084, 2015 25920013

Peters M: Handedness and its relation to other indices of cerebral lateralization, in Brain Asymmetry. Edited by Davidson RJ, Hugdahl K. Cambridge, MA, MIT Press, 1995, pp 183–214

Peters SG, Wochos DN, Peterson GC: Status epilepticus as a complication of concurrent electroconvulsive and theophylline therapy. Mayo Clin Proc 59(8):568–570, 1984 6748746

Petersen JZ, Porter RJ, Miskowiak KW: Clinical characteristics associated with the discrepancy between subjective and objective cognitive impairment in depression. J Affect Disord 246:763–774, 2019 30623822

Petit AC, Hozer F, Youssov K, et al: Differential response to ECT of psychotic and affective symptoms in Huntington's disease: a case report. J Neuropsychiatry Clin Neurosci 28(1):e3–e5, 2016 26844968

Petrides G: Continuation ECT: a review. Psychiatr Ann 28:517–523, 1998

Petrides G, Fink M: Atrial fibrillation, anticoagulation, and electroconvulsive therapy. Convuls Ther 12(2):91–98, 1996a 8744168

Petrides G, Fink M: The "half-age" stimulation strategy for ECT dosing. Convuls Ther 12(3):138–146, 1996b 8872401

Petrides G, Dhossche D, Fink M, et al: Continuation ECT: relapse prevention in affective disorders. Convuls Ther 10(3):189–194, 1994 7834255

Petrides G, Divadeenam KM, Bush G, et al: Synergism of lorazepam and electroconvulsive therapy in the treatment of catatonia. Biol Psychiatry 42(5):375–381, 1997 9276078

Petrides G, Fink M, Husain MM, et al: ECT remission rates in psychotic versus nonpsychotic depressed patients: a report from CORE. J ECT 17(4):244–253, 2001 11731725

Petrides G, Braga RJ, Fink M, et al: Seizure threshold in a large sample: implications for stimulus dosing strategies in bilateral electroconvulsive therapy: a report from CORE. J ECT 25(4):232–237, 2009 19972637

Petrides G, Tobias KG, Kellner CH, Rudorfer MV: Continuation and maintenance electroconvulsive therapy for mood disorders: review of the literature. Neuropsychobiology 64(3):129–140, 2011 21811083

Petrides G, Malur C, Braga RJ, et al: Electroconvulsive therapy augmentation in clozapine-resistant schizophrenia: a prospective, randomized study. Am J Psychiatry 172(1):52–58, 2015 25157964

Pettinati HM, Mathisen KS, Rosenberg J, et al: Meta-analytical approach to reconciling discrepancies in efficacy between bilateral and unilateral electroconvulsive therapy. Convuls Ther 2(1):7–17, 1986 11940840

Pettinati HM, Stephens SM, Willis KM, et al: Evidence for less improvement in depression in patients taking benzodiazepines during unilateral ECT. Am J Psychiatry 147(8):1029–1035, 1990 2375437

Philibert RA, Richards L, Lynch CF, et al: Effect of ECT on mortality and clinical outcome in geriatric unipolar depression. J Clin Psychiatry 56(9):390–394, 1995 7665536

Phillips JL, Norris S, Talbot J, et al: Single, repeated, and maintenance ketamine infusions for treatment-resistant depression: a randomized controlled trial. Am J Psychiatry 176(5):401–409, 2019 30922101

Phutane VH, Thirthalli J, Muralidharan K, et al: Double-blind randomized controlled study showing symptomatic and cognitive superiority of bifrontal over bitemporal electrode placement during electroconvulsive therapy for schizophrenia. Brain Stimul 6(2):210–217, 2013 22560048

Picardi A: Rating scales in bipolar disorder. Curr Opin Psychiatry 22(1):42–49, 2009 19122534

Picot C, Berard A, Grenet G, et al: Risk of malformation after ondansetron in pregnancy: an updated systematic review and meta-analysis. Birth Defects Res 112(13):996–1013, 2020 32420702

Pier KS, Briggs MC, Pasculli RM, et al: Successful electroconvulsive therapy for major depression misdiagnosed as Alzheimer dementia. Am J Geriatr Psychiatry 20(10):909–910, 2012 22771953

Pigot M, Andrade C, Loo C: Pharmacological attenuation of electroconvulsive therapy–induced cognitive deficits: theoretical background and clinical findings. J ECT 24(1):57–67, 2008 18379337

Pinchotti DM, Abbott C, Quinn DK: Targeted electroconvulsive therapy for super refractory status epilepticus: a case report and literature review. Psychosomatics 59(3):302–305, 2018 29150213

Pinna M, Manchia M, Oppo R, et al: Clinical and biological predictors of response to electroconvulsive therapy (ECT): a review. Neurosci Lett 669:32–42, 2018 27793702

Pisvejc J, Hyrman V, Sikora J, et al: A comparison of brief and ultrabrief pulse stimuli in unilateral ECT. J ECT 14(2):68–75, 1998 9641801

Pitts FJ: Medical physiology of ECT, in Electroconvulsive Therapy: Biological Foundations and Clinical Applications. Edited by Abrams R, Essman W. New York, Spectrum, 1982, pp 57–90

Plahouras JE, Konstantinou G, Kaster TS, et al: Treatment capacity and clinical outcomes for patients with schizophrenia who were treated with electroconvulsive therapy: a retrospective cohort study. Schizophr Bull 47(2):424–432, 2021 33145601

Pluijms EM, Birkenhäger TK, Mulder PG, et al: Influence of episode duration of major depressive disorder on response to electroconvulsive therapy. J Affect Disord 90(2-3):233–237, 2006 16376432

Pluijms EM, Kamperman AM, Hoogendijk WJ, et al: Influence of an adjuvant antidepressant on the efficacy of electroconvulsive therapy: a systematic review and meta-analysis. Aust N Z J Psychiatry 55(4):366–380, 2021 32900217

Pluijms EM, Kamperman AM, Hoogendijk WJG, et al: Influence of adjuvant nortriptyline on the efficacy of electroconvulsive therapy: a randomized controlled trial and 1-year follow-up. Acta Psychiatr Scand 145(5):517–528, 2022 35152416

Pompili M, Lester D, Dominici G, et al: Indications for electroconvulsive treatment in schizophrenia: a systematic review. Schizophr Res 146(1-3):1–9, 2013 23499244

Pope HG Jr, Lipinski JF, Cohen BM, et al: "Schizoaffective disorder": an invalid diagnosis? A comparison of schizoaffective disorder, schizophrenia, and affective disorder. Am J Psychiatry 137(8):921–927, 1980 6106396

Popeo D, Kellner CH: ECT for Parkinson's disease. Med Hypotheses 73(4):468–469, 2009 19660875

Popiolek K, Bejerot S, Brus O, et al: Electroconvulsive therapy in bipolar depression: effectiveness and prognostic factors. Acta Psychiatr Scand 140(3):196–204, 2019 31334829

Popova V, Daly EJ, Trivedi M, et al: Efficacy and safety of flexibly dosed esketamine nasal spray combined with a newly initiated oral antidepressant in treatment-resistant depression: a randomized double-blind active-controlled study. Am J Psychiatry 176(6):428–438, 2019 31109201

Porac C, Coren S: Lateral Preferences and Human Behavior. New York, Springer Verlag, 1981

Pornnoppadol C, Isenberg K: ECT with implantable cardioverter defibrillator. J ECT 14(2):124–126, 1998 9641812

Porquez JM, Thompson TR, McDonald WM: Administration of ECT in a patient with an inoperable abdominal aortic aneurysm: serial imaging of the aorta during maintenance. J ECT 19(2):118–120, 2003 12792463

Porter E, Chambless DL, McCarthy KS, et al: Psychometric properties of the reconstructed Hamilton Depression and Anxiety scales. J Nerv Ment Dis 205(8):656–664, 2017 28225509

Porter R, Booth D, Gray H, et al: Effects of the addition of remifentanil to propofol anesthesia on seizure length and postictal suppression index in electroconvulsive therapy. J ECT 24(3):203–207, 2008a 18772705

Porter R, Heenan H, Reeves J: Early effects of electroconvulsive therapy on cognitive function. J ECT 24(1):35–39, 2008b 18379333

Postaci A, Tiryaki C, Sacan O, et al: Rocuronium-sugammadex decreases the severity of post-electroconvulsive therapy agitation. J ECT 29(1):e2–e3, 2013 23422529

Potokar J, Wilson S, Nutt DJ: Do SSRIs prolong seizure duration during ECT? Int J Psychiatry Clin Pract 1(4):277–280, 1997 24946194

Potvin S, Charbonneau G, Juster RP, et al: Self-evaluation and objective assessment of cognition in major depression and attention deficit disorder: implications for clinical practice. Compr Psychiatry 70:53–64, 2016 27624423

Practice Guidelines for Obstetric Anesthesia: An Updated Report by the American Society of Anesthesiologists Task Force on Obstetric Anesthesia and the Society for Obstetric Anesthesia and Perinatology. Anesthesiology 124(2):270–300, 2016 26580836

Pradhan BK, van Helmond N, Mitrev LV, et al: Hereditary pseudocholinesterase deficiency discovery after electroconvulsive therapy. BMJ Case Rep 14(1):14, 2021 33462045

Prakash J, Kotwal A, Prabhu H: Therapeutic and prophylactic utility of the memory-enhancing drug donepezil hydrochloride on cognition of patients undergoing electroconvulsive therapy: a randomized controlled trial. J ECT 22(3):163–168, 2006 16957530

Prakash J, Chaudhury S, Chatterjee K, et al: Therapeutic and prophylactic role of cognitive enhancers in electroconvulsive therapy-induced cognitive deficits. Ind Psychiatry J 28(2):286–293, 2019 33223724

Pratt RT, Warrington EK, Halliday AM: Unilateral ECT as a test for cerebral dominance, with a strategy for treating left-handers. Br J Psychiatry 119(548):79–83, 1971 5556664

Price JW, Price JR, Perry TL: Excessive hypertension and pulmonary edema after electroconvulsive therapy. J ECT 21(3):174–177, 2005 16127308

Price TR, McAllister TW: Response of depressed patients to sequential unilateral nondominant brief-pulse and bilateral sinusoidal ECT. J Clin Psychiatry 47(4):182–186, 1986 3957877

Price TR, McAllister TW: Safety and efficacy of ECT in depressed patients with dementia: a review of clinical experience. Convuls Ther 5(1):61–74, 1989 11940996

Pridmore S, May T: Relapse prevention (RP) TMS. Brain Stimul 11(6):1391–1392, 2018 30143418

Pridmore S, Erger S, Rybak M, et al: Early relapse (ER) transcranial magnetic stimulation (TMS) in treatment resistant major depression. Brain Stimul 11(5):1098–1102, 2018 29805096

Pritchett JT, Bernstein HJ, Kellner CH: Combined ECT and antidepressant drug therapy. Convuls Ther 9(4):256–261, 1993 11941221

Proakis AG, Harris GB: Comparative penetration of glycopyrrolate and atropine across the blood-brain and placental barriers in anesthetized dogs. Anesthesiology 48(5):339–344, 1978 646152

Próchnicki M, Rudzki G, Dzikowski M, et al: The impact of electroconvulsive therapy on the spatial QRS-T angle and cardiac troponin T concentration in psychiatric patients. PLoS One 14(10):e0224020, 2019 31644576

Protheroe C: Puerperal psychoses: a long term study 1927–1961. Br J Psychiatry 115(518):9–30, 1969 5781966

Prudic J: Strategies to minimize cognitive side effects with ECT: aspects of ECT technique. J ECT 24(1):46–51, 2008 18379335

Prudic J, Sackeim HA, Decina P, et al: Acute effects of ECT on cardiovascular functioning: relations to patient and treatment variables. Acta Psychiatr Scand 75(4):344–351, 1987 3591419

Prudic J, Devanand DP, Sackeim HA, et al: Relative response of endogenous and non-endogenous symptoms to electroconvulsive therapy. J Affect Disord 16(1):59–64, 1989 2521653

Prudic J, Sackeim HA, Devanand DP: Medication resistance and clinical response to electroconvulsive therapy. Psychiatry Res 31(3):287–296, 1990 1970656

Prudic J, Sackeim HA, Devanand DP, et al: The efficacy of ECT in double depression. Depression 1:38–44, 1993

Prudic J, Sackeim HA, Devanand DP, et al: Acute cognitive effects of subconvulsive electrical stimulation. Convuls Ther 10(1):4–24, 1994 8055291

Prudic J, Haskett RF, Mulsant B, et al: Resistance to antidepressant medications and short-term clinical response to ECT. Am J Psychiatry 153(8):985–992, 1996 8678194

Prudic J, Peyser S, Sackeim HA: Subjective memory complaints: a review of patient self-assessment of memory after electroconvulsive therapy. J ECT 16(2):121–132, 2000 10868322

Prudic J, Olfson M, Marcus SC, et al: Effectiveness of electroconvulsive therapy in community settings. Biol Psychiatry 55(3):301–312, 2004 14744473

Prudic J, Haskett RF, McCall WV, et al: Pharmacological strategies in the prevention of relapse after electroconvulsive therapy. J ECT 29(1):3–12, 2013 23303417

Puffer CC, Wall CA, Huxsahl JE, et al: A 20 year practice review of electroconvulsive therapy for adolescents. J Child Adolesc Psychopharmacol 26(7):632–636, 2016 26784386

Pullen SJ, Rasmussen KG, Angstman ER, et al: The safety of electroconvulsive therapy in patients with prolonged QTc intervals on the electrocardiogram. J ECT 27(3):192–200, 2011 21681107

Puri BK, Langa A, Coleman RM, et al: The clinical efficacy of maintenance electroconvulsive therapy in a patient with a mild mental handicap. Br J Psychiatry 161:707–709, 1992 1422626

Purohith AN, Vaidyanathan S, Udupa ST, et al: Electroconvulsive therapy in patients with cardiac implantable electronic devices: a case report and systematic review of published cases. J ECT 39(1):46–52, 2023 35482902

Qaseem A, Wilt TJ, Weinberger SE, et al: Diagnosis and management of stable chronic obstructive pulmonary disease: a clinical practice guideline update from the American College of Physicians, American College of Chest Physicians, American Thoracic Society, and European Respiratory Society. Ann Intern Med 155(3):179–191, 2011 21810710

Qiu Z, Zhou S, Zhang M, et al: Preventive effect of dexmedetomidine on postictal delirium after electroconvulsive therapy: a randomised controlled study. Eur J Anaesthesiol 37(1):5–13, 2020 31688331

Quitkin FM: The importance of dosage in prescribing antidepressants. Br J Psychiatry 147:593–597, 1985 3913485

Quitkin FM, Rabkin JG, Ross D, et al: Duration of antidepressant drug treatment: what is an adequate trial? Arch Gen Psychiatry 41(3):238–245, 1984 6367689

Quitkin FM, McGrath PJ, Stewart JW, et al: Can the effects of antidepressants be observed in the first two weeks of treatment? Neuropsychopharmacology 15(4):390–394, 1996 8887993

Rabheru K, Persad E: A review of continuation and maintenance electroconvulsive therapy. Can J Psychiatry 42(5):476–484, 1997 9220110

Rabheru K, Wiens A, Ramprasad B, et al: Comparison of traditional didactic seminar to high-fidelity simulation for teaching electroconvulsive therapy technique to psychiatry trainees. J ECT 29(4):291–296, 2013 24263274

Rabie N, Shah R, Ray-Griffith S, et al: Continuous fetal monitoring during electroconvulsive therapy: a prospective observation study. Int J Womens Health 13:1–7, 2021 33442300

Rachlin HL, Goldman GS, Gurvitz M, et al: Follow-up study of 317 patients discharged from Hillside Hospital in 1950. J Hillside Hosp 5:17–40, 1956

Rackowski D, Kalat JW, Nebes R: Reliability and validity of some handedness questionnaire items. Neuropsychologia 8:523–526, 1976

Raffin M, Zugaj-Bensaou L, Bodeau N, et al: Treatment use in a prospective naturalistic cohort of children and adolescents with catatonia. Eur Child Adolesc Psychiatry 24(4):441–449, 2015 25159089

Rajagopal R, Chakrabarti S, Grover S: Satisfaction with electroconvulsive therapy among patients and their relatives. J ECT 29(4):283–290, 2013 23670027

Rakesh G, Thirthalli J, Kumar CN, et al: Concomitant anticonvulsants with bitemporal electroconvulsive therapy: a randomized controlled trial with clinical and neurobiological application. J ECT 33(1):16–21, 2017 27668943

Rakesh G, Mischel NA, Gunderson-Falcone G, et al: Effect of extended release bupropion on unilateral ultrabrief electroconvulsive therapy seizure parameters in major depressive disorder. J ECT 36(4):e45–e46, 2020 32243338

Ramalingam J, Elias A, George K, et al: Retrospective comparison of effectiveness of right unilateral ultra-brief pulse with brief pulse ECT in older adults (over 65) with depression. Int Psychogeriatr 28(3):469–475, 2016 26344656

Randolph C, Tierney MC, Mohr E, et al: The Repeatable Battery for the Assessment of Neuropsychological Status (RBANS): preliminary clinical validity. J Clin Exp Neuropsychol 20(3):310–319, 1998 9845158

Randt CT, Brown ER: Randt Memory Test. Bayport, NY, Life Science, 1983

Randt CT, Brown ER, Osbourne DP: A memory test for longitudinal measurement of mild to moderate deficits. Clin Neuropsychol 2:184–194, 1980

Ranen NG, Peyser CE, Folstein SE: ECT as a treatment for depression in Huntington's disease. J Neuropsychiatry Clin Neurosci 6(2):154–159, 1994 8044037

Rao KM, Gangadhar BN, Janakiramaiah N: Nonconvulsive status epilepticus after the ninth electroconvulsive therapy. Convuls Ther 9(2):128–129, 1993 11941202

Rao NP, Palaniyappan P, Chandur J, et al: Successful use of donepezil in treatment of cognitive impairment caused by maintenance electroconvulsive therapy: a case report. J ECT 25(3):216–218, 2009 19190508

Rao VR, Sellers KK, Wallace DL, et al: Direct electrical stimulation of lateral orbitofrontal cortex acutely improves mood in individuals with symptoms of depression. Curr Biol 28(24):3893.e4–3902.e4, 2018 30503621

Rapinesi C, Kotzalidis GD, Serata D, et al: Prevention of relapse with maintenance electroconvulsive therapy in elderly patients with major depressive episode. J ECT 29(1):61–64, 2013 23011573

Rasheed HA, Cohenmehr J, Chen ST: Electroconvulsive therapy with titanium-based uveoscleral stents. J ECT 38(4):262–263, 2022 35700965

Rask O, Nordenskjöld A, Johansson BA, et al: Electroconvulsive therapy in children and adolescents: results from a population-based study utilising the Swedish National Quality Register. Eur Child Adolesc Psychiatry 32(12):2649–2656, 2023 36513894

Rasmussen KG: Some considerations in choosing electroconvulsive therapy versus transcranial magnetic stimulation for depression. J ECT 27(1):51–54, 2011 21343711

Rasmussen KG: Propofol for ECT anesthesia a review of the literature. J ECT 30(3):210–215, 2014 24820943

Rasmussen KG: Do patients with personality disorders respond differentially to electroconvulsive therapy? A review of the literature and consideration of conceptual issues. J ECT 31(1):6–12, 2015 25054362

Rasmussen KG: What type of cognitive testing should be part of routine electroconvulsive therapy practice? J ECT 32(1):7–12, 2016 26075697

Rasmussen KG: Principles and Practice of Electroconvulsive Therapy. Washington, DC, American Psychiatric Association Publishing, 2019

Rasmussen KG, Keegan BM: Electroconvulsive therapy in patients with multiple sclerosis. J ECT 23(3):179–180, 2007 17804994

Rasmussen T, Milner B: The role of early left-brain injury in determining lateralization of cerebral speech functions. Ann N Y Acad Sci 299:355–369, 1977 101116

Rasmussen KG, Ritter MJ: Some considerations of the tolerability of ketamine for ECT anesthesia: a case series and review of the literature. J ECT 30(4):283–286, 2014 24820945

Rasmussen KG, Ryan DA: The effect of electroconvulsive therapy treatments on blood sugar in nondiabetic patients. J ECT 21(4):232–234, 2005 16301883

Rasmussen KG, Zorumski CF: Electroconvulsive therapy in patients taking theophylline. J Clin Psychiatry 54(11):427–431, 1993 8270586

Rasmussen KG, Zorumski CF, Jarvis MR: Possible impact of stimulus duration on seizure threshold in ECT. Convuls Ther 10(2):177–180, 1994 8069644

Rasmussen KG, Jarvis MR, Zorumski CF: Ketamine anesthesia in electroconvulsive therapy. Convuls Ther 12(4):217–223, 1996 9034696

Rasmussen KG, Jarvis MR, Zorumski CF, et al: Low-dose atropine in electroconvulsive therapy. J ECT 15(3):213–221, 1999 10492860

Rasmussen KG, Rummans TA, Richardson JW: Electroconvulsive therapy in the medically ill. Psychiatr Clin North Am 25(1):177–193, 2002 11912939

Rasmussen KG, Ryan DA, Mueller PS: Blood glucose before and after ECT treatments in Type 2 diabetic patients. J ECT 22(2):124–126, 2006 16801828

Rasmussen P, Andersson JE, Koch P, et al: Glycopyrrolate prevents extreme bradycardia and cerebral deoxygenation during electroconvulsive therapy. J ECT 23(3):147–152, 2007a 17804987

Rasmussen KG, Hooten WM, Dodd ML, et al: QTc dispersion on the baseline ECG predicts arrhythmias during electroconvulsive therapy. Acta Cardiol 62(4):345–347, 2007b 17824294

Rasmussen KG, Mueller M, Knapp RG, et al: Antidepressant medication treatment failure does not predict lower remission with ECT for major depressive disorder: a report from the consortium for research in electroconvulsive therapy. J Clin Psychiatry 68(11):1701–1706, 2007c 18052563

Rasmussen KG, Perry CL, Sutor B, et al: ECT in patients with intracranial masses. J Neuropsychiatry Clin Neurosci 19(2):191–193, 2007d 17431067

Rasmussen KG, Petersen KN, Sticka JL, et al: Correlates of myalgia in electroconvulsive therapy. J ECT 24(1):84–87, 2008 18379340

Rasmussen KG, Mueller M, Rummans TA, et al: Is baseline medication resistance associated with potential for relapse after successful remission of a depressive episode with ECT? Data from the Consortium for Research on Electroconvulsive Therapy (CORE). J Clin Psychiatry 70(2):232–237, 2009 19192459

Rasmussen KG, Kung S, Lapid MI, et al: A randomized comparison of ketamine versus methohexital anesthesia in electroconvulsive therapy. Psychiatry Res 215(2):362–365, 2014 24388729

Rasmussen SA, Mazurek MF, Rosebush PI: Catatonia: our current understanding of its diagnosis, treatment and pathophysiology. World J Psychiatry 6(4):391–398, 2016 28078203

Ravanić DB, Pantović MM, Milovanović DR, et al: Long-term efficacy of electroconvulsive therapy combined with different antipsychotic drugs in previously resistant schizophrenia. Psychiatr Danub 21(2):179–186, 2009 19556946

Raveendranathan D, Narayanaswamy JC, Reddi SV: Response rate of catatonia to electroconvulsive therapy and its clinical correlates. Eur Arch Psychiatry Clin Neurosci 262(5):425–430, 2012 22207031

Ray AK: Does electroconvulsive therapy cause epilepsy? J ECT 29(3):201–205, 2013 23291703

Ray SD: Relative efficacy of ECT and CPZ in schizophrenia. J Indian Med Assoc 38:332–333, 1962 14490710

Rayburn BK: Electroconvulsive therapy in patients with heart failure or valvular heart disease. Convuls Ther 13(3):145–156, 1997 9342130

Ray-Griffith SL, Coker JL, Rabie N, et al: Pregnancy and electroconvulsive therapy: a multidisciplinary approach. J ECT 32(2):104–112, 2016 26796501

Raysin A, Gillett B, Carmody J, et al: From information to simulation: Improving competency in ECT training using high-fidelity simulation. Acad Psychiatry 42(5):653–658, 2018 29256032

Recart A, Rawal S, White PF, et al: The effect of remifentanil on seizure duration and acute hemodynamic responses to electroconvulsive therapy. Anesth Analg 96(4):1047–1050, 2003 12651657

Reddy BK, Pizer B, Bull PT: Neonatal serum cortisol suppression by etomidate compared with thiopentone, for elective caesarean section. Eur J Anaesthesiol 5(3):171–176, 1988 3181146

Reddy S, Nobler MS: Dangerous hyperglycemia associated with electroconvulsive therapy. Convuls Ther 12(2):99–103, 1996 8744169

Redlich R, Opel N, Grotegerd D, et al: Prediction of individual response to electroconvulsive therapy via machine learning on structural magnetic resonance imaging data. JAMA Psychiatry 73(6):557–564, 2016 27145449

Reed P, Sermin N, Appleby L, et al: A comparison of clinical response to electroconvulsive therapy in puerperal and non-puerperal psychoses. J Affect Disord 54(3):255–260, 1999 10467968

Regenold WT, Weintraub D, Taller A: Electroconvulsive therapy for epilepsy and major depression. Am J Geriatr Psychiatry 6(2):180–183, 1998 9581214

Regenold WT, Noorani RJ, Piez D, et al: Nonconvulsive electrotherapy for treatment resistant unipolar and bipolar major depressive disorder: a proof-of-concept trial. Brain Stimul 8(5):855–861, 2015 26187603

Reid WH, Keller S, Leatherman M, et al: ECT in Texas: 19 months of mandatory reporting. J Clin Psychiatry 59(1):8–13, 1998 9491059

Reinfeld S, Yacoub A: A case of delirious mania induced by COVID-19 treated with electroconvulsive therapy. J ECT 37(4):e38–e39, 2021 34294651

Reinfeld S, Williams R, Yacoub A: Electroconvulsive therapy 1 week after the removal of a deep brain stimulator. J ECT 39(2):124–125, 2023 36897196

Reiter-Theil S: Autonomy and beneficence: ethical issues in electroconvulsive therapy. Convuls Ther 8(4):237–244, 1992 11659608

Remick RA, Jewesson P, Ford RWJ: Monoamine oxidase inhibitors in general anesthesia: a reevaluation. Convuls Ther 3(3):196–203, 1987 11940916

Ren J, Li H, Palaniyappan L, et al: Repetitive transcranial magnetic stimulation versus electroconvulsive therapy for major depression: a systematic review and meta-analysis. Prog Neuropsychopharmacol Biol Psychiatry 51:181–189, 2014 24556538

Ren L, Deng J, Min S, et al: Ketamine in electroconvulsive therapy for depressive disorder: a systematic review and meta-analysis. J Psychiatr Res 104:144–156, 2018 30077114

Reti IM, Walker M, Pulia K, et al: Safety considerations for outpatient electroconvulsive therapy. J Psychiatr Pract 18(2):130–136, 2012 22418405

Réus GZ, de Moura AB, Borba LA, et al: Strategies for treatment-resistant depression: lessons learned from animal models. Mol Neuropsychiatry 5(4):178–189, 2019 31768371

Reveles Jensen KH, Navntoft CA, Sindahl CH, et al: Cochlear implant should not be absolute contraindication for electroconvulsive therapy and transcranial magnetic stimulation. Brain Stimul 13(5):1464–1466, 2020 32800965

Rey A: L'Examen Clinique en Psychologie. Paris, Press Universitaire de France, 1964

Rey JM, Walter G: Half a century of ECT use in young people. Am J Psychiatry 154(5):595–602, 1997 9137112

Rhee TG, Sint K, Olfson M, et al: Association of ECT with risks of all-cause mortality and suicide in older Medicare patients. Am J Psychiatry 178(12):1089–1097, 2021 34503341

Rhee TG, Shim SR, Forester BP, et al: Efficacy and safety of ketamine vs electroconvulsive therapy among patients with major depressive episode: a systematic review and meta-analysis. JAMA Psychiatry 79(12):1162–1172, 2022 36260324

Rice EH, Sombrotto LB, Markowitz JC, et al: Cardiovascular morbidity in high-risk patients during ECT. Am J Psychiatry 151(11):1637–1641, 1994 7943453

Ricken R, Ulrich S, Schlattmann P, et al: Tranylcypromine in mind (Part II): review of clinical pharmacology and meta-analysis of controlled studies in depression. Eur Neuropsychopharmacol 27(8):714–731, 2017 28579071

Riddle M, Potter GG, McQuoid DR, et al: Longitudinal cognitive outcomes of clinical phenotypes of late-life depression. Am J Geriatr Psychiatry 25(10):1123–1134, 2017 28479153

Riddle WJ, Scott AI, Bennie J, et al: Current intensity and oxytocin release after electroconvulsive therapy. Biol Psychiatry 33(11-12):839–841, 1993 8373922

Riedel M, Möller HJ, Obermeier M, et al: Clinical predictors of response and remission in inpatients with depressive syndromes. J Affect Disord 133(1-2):137–149, 2011 21555156

Ries R, Bokan J: Electroconvulsive therapy following pituitary surgery. J Nerv Ment Dis 167(12):767–768, 1979 41885

Ries RK, Wilson L, Bokan JA, et al: ECT in medication resistant schizoaffective disorder. Compr Psychiatry 22(2):167–173, 1981 7214880

Rifkin A: ECT versus tricyclic antidepressants in depression: a review of the evidence. J Clin Psychiatry 49(1):3–7, 1988 3275634

Riva-Posse P, Hermida AP, McDonald WM: The role of electroconvulsive and neuromodulation therapies in the treatment of geriatric depression. Psychiatr Clin North Am 36(4):607–630, 2013 24229660

Rivera FA, Lapid MI, Sampson S, et al: Safety of electroconvulsive therapy in patients with a history of heart failure and decreased left ventricular systolic heart function. J ECT 27(3):207–213, 2011 21865957

Roberts JM: Prognostic factors in the electroshock treatment of depressive states I: clinical features from history and examination. J Ment Sci 105:693–702, 1959a 14437823

Roberts JM: Prognostic factors in the electro-shock treatment of depressive states II: the application of specific tests. J Ment Sci 105:703–713, 1959b 14437822

Robertson GS: Serum cholinesterase deficiency. I. Disease and inheritance. Br J Anaesth 38(5):355–360, 1966 5328263

Robin A, de Tissera S: A double-blind controlled comparison of the therapeutic effects of low and high energy electroconvulsive therapies. Br J Psychiatry 141:357–366, 1982 6756529

Robin AA, Harris JA: A controlled comparison of imipramine and electroplexy. J Ment Sci 108:217–219, 1962 14492854

Robinson GE, Stewart DE: Postpartum psychiatric disorders. CMAJ 134(1):31–37, 1986 3510069

Robinson M, Lighthall G: Asystole during successive electroconvulsive therapy sessions: a report of two cases. J Clin Anesth 16(3):210–213, 2004 15217662

Rodenbach KE, Varon D, Denko T, et al: Use of ECT in major vascular neurocognitive disorder with treatment-resistant behavioral disturbance following an acute stroke in a young patient. Case Rep Psychiatry 2019:9694765, 2019 31139486

Roebuck-Spencer TM, Glen T, Puente AE, et al: Cognitive screening tests versus comprehensive neuropsychological test batteries: a National Academy of Neuropsychology education paper. Arch Clin Neuropsychol 32(4):491–498, 2017 28334244

Roemer RA, Dubin WR, Jaffe R, et al: An efficacy study of single- versus double-seizure induction with ECT in major depression. J Clin Psychiatry 51(11):473–478, 1990 2228983

Rogan T, Wilkinson ST: The role of psychotherapy in the management of treatment-resistant depression. Psychiatr Clin North Am 46(2):349–358, 2023 37149349

Rogers JP, Pollak TA, Blackman G, et al: Catatonia and the immune system: a review. Lancet Psychiatry 6(7):620–630, 2019 31196793

Rogers JP, Oldham MA, Fricchione G, et al: Evidence-based consensus guidelines for the management of catatonia: recommendations from the British Association for Psychopharmacology. J Psychopharmacol 37(4):327–369, 2023 37039129

Rohde P, Sargant W: Treatment of schizophrenia in general hospitals. BMJ 2(5244):67–70, 1961 13742822

Rohland BM, Carroll BT, Jacoby RG: ECT in the treatment of the catatonic syndrome. J Affect Disord 29(4):255–261, 1993 8126312

Rönnqvist I, Nilsson FK, Nordenskjöld A: Electroconvulsive therapy and the risk of suicide in hospitalized patients with major depressive disorder. JAMA Netw Open 4(7):e2116589, 2021 34287633

Roose SP, Glassman AH, Walsh BT, et al: Depression, delusions, and suicide. Am J Psychiatry 140(9):1159–1162, 1983 6614220

Rootes-Murdy K, Carlucci M, Tibbs M, et al: Non-suicidal self-injury and electroconvulsive therapy: outcomes in adolescent and young adult populations. J Affect Disord 250:94–98, 2019 30844603

Rosa MA, Rosa MO, Marcolin MA, et al: Cardiovascular effects of anesthesia in ECT: a randomized, double-blind comparison of etomidate, propofol, and thiopental. J ECT 23(1):6–8, 2007 17435563

Rosa MA, Rosa MO, Belegarde IM, et al: Recovery after ECT: comparison of propofol, etomidate and thiopental. Rev Bras Psiquiatr 30(2):149–151, 2008 18470404

Rosa MA, Abdo GL, Lisanby SH, et al: Seizure induction with low-amplitude-current (0.5 A) electroconvulsive therapy. J ECT 27(4):341–342, 2011 22124222

Rose JT: Reactive and endogenous depressions—response to E.C.T. Br J Psychiatry 109:213–217, 1963 13974791

Rose S, Dotters-Katz SK, Kuller JA: Electroconvulsive therapy in pregnancy: safety, best practices, and barriers to care. Obstet Gynecol Surv 75(3):199–203, 2020 32232498

Rosen AM, Mukherjee S, Shinbach K: The efficacy of ECT in phencyclidine-induced psychosis. J Clin Psychiatry 45(5):220–222, 1984 6144671

Rosenberg O, Zangen A, Stryjer R, et al: Response to deep TMS in depressive patients with previous electroconvulsive treatment. Brain Stimul 3(4):211–217, 2010 20965450

Rosenquist PB, Miller B, Pillai A: The antipsychotic effects of ECT: a review of possible mechanisms. J ECT 30(2):125–131, 2014 24810776

Rosenquist PB, Youssef NA, Surya S, et al: When all else fails: the use of electroconvulsive therapy for conditions other than major depressive episode. Psychiatr Clin North Am 41(3):355–371, 2018 30098650

Ross AF, Tucker JH: Anesthesia risk, in Anesthesia, 3rd Edition. Edited by Miller RD. New York, Churchill Livingstone, 1990, pp 715–742

Ross CA, Tabrizi SJ: Huntington's disease: from molecular pathogenesis to clinical treatment. Lancet Neurol 10(1):83–98, 2011 21163446

Ross JR, Malzberg B: A review of the results of the pharmacological shock therapy and the metrazol convulsive therapy in New York State. Am J Psychiatry 96:297–316, 1939

Rossi S, Antal A, Bestmann S, et al: Safety and recommendations for TMS use in healthy subjects and patient populations, with updates on training, ethical and regulatory issues: expert guidelines. Clin Neurophysiol 132(1):269–306, 2021 33243615

Roth LH: Data on informed consent for ECT. Psychopharmacol Bull 22:494–495, 1986

Roth LH, Meisel A, Lidz CW: Tests of competency to consent to treatment. Am J Psychiatry 134(3):279–284, 1977 842704

Roth LH, Lidz CW, Meisel A, et al: Competency to decide about treatment and research: an overview of some empirical data. Int J Law Psychiatry 5:29–50, 1982

Rothschild AJ: Challenges in the treatment of major depressive disorder with psychotic features. Schizophr Bull 39(4):787–796, 2013 23599251

Royal Australian and New Zealand College of Psychiatrists: Electroconvulsive therapy (Clinical Memorandum #12). Melbourne, Australia, Royal Australian and New Zealand College of Psychiatrists, 1992

Royal College of Psychiatrists: The ECT Handbook: The Second Report of the Royal College of Psychiatrists' Special Committee on ECT. London, Royal College of Psychiatrists, 1995

Roy-Byrne P, Gerner RH: Legal restrictions on the use of ECT in California: clinical impact on the incompetent patient. J Clin Psychiatry 42(8):300–303, 1981 7251565

Rozing MP, Jørgensen MB, Osler M: Electroconvulsive therapy and later stroke in patients with affective disorders. Br J Psychiatry 214(3):168–170, 2019 30106358

Rubner P, Koppi S, Conca A: Frequency of and rationales for the combined use of electroconvulsive therapy and antiepileptic drugs in Austria and the literature. World J Biol Psychiatry 10(4 Pt 3):836–845, 2009 19995220

Rucker J, Cook M: A case of prolonged seizure after ECT in a patient treated with clomipramine, lithium, L-tryptophan, quetiapine, and thyroxine for major depression. J ECT 24(4):272–274, 2008 18648320

Rudorfer MV, Linnoila M, Potter WZ: Combined lithium and electroconvulsive therapy: pharmacokinetic and pharmacodynamic interactions. Convuls Ther 3(1):40–45, 1987 11940888

Rudorfer MV, Manji HK, Potter WZ: Bupropion, ECT, and dopaminergic overdrive. Am J Psychiatry 148(8):1101–1102, 1991 1906685

Rudorfer MV, Manji HK, Potter WZ: ECT and delirium in Parkinson's disease. Am J Psychiatry 149(12):1758–1759, author reply 1759–1760, 1992 1443266

Rummans TA, Bassingthwaighte ME: Severe medical and neurologic complications associated with near-lethal catatonia treated with electroconvulsive therapy. Convuls Ther 7(2):121–124, 1991 11941111

Rundgren S, Brus O, Båve U, et al: Improvement of postpartum depression and psychosis after electroconvulsive therapy: a population-based study with a matched comparison group. J Affect Disord 235:258–264, 2018 29660641

Rush AJ, Gullion CM, Basco MR, et al: The Inventory of Depressive Symptomatology (IDS): psychometric properties. Psychol Med 26(3):477–486, 1996 8733206

Rush AJ, George MS, Sackeim HA, et al: Vagus nerve stimulation (VNS) for treatment-resistant depressions: a multicenter study. Biol Psychiatry 47(4):276–286, 2000 10686262

Rush AJ, Trivedi MH, Ibrahim HM, et al: The 16-Item Quick Inventory of Depressive Symptomatology (QIDS), clinician rating (QIDS-C), and self-report (QIDS-SR): a psychometric evaluation in patients with chronic major depression. Biol Psychiatry 54(5):573–583, 2003 12946886

Rush AJ, Marangell LB, Sackeim HA, et al: Vagus nerve stimulation for treatment-resistant depression: a randomized, controlled acute phase trial. Biol Psychiatry 58(5):347–354, 2005a 16139580

Rush AJ, Sackeim HA, Marangell LB, et al: Effects of 12 months of vagus nerve stimulation in treatment-resistant depression: a naturalistic study. Biol Psychiatry 58(5):355–363, 2005b 16139581

Rush AJ, Trivedi MH, Wisniewski SR, et al: Bupropion-SR, sertraline, or venlafaxine-XR after failure of SSRIs for depression. N Engl J Med 354(12):1231–1242, 2006 16554525

Saad DA, Black JL III, Krahn LE, et al: ECT post eye surgery: two cases and a review of the literature. J ECT 16(4):409–414, 2000 11314879

Sackeim HA: Acute cognitive side effects of ECT. Psychopharmacol Bull 22:482–484, 1986

Sackeim HA: The cognitive effects of electroconvulsive therapy, in Cognitive Disorders: Pathophysiology and Treatment. Edited by Moos WH, Gamzu ER, Thal LJ. New York, Marcel Dekker, 1992, pp 183–228

Sackeim HA: Continuation therapy following ECT: directions for future research. Psychopharmacol Bull 30(3):501–521, 1994 7878189

Sackeim HA: The use of electroconvulsive therapy in late-life depression, in Geriatric Psychopharmacology, 3rd Edition. Edited by Salzman C. Baltimore, MD, Williams & Wilkins, 1998, pp 262–309

Sackeim HA: The anticonvulsant hypothesis of the mechanisms of action of ECT: current status. J ECT 15(1):5–26, 1999 10189616

Sackeim HA: Memory and ECT: from polarization to reconciliation. J ECT 16(2):87–96, 2000 10868319

Sackeim HA: Autobiographical memory and electroconvulsive therapy: do not throw out the baby. J ECT 30(3):177–186, 2014 24755727

Sackeim HA, Rush AJ: Melancholia and response to ECT. Am J Psychiatry 152(8):1242–1243, 1995 7625490

Sackeim HA, Stern Y: The neuropsychiatry of memory and amnesia, in The American Psychiatric Press Textbook of Neuropsychiatry, 3rd Edition. Edited by Yudofsky SC, Hales RE. Washington, DC, American Psychiatric Press, 1997, pp 501–518

Sackeim HA, Decina P, Prohovnik I, et al: Anticonvulsant and antidepressant properties of electroconvulsive therapy: a proposed mechanism of action. Biol Psychiatry 18(11):1301–1310, 1983 6317065

Sackeim HA, Portnoy S, Neeley P, et al: Cognitive consequences of low-dosage electroconvulsive therapy. Ann N Y Acad Sci 462:326–340, 1986 3458413

Sackeim HA, Decina P, Kanzler M, et al: Effects of electrode placement on the efficacy of titrated, low-dose ECT. Am J Psychiatry 144(11):1449–1455, 1987a 3314538

Sackeim HA, Decina P, Portnoy S, et al: Studies of dosage, seizure threshold, and seizure duration in ECT. Biol Psychiatry 22(3):249–268, 1987b 3814678

Sackeim HA, Decina P, Prohovnik I, et al: Seizure threshold in electroconvulsive therapy: effects of sex, age, electrode placement, and number of treatments. Arch Gen Psychiatry 44(4):355–360, 1987c 3566457

Sackeim HA, Ross FR, Hopkins N, et al: Subjective side effects acutely following ECT: associations with treatment modality and clinical response. Convuls Ther 3(2):100–110, 1987d 11940903

Sackeim HA, Prudic J, Devanand DP, et al: The impact of medication resistance and continuation pharmacotherapy on relapse following response to electroconvulsive therapy in major depression. J Clin Psychopharmacol 10(2):96–104, 1990 2341598

Sackeim HA, Devanand DP, Prudic J: Stimulus intensity, seizure threshold, and seizure duration: impact on the efficacy and safety of electroconvulsive therapy. Psychiatr Clin North Am 14(4):803–843, 1991 1771150

Sackeim HA, Nobler MS, Prudic J, et al: Acute effects of electroconvulsive therapy on hemispatial neglect. Neuropsychiatry Neuropsychol Behav Neurol 5:151–160, 1992

Sackeim HA, Prudic J, Devanand DP, et al: Effects of stimulus intensity and electrode placement on the efficacy and cognitive effects of electroconvulsive therapy. N Engl J Med 328(12):839–846, 1993 8441428

Sackeim HA, Long J, Luber B, et al: Physical properties and quantification of the ECT stimulus: I. Basic principles. Convuls Ther 10(2):93–123, 1994 8069647

Sackeim HA, Prudic J, Devanand DP, et al: A prospective, randomized, double-blind comparison of bilateral and right unilateral ECT at different stimulus intensities. Arch Gen Psychiatry 57:425–434, 2000 10807482

Sackeim HA, Haskett RF, Mulsant BH, et al: Continuation pharmacotherapy in the prevention of relapse following electroconvulsive therapy: a randomized controlled trial. JAMA 285(10):1299–1307, 2001a 11255384

Sackeim HA, Keilp JG, Rush AJ, et al: The effects of vagus nerve stimulation on cognitive performance in patients with treatment-resistant depression. Neuropsychiatry Neuropsychol Behav Neurol 14(1):53–62, 2001b 11234909

Sackeim HA, Rush AJ, George MS, et al: Vagus nerve stimulation (VNS) for treatment-resistant depression: efficacy, side effects, and predictors of outcome. Neuropsychopharmacology 25(5):713–728, 2001c 11682255

Sackeim HA, Prudic J, Fuller R, et al: The cognitive effects of electroconvulsive therapy in community settings. Neuropsychopharmacology 32(1):244–254, 2007 16936712

Sackeim HA, Prudic J, Nobler MS, et al: Effects of pulse width and electrode placement on the efficacy and cognitive effects of electroconvulsive therapy. Brain Stimul 1(2):71–83, 2008 19756236

Sackeim HA, Dillingham EM, Prudic J, et al: Effect of concomitant pharmacotherapy on electroconvulsive therapy outcomes: short-term efficacy and adverse effects. Arch Gen Psychiatry 66(7):729–737, 2009 19581564

Sackeim HA, Prudic J, Devanand DP, et al: The benefits and costs of changing treatment technique in electroconvulsive therapy due to insufficient improvement of a major depressive episode. Brain Stimul 13(5):1284–1295, 2020 32585354

Sadananda SK, Narayanaswamy JC, Srinivasaraju R, et al: Delirium during the course of electroconvulsive therapy in a patient on lithium carbonate treatment. Gen Hosp Psychiatry 35(6):e678e–129535:678 e671–672, 2013

Saffer BY, Lanting SC, Koehle MS, et al: Assessing cognitive impairment using PROMIS® applied cognition-abilities scales in a medical outpatient sample. Psychiatry Res 226(1):169–172, 2015 25639374

Saffer S, Berk M: Anesthetic induction for ECT with etomidate is associated with longer seizure duration than thiopentone. J ECT 14(2):89–93, 1998 9641804

Safferman AZ, Munne R: Combining clozapine with ECT. Convuls Ther 8(2):141–143, 1992 11941161

Sahlem GL, McCall WV, Short EB, et al: A two-site, open-label, non-randomized trial comparing Focal Electrically-Administered Seizure Therapy (FEAST) and right unilateral ultrabrief pulse electroconvulsive therapy (RUL-UBP ECT). Brain Stimul 13(5):1416–1425, 2020 32735987

Saito N, Shioda K, Nisijima K, et al: Second case report of successful electroconvulsive therapy for a patient with schizophrenia and severe hemophilia A. Neuropsychiatr Dis Treat 10:865–867, 2014 24876778

Saito S: Anesthesia management for electroconvulsive therapy: hemodynamic and respiratory management. J Anesth 19(2):142–149, 2005 15875132

Saito S, Miyoshi S, Yoshikawa D, et al: Regional cerebral oxygen saturation during electroconvulsive therapy: monitoring by near-infrared spectrophotometry. Anesth Analg 83(4):726–730, 1996 8831310

Saito T, Saito R, Suwa H, et al: Differences in the treatment response to antithyroid drugs versus electroconvulsive therapy in a case of recurrent catatonia due to Graves' disease. Case Rep Psychiatry 2012:868490, 2012 22937417

Sajatovic M, Meltzer HY: The effect of short-term electroconvulsive treatment plus neuroleptics in treatment-resistant schizophrenia and schizoaffective disorder. Convuls Ther 9(3):167–175, 1993 11941209

Salaris S, Szuba MP, Traber K: ECT and intracranial vascular masses. J ECT 16(2):198–203, 2000 10868330

Saltychev M, Katajapuu N, Bärlund E, et al: Psychometric properties of 12-item self-administered World Health Organization disability assessment schedule 2.0 (WHODAS 2.0) among general population and people with nonacute physical causes of disability: systematic review. Disabil Rehabil 43(6):789–794, 2021 31335215

Salzman C: ECT and ethical psychiatry. Am J Psychiatry 134(9):1006–1009, 1977 900283

Salzman C, Schneider L, Alexopoulos G: Pharmacological treatment of depression in late life, in Psychopharmacology: Fourth Generation of Progress. Edited by Bloom F, Kupfer D. New York, Raven, 1995, pp 1471–1477

Sanghani SN, Petrides G, Kellner CH: Electroconvulsive therapy (ECT) in schizophrenia: a review of recent literature. Curr Opin Psychiatry 31(3):213–222, 2018 29528902

San-Juan D, Dávila-Rodríguez DO, Jiménez CR, et al: Neuromodulation techniques for status epilepticus: a review. Brain Stimul 12(4):835–844, 2019 31053521

Santor DA, Gregus M, Welch A: Eight decades of measurement in depression. Measurement 4:135–155, 2006

Sargant W, Slater E: An Introduction to Physical Methods of Treatment in Psychiatry. Baltimore, MD, Williams & Wilkins, 1954

Sargent N, Allen RM: Long-term management of schizophrenia with maintenance rTMS: a case report. J ECT 39(3):e11–e12, 2023 37145920

Sargent P, Reeves J: Pulmonary edema after electroconvulsive therapy. J ECT 24(4):283–285, 2008 18617864

Saricicek V, Sahin L, Bulbul F, et al: Does rocuronium-sugammadex reduce myalgia and headache after electroconvulsive therapy in patients with major depression? J ECT 30(1):30–34, 2014 23812022

Sarkar P, Andrade C, Kapur B, et al: An exploratory evaluation of ECT in haloperidol-treated DSM-IIIR schizophreniform disorder. Convuls Ther 10(4):271–278, 1994 7850397

Sarkis RA, Coffey MJ, Cooper JJ, et al: Anti-N-methyl-D-aspartate receptor encephalitis: a review of psychiatric phenotypes and management considerations: a report of the American Neuropsychiatric Association Committee on Research. J Neuropsychiatry Clin Neurosci 31(2):137–142, 2019 30561283

Sartorius A, Wolf J, Henn FA: Lithium and ECT: concurrent use still demands attention: three case reports. World J Biol Psychiatry 6(2):121–124, 2005 16156485

Saucedo CL, Courtois EC, Wade ZS, et al: Transcranial laser stimulation: mitochondrial and cerebrovascular effects in younger and older healthy adults. Brain Stimul 14(2):440–449, 2021 33636401

Sawayama E, Takahashi M, Inoue A, et al: Moderate hyperventilation prolongs electroencephalogram seizure duration of the first electroconvulsive therapy. J ECT 24(3):195–198, 2008 18772703

Scangos KW, Makhoul GS, Sugrue LP, et al: State-dependent responses to intracranial brain stimulation in a patient with depression. Nat Med 27(2):229–231, 2021 33462446

Schaerf FW, Miller RR, Lipsey JR, et al: ECT for major depression in four patients infected with human immunodeficiency virus. Am J Psychiatry 146(6):782–784, 1989 2729429

Schak KM, Mueller PS, Barnes RD, et al: The safety of ECT in patients with chronic obstructive pulmonary disease. Psychosomatics 49(3):208–211, 2008 18448774

Scheiner NS, Smith AK, Wohlleber M, et al: COVID-19 and catatonia: a case series and systematic review of existing literature. J Acad Consult Liaison Psychiatry 62(6):645–656, 2021 33992595

Schneegans H, Stetefeld H, Dohmen C, et al: Successful treatment of superrefractory status epilepticus with high-intensity electroconvulsive therapy: a case report and review of the current literature. J Epilepsy Res 9(1):76–82, 2019 31482059

Schnur DB, Mukherjee S, Silver J, et al: Electroconvulsive therapy in the treatment of episodic aggressive dyscontrol in psychotic patients. Convuls Ther 5(4):353–361, 1989 11941035

Schnur DB, Mukherjee S, Sackeim HA, et al: Symptomatic predictors of ECT response in medication-nonresponsive manic patients. J Clin Psychiatry 53(2):63–66, 1992 1347293

Schooler NR: Precursors to the PANSS: the BPRS and its progenitors. Innov Clin Neurosci 14(11-12):10–11, 2017 29410931

Schwarz T, Loewenstein J, Isenberg KE: Maintenance ECT: indications and outcome. Convuls Ther 11(1):14–23, 1995 7796063

Scott AI, Riddle W: Status epilepticus after electroconvulsive therapy. Br J Psychiatry 155:119–121, 1989 2605416

Scott AI, Weeks DJ, McDonald CF: Continuation electroconvulsive therapy: preliminary guidelines and an illustrative case report. Br J Psychiatry 159:867–870, 1991 1790461

Scott AI, Rodger CR, Stocks RH, et al: Is old-fashioned electroconvulsive therapy more efficacious? A randomised comparative study of bilateral brief-pulse and bilateral sine-wave treatments. Br J Psychiatry 160:360–364, 1992 1562862

Scott G, Semple DM: Survey of core trainees' confidence in electroconvulsive therapy. J ECT 34(2):113–116, 2018 29424757

Seager CP, Bird RL: Imipramine with electrical treatment in depression: a controlled trial. J Ment Sci 108:704–707, 1962 13987497

Sedgwick JV, Lewis IH, Linter SP: Anesthesia and mental illness. Int J Psychiatry Med 20(3):209–225, 1990 2265884

Segman RH, Shapira B, Gorfine M, et al: Onset and time course of antidepressant action: psychopharmacological implications of a controlled trial of electroconvulsive therapy. Psychopharmacology (Berl) 119(4):440–448, 1995 7480524

Sekimoto Y, Suzuki Y, Kanamori K, et al: A case of negative-pressure pulmonary oedema after first-time electroconvulsive therapy. Respirol Case Rep 10(6):e0956, 2022 35582342

Selvadurai C, Farahmand P, Jain N, et al: New onset seizure disorder following electroconvulsive therapy. Conn Med 80(8):479–481, 2016 29782784

Semkovska M, McLoughlin DM: Objective cognitive performance associated with electroconvulsive therapy for depression: a systematic review and meta-analysis. Biol Psychiatry 68(6):568–577, 2010 20673880

Semkovska M, McLoughlin DM: Measuring retrograde autobiographical amnesia following electroconvulsive therapy: historical perspective and current issues. J ECT 29(2):127–133, 2013 23303426

Semkovska M, McLoughlin DM: Retrograde autobiographical amnesia after electroconvulsive therapy: on the difficulty of finding the baby and clearing murky bathwater. J ECT 30(3):187–188, discussion 189–190, 2014 24755723

Semkovska M, Keane D, Babalola O, et al: Unilateral brief-pulse electroconvulsive therapy and cognition: effects of electrode placement, stimulus dosage and time. J Psychiatr Res 45(6):770–780, 2011 21109254

Semkovska M, Noone M, Carton M, et al: Measuring consistency of autobiographical memory recall in depression. Psychiatry Res 197(1–2):41–48, 2012 22397910

Semkovska M, Landau S, Dunne R, et al: Bitemporal versus high-dose unilateral twice-weekly electroconvulsive therapy for depression (EFFECT-Dep): a pragmatic, randomized, non-inferiority trial. Am J Psychiatry 173(4):408–417, 2016 26892939

Semkovska M, Knittle H, Leahy J, et al: Subjective cognitive complaints and subjective cognition following electroconvulsive therapy for depression: a systematic review and meta-analysis. Aust N Z J Psychiatry 57(1):21–33, 2023 35362328

Serra-Blasco M, Torres IJ, Vicent-Gil M, et al: Discrepancy between objective and subjective cognition in major depressive disorder. Eur Neuropsychopharmacol 29(1):46–56, 2019 30503099

Serra-Mestres J, Villagrasa-Blasco B, Thacker V, et al: Catatonia in N-methyl-D-aspartate receptor antibody encephalitis: phenomenological characteristics from a systematic review of case reports. Gen Hosp Psychiatry 64:9–16, 2020 32070914

Shafer A: Meta-analysis of the brief psychiatric rating scale factor structure. Psychol Assess 17(3):324–335, 2005 16262458

Shafer A, Dazzi F: Meta-analysis of the Positive and Negative Syndrome Scale (PANSS) factor structure. J Psychiatr Res 115:113–120, 2019 31128501

Shah N, Pande N, Bhat T, et al: Maintenance ECT as a therapeutic approach to medication-refractory epilepsy in an adult with mental retardation: case report and review of literature. J ECT 28(2):136–140, 2012 22531207

Shah RP, Alluri V, Sharma S: Treatment of agitation in Huntington's disease with electroconvulsive therapy. J Neuropsychiatry Clin Neurosci 29(3):293–294, 2017 28121260

Shanechi MM: Brain-machine interfaces from motor to mood. Nat Neurosci 22(10):1554–1564, 2019 31551595

Shapira B, Zohar J, Newman M, et al: Potentiation of seizure length and clinical response to electroconvulsive therapy by caffeine pretreatment: a case report. Convuls Ther 1(1):58–60, 1985 11940806

Shapira B, Lerer B, Gilboa D, et al: Facilitation of ECT by caffeine pretreatment. Am J Psychiatry 144(9):1199–1202, 1987 3631318

Shapira B, Kindler S, Lerer B: Medication outcome in ECT-resistant depression. Convuls Ther 4(3):192–198, 1988 11940964

Shapira B, Gorfine M, Lerer B: A prospective study of lithium continuation therapy in depressed patients who have responded to electroconvulsive therapy. Convuls Ther 11(2):80–85, 1995 7552058

Shapira B, Lidsky D, Gorfine M, et al: Electroconvulsive therapy and resistant depression: clinical implications of seizure threshold. J Clin Psychiatry 57(1):32–38, 1996 8543545

Shapira B, Tubi N, Drexler H, et al: Cost and benefit in the choice of ECT schedule: twice versus three times weekly ECT. Br J Psychiatry 172:44–48, 1998 9534831

Sharma A, Ramaswamy S, Bhatia SC: Electroconvulsive therapy after repair of cerebral aneurysm. J ECT 21(3):180–181, 2005 16127310

Sharma A, Chaturvedi R, Sharma A, et al: Electroconvulsive therapy in patients with vagus nerve stimulation. J ECT 25(2):141–143, 2009 18665100

Shaw IH, McKeith IG: Propofol and electroconvulsive therapy in a patient at risk from acute intermittent porphyria. Br J Anaesth 80(2):260–262, 1998 9602601

Shelef A, Mazeh D, Berger U, et al: Acute electroconvulsive therapy followed by maintenance electroconvulsive therapy decreases hospital re-admission rates of older patients with severe mental illness. J ECT 31(2):125–128, 2015 25373561

Shettar SM, Grunhaus L, Pande AC, et al: Protective effects of intramuscular glycopyrrolate on cardiac conduction during ECT. Convuls Ther 5(4):349–352, 1989 11941034

Shilton T, Enoch-Levy A, Giron Y, et al: A retrospective case series of electroconvulsive therapy in the management of comorbid depression and anorexia nervosa. Int J Eat Disord 53(2):210–218, 2020 31639233

Shin HW, O'Donovan CA, Boggs JG, et al: Successful ECT treatment for medically refractory nonconvulsive status epilepticus in pediatric patient. Seizure 20(5):433–436, 2011 21333551

Shiwach RS, Reid WH, Carmody TJ: An analysis of reported deaths following electroconvulsive therapy in Texas, 1993–1998. Psychiatr Serv 52(8):1095–1097, 2001 11474057

Shrestha S, Shrestha BR, Thapa C, et al: Comparative study of esmolol and labetalol to attenuate haemodynamic responses after electroconvulsive therapy. Kathmandu Univ Med J (KUMJ) 5(3):318–323, 2007 18604047

Shugar G, Schertzer S, Toner BB, et al: Development, use, and factor analysis of a self-report inventory for mania. Compr Psychiatry 33(5):325–331, 1992 1395552

Shulman KI, Fischer HD, Herrmann N, et al: Current prescription patterns and safety profile of irreversible monoamine oxidase inhibitors: a population-based cohort study of older adults. J Clin Psychiatry 70(12):1681–1686, 2009 19852903

Sienaert P, Peuskens J: Anticonvulsants during electroconvulsive therapy: review and recommendations. J ECT 23(2):120–123, 2007 17548985

Sienaert PA, Vanholst C: Electroconvulsive therapy after eye surgery. J ECT 29(2):139–141, 2013 23303425

Sienaert P, Dierick M, Degraeve G, et al: Electroconvulsive therapy in Belgium: a nationwide survey on the practice of electroconvulsive therapy. J Affect Disord 90(1):67–71, 2006 16337689

Sienaert P, Vansteelandt K, Demyttenaere K, et al: Randomized comparison of ultra-brief bifrontal and unilateral electroconvulsive therapy for major depression: clinical efficacy. J Affect Disord 116(1-2):106–112, 2009 19081638

Sienaert P, Vansteelandt K, Demyttenaere K, et al: Randomized comparison of ultra-brief bifrontal and unilateral electroconvulsive therapy for major depression: cognitive side-effects. J Affect Disord 122(1-2):60–67, 2010 19577808

Sienaert P, Roelens Y, Demunter H, et al: Concurrent use of lamotrigine and electroconvulsive therapy. J ECT 27(2):148–152, 2011a 20562637

Sienaert P, Rooseleer J, De Fruyt J: Measuring catatonia: a systematic review of rating scales. J Affect Disord 135(1-3):1–9, 2011b 21420736

Sienaert P, Dhossche DM, Vancampfort D, et al: A clinical review of the treatment of catatonia. Front Psychiatry 5:181, 2014 25538636

Sienaert P, Lambrichts S, Popleu L, et al: Electroconvulsive therapy during COVID-19-times: our patients cannot wait. Am J Geriatr Psychiatry 28(7):772–775, 2020 32345550

Sienaert P, Brus O, Lambrichts S, et al: Suicidal ideation and ECT, ECT and suicidal ideation: a register study. Acta Psychiatr Scand 146(1):74–84, 2022 35279825

Sikdar S, Kulhara P, Avasthi A, et al: Combined chlorpromazine and electroconvulsive therapy in mania. Br J Psychiatry 164(6):806–810, 1994 7952988

Silberstein SD, Mechtler LL, Kudrow DB, et al: Non-invasive vagus nerve stimulation for the ACute Treatment of cluster headache: findings from the randomized, double-blind, sham-controlled ACT1 study. Headache 56(8):1317–1332, 2016 27593728

Simon JS, Evans D: Pheochromocytoma, depression, and electroconvulsive therapy. Convuls Ther 2(4):296–298, 1986 11940881

Simpson KH, Smith RJ, Davies LF: Comparison of the effects of atropine and glycopyrrolate on cognitive function following general anaesthesia. Br J Anaesth 59(8):966–969, 1987 3651279

Sinclair DJM, Zhao S, Qi F, et al: Electroconvulsive therapy for treatment-resistant schizophrenia. Schizophr Bull 45(4):730–732, 2019 31150556

Singh G, Wahi S: Pulmonary embolism in the ECT patient: a case report and discussion. Gen Hosp Psychiatry 30(1):87–89, 2008 18164948

Singh MM, Kay SR: A comparative study of haloperidol and chlorpromazine in terms of clinical effects and therapeutic reversal with benztropine in schizophrenia: theoretical implications for potency differences among neuroleptics. Psychopharmacology (Berl) 43(2):103–113, 1975 1103205

Singh PM, Arora S, Borle A, et al: Evaluation of etomidate for seizure duration in electroconvulsive therapy: a systematic review and meta-analysis. J ECT 31(4):213–225, 2015 25634566

Singla L, Shah M, Moore-Hill D, et al: Electroconvulsive therapy for super refractory status epilepticus in pregnancy: case report and review of literature. Int J Neurosci 133(10):1109–1119, 2022 35287528

Sinha P, Goyal P, Andrade C: A meta-review of the safety of electroconvulsive therapy in pregnancy. J ECT 33(2):81–88, 2017 28009621

Sivan AB: Benton Visual Retention Test, 5th Edition. San Antonio, TX, Psychological Corporation, 1992

Sjonnesen K, Bulloch AG, Williams J, et al: Characterization of disability in Canadians with mental disorders using an abbreviated version of a DSM-5 emerging measure: the 12-item WHO Disability Assessment Schedule (WHODAS) 2.0. Can J Psychiatry 61(4):227–235, 2016 27254415

Small JG, Kellams JJ, Milstein V, et al: Complications with electroconvulsive treatment combined with lithium. Biol Psychiatry 15(1):103–112, 1980 7357049

Small JG, Klapper MH, Kellams JJ, et al: Electroconvulsive treatment compared with lithium in the management of manic states. Arch Gen Psychiatry 45(8):727–732, 1988 2899425

Small JG, Milstein V: Lithium interactions: lithium and electroconvulsive therapy. J Clin Psychopharmacol 10(5):346–350, 1990 2258451

Smesny S, Volz HP, Liepert J, et al: Repetitive transcranial magnetic stimulation (rTMS) in the acute and long-term therapy of refractory depression—a case report [in German]. Nervenarzt 72(9):734–738, 2001 11572108

Smetana GW: Preoperative pulmonary evaluation. N Engl J Med 340(12):937–944, 1999 10089188

Smilowitz NR, Berger JS: Perioperative cardiovascular risk assessment and management for noncardiac surgery: a review. JAMA 324(3):279–290, 2020 32692391

Smith DL, Angst MS, Brock-Utne JG, et al: Seizure duration with remifentanil/methohexital vs. methohexital alone in middle-aged patients undergoing electroconvulsive therapy. Acta Anaesthesiol Scand 47(9):1064–1066, 2003 12969096

Smith GE, Rasmussen KG Jr, Cullum CM, et al: A randomized controlled trial comparing the memory effects of continuation electroconvulsive therapy versus continuation pharmacotherapy: results from the Consortium for Research in ECT (CORE) study. J Clin Psychiatry 71(2):185–193, 2010 20193646

Smith LH, Hastings DW, Hughes J: Immediate and follow up results of electroshock therapy. Am J Psychiatry 99:351–354, 1943

Sobin C, Sackeim HA, Prudic J, et al: Predictors of retrograde amnesia following ECT. Am J Psychiatry 152(7):995–1001, 1995 7793470

Sobin C, Prudic J, Devanand DP, et al: Who responds to electroconvulsive therapy? A comparison of effective and ineffective forms of treatment. Br J Psychiatry 169(3):322–328, 1996 8879718

Society for Obstetric Anesthesia and Perinatology: Statement on Sugammadex During Pregnancy and Lactation. April 22, 2019. Available at: www.soap.org/assets/docs/SOAP_Statement_Sugammadex_During_Pregnancy_Lactation_APPROVED.pdf. Accessed January 22, 2021.

Soda T, McLoughlin DM, Clark SR, et al: International Consortium on the Genetics of Electroconvulsive Therapy and Severe Depressive Disorders (Gen-ECT-ic). Eur Arch Psychiatry Clin Neurosci 270(7):921–932, 2020 31802253

Sommer BR, Satlin A, Friedman L, et al: Glycopyrrolate versus atropine in post-ECT amnesia in the elderly. J Geriatr Psychiatry Neurol 2(1):18–21, 1989 2663013

Song J, Lee PP, Weiner R, Challa P: The effect of surgery on intraocular pressure fluctuations with electroconvulsive therapy in a patient with severe glaucoma. J ECT 20(4):264–266, 2004 15591863

Spaans H-P, Verwijk E, Comijs HC, et al: Efficacy and cognitive side effects after brief pulse and ultrabrief pulse right unilateral electroconvulsive therapy for major depression: a randomized, double-blind, controlled study. J Clin Psychiatry 74(11):e1029–e1036, 2013 24330903

Spashett R, Fernie G, Reid IC, et al: MADRS symptom subtypes in ECT-treated depressed patients: relationship to response and subsequent ECT. J ECT 30(3):227–231, 2014 24831998

Spellman T, Peterchev AV, Lisanby SH: Focal electrically administered seizure therapy: a novel form of ECT illustrates the roles of current directionality, polarity, and electrode configuration in seizure induction. Neuropsychopharmacology 34(8):2002–2010, 2009 19225453

Spielberger CD, Gorsuch RL, Lushene RE: STAI: Manual for the State-Trait Anxiety Inventory. Palo Alto, CA, Consulting Psychologists Press, 1970

Spielberger CD, Gorsuch RL, Lushene RE, et al: Manual for the State-Trait Anxiety Inventory STAI (Form Y). Palo Alto, CA, Consulting Psychologists Press, 1983

Spiker DG, Weiss JC, Dealy RS, et al: The pharmacological treatment of delusional depression. Am J Psychiatry 142(4):430–436, 1985 3883815

Spitzer RL, Kroenke K, Williams JBW, et al: A brief measure for assessing generalized anxiety disorder: the GAD-7. Arch Intern Med 166(10):1092–1097, 2006 16717171

Sprung J, Distel D, Grass J, et al: Cardiovascular collapse during anesthesia in a patient with preoperatively discontinued chronic MAO inhibitor therapy. J Clin Anesth 8(8):662–665, 1996 8982896

Squire LR: Memory functions as affected by electroconvulsive therapy. Ann N Y Acad Sci 462:307–314, 1986 3458411

Squire LR, Chace PM: Memory functions six to nine months after electroconvulsive therapy. Arch Gen Psychiatry 32(12):1557–1564, 1975 1200774

Squire LR, Slater PC: Electroconvulsive therapy and complaints of memory dysfunction: a prospective three-year follow-up study. Br J Psychiatry 142:1–8, 1983 6831121

Squire LR, Zouzounis JA: Self-ratings of memory dysfunction: different findings in depression and amnesia. J Clin Exp Neuropsychol 10(6):727–738, 1988 3235647

Squire LR, Wetzel CD, Slater PC: Memory complaint after electroconvulsive therapy: assessment with a new self-rating instrument. Biol Psychiatry 14(5):791–801, 1979 497304

Stack CG, Abernethy MH, Thacker M: Atracurium for ECT in plasma cholinesterase deficiency. Br J Anaesth 60(2):244–245, 1988 3345286

Stadtland C, Erfurth A, Ruta U, et al: A switch from propofol to etomidate during an ECT course increases EEG and motor seizure duration. J ECT 18(1):22–25, 2002 11925517

Stallwood E, Monsour A, Rodrigues C, et al: Systematic review: the measurement properties of the Children's Depression Rating Scale-Revised in adolescents with major depressive disorder. J Am Acad Child Adolesc Psychiatry 60(1):119–133, 2021 33130251

Standish-Barry HM, Deacon V, Snaith RP: The relationship of concurrent benzodiazepine administration to seizure duration in ECT. Acta Psychiatr Scand 71(3):269–271, 1985 3984767

Stanley WJ, Fleming H: A clinical comparison of phenelzine and electro-convulsive therapy in the treatment of depressive illness. J Ment Sci 108:708–710, 1962 13983404

Stead M, Josephs KA: Successful treatment of status migrainosus after electroconvulsive therapy with dihydroergotamine. Headache 45(4):378–380, 2005 15836577

Steen K, Narang P, Lippmann S: Electroconvulsive therapy in multiple sclerosis. Innov Clin Neurosci 12(7-8):28–30, 2015 26351621

Steffens DC, Krystal AD, Sibert TE, et al: Cost effectiveness of maintenance ECT. Convuls Ther 11(4):283–284, 1995 8919583

Steffens DC, Conway CR, Dombeck CB, et al: Severity of subcortical gray matter hyperintensity predicts ECT response in geriatric depression. J ECT 17(1):45–49, 2001 11281515

Steif BL, Sackeim HA, Portnoy S, et al: Effects of depression and ECT on anterograde memory. Biol Psychiatry 21(10):921–930, 1986 3741909

Stein ALS, Sacks SM, Roth JR, et al: Anesthetic management during electroconvulsive therapy in children: a systematic review of the available literature. Anesth Analg 130(1):126–140, 2020 31425262

Stenmark L, Kellner CH, Landén M, et al: Electroconvulsive therapy and psychiatric readmission in major depressive disorder: a population-based register study. Acta Psychiatr Scand 144(6):599–625, 2021 34523119

Stephens SM, Pettinati HM, Greenberg RM, et al: Continuation and maintenance therapy with outpatient ECT, in The Clinical Science of Electroconvulsive Therapy. Edited by Coffey CE. Washington, DC, American Psychiatric Press, 1993, pp 143–164

Sterina E, Gregory N, Hermida AP: Acute and prophylactic management of postictal agitation in electroconvulsive therapy. J ECT 39(3):136–140, 2023 36215425

Sternberg DE, Jarvik ME: Memory functions in depression. Arch Gen Psychiatry 33(2):219–224, 1976 1252098

Sternhell PS, Corr MJ: Psychiatric morbidity and adherence to antiretroviral medication in patients with HIV/AIDS. Aust N Z J Psychiatry 36(4):528–533, 2002 12169154

Stockings E, Degenhardt L, Lee YY, et al: Symptom screening scales for detecting major depressive disorder in children and adolescents: a systematic review and meta-analysis of reliability, validity and diagnostic utility. J Affect Disord 174:447–463, 2015 25553406

Stoudemire A, Hill CD, Dalton ST, et al: Rehospitalization rates in older depressed adults after antidepressant and electroconvulsive therapy treatment. J Am Geriatr Soc 42(12):1282–1285, 1994 7983293

Strain JJ, Bidder TG: Transient cerebral complication associated with multiple monitored electroconvulsive therapy. Dis Nerv Syst 32(2):95–100, 1971 5547041

Streckenbach SC, Benedetto WJ, Fitzsimons MG: Implantable cardioverter-defibrillator shock delivered during electroconvulsive therapy despite magnet application: a case report. A A Pract 14(11):e01284, 2020 32985853

Stripp TK, Jorgensen MB, Olsen NV: Anaesthesia for electroconvulsive therapy—new tricks for old drugs: a systematic review. Acta Neuropsychiatr 30(2):61–69, 2018 28462732

Strömgren LS: Unilateral versus bilateral electroconvulsive therapy: investigations into the therapeutic effect in endogenous depression. Acta Psychiatr Scand Suppl 240:8–65, 1973 4515575

Strömgren LS: Is bilateral ECT ever indicated? Acta Psychiatr Scand 69(6):484–490, 1984 6741598

Strömgren LS: ECT in acute delirium and related clinical states. Convuls Ther 13(1):10–17, 1997 9152583

Strömgren LS, Juul-Jensen P: EEG in unilateral and bilateral electroconvulsive therapy. Acta Psychiatr Scand 51(5):340–360, 1975 1096539

Strömgren LS, Dahl J, Fjeldborg N, et al: Factors influencing seizure duration and number of seizures applied in unilateral electroconvulsive therapy: anaesthetics and benzodiazepines. Acta Psychiatr Scand 62(2):158–165, 1980 6110313

Subsoontorn P, Lekprasert V, Waleeprakhon P, et al: Premedication with dexmedetomidine for prevention of hyperdynamic response after electroconvulsive therapy: a cross-over, randomized controlled trial. BMC Psychiatry 21(1):408, 2021 34404384

Sullivan CRP, Olsen S, Widge AS: Deep brain stimulation for psychiatric disorders: from focal brain targets to cognitive networks. Neuroimage 225:117515, 2021 33137473

Sundsted KK, Burton MC, Shah R, et al: Preanesthesia medical evaluation for electroconvulsive therapy: a review of the literature. J ECT 30(1):35–42, 2014 24091900

Suppes T, Webb A, Carmody T, et al: Is postictal electrical silence a predictor of response to electroconvulsive therapy? J Affect Disord 41(1):55–58, 1996 8938205

Suri R, Lin AS, Cohen LS, et al: Acute and long-term behavioral outcome of infants and children exposed in utero to either maternal depression or antidepressants: a review of the literature. J Clin Psychiatry 75(10):e1142–e1152, 2014 25373125

Suzuki K, Takamatsu K, Takano T, et al: Safety of electroconvulsive therapy in psychiatric patients shortly after the occurrence of pulmonary embolism. J ECT 24(4):286–288, 2008 18617865

Suzuki Y, Miyajima M, Ohta K, et al: Is prolongation of corrected QT interval associated with seizures induced by electroconvulsive therapy reduced by atropine sulfate? Pacing Clin Electrophysiol 40(11):1246–1253, 2017 28862317

Swan HD, Borshoff DC: Informed consent—recall of risk information following epidural analgesia in labour. Anaesth Intensive Care 22(2):139–141, 1994 8210014

Swartz CM: Propofol anesthesia in ECT. Convuls Ther 8(4):262–266, 1992 11941177

Swartz CM: Asymmetric bilateral right frontotemporal left frontal stimulus electrode placement for electroconvulsive therapy. Neuropsychobiology 29(4):174–178, 1994 8047243

Swartz CM, Larson G: ECT stimulus duration and its efficacy. Ann Clin Psychiatry 1:147–152, 1989

Swartz CM, Lewis RK: Theophylline reversal of electroconvulsive therapy (ECT) seizure inhibition. Psychosomatics 32(1):47–51, 1991 2003137

Swartz CM, Manly DT: Efficiency of the stimulus characteristics of ECT. Am J Psychiatry 157(9):1504–1506, 2000 10964870

Swartz CM, Saheba NC: Comparison of atropine with glycopyrrolate for use in ECT. Convuls Ther 5(1):56–60, 1989 11940995

Swartz CM, Acosta D, Bashir A: Diminished ECT response in catatonia due to chronic neurologic condition. J ECT 19(2):110–114, 2003 12792461

Swindells SR, Simpson KH: Oxygen saturation during electroconvulsive therapy. Br J Psychiatry 150:695–697, 1987 3651707

Taieb O, Flament MF, Corcos M, et al: Electroconvulsive therapy in adolescents with mood disorder: patients' and parents' attitudes. Psychiatry Res 104(2):183–190, 2001 11711171

Takada JY, Solimene MC, da Luz PL, et al: Assessment of the cardiovascular effects of electroconvulsive therapy in individuals older than 50 years. Braz J Med Biol Res 38(9):1349–1357, 2005 16138218

Takahashi T, Kinoshita K, Fuke T, et al: Acute neurogenic pulmonary edema following electroconvulsive therapy: a case report. Gen Hosp Psychiatry 34(6):703.e9–703.e11, 2012 22516213

Takala CR, Leung JG, Murphy LL, et al: Concurrent electroconvulsive therapy and bupropion treatment. J ECT 33(3):185–189, 2017 28570500

Takamiya A, Seki M, Kudo S, et al: Electroconvulsive therapy for Parkinson's disease: a systematic review and meta-analysis. Mov Disord 36(1):50–58, 2021 33280168

Tan HJ, Tee TY, Husin M, et al: A case series of super-refractory status epilepticus successfully treated with electroconvulsive therapy. Epileptic Disord 22(6):828–833, 2020 33337333

Tang YL, Jiang W, Ren YP, et al: Electroconvulsive therapy in China: clinical practice and research on efficacy. J ECT 28(4):206–212, 2012 22801297

Tanguturi YC, Cundiff AW, Fuchs C: Anti-N-methyl-D-aspartate receptor encephalitis and electroconvulsive therapy: literature review and future directions. Child Adolesc Psychiatr Clin N Am 28(1):79–89, 2019 30389078

Taub S: Electroconvulsive therapy, malpractice, and informed consent. J Psychiatry Law 15(1):7–54, 1987 11659244

Taye T, Dobranici L, Fisher M, Cullum S: Use of ECT in the presence of acute bilateral posterior vitreous detachment. Australas Psychiatry 26(2):193–195, 2018 29334228

Taylor MA, Fink M: Catatonia in psychiatric classification: a home of its own. Am J Psychiatry 160(7):1233–1241, 2003 12832234

Taylor P, Fleminger JJ: ECT for schizophrenia. Lancet 1(8183):1380–1382, 1980 6104172

Taylor RW, Marwood L, Oprea E, et al: Pharmacological augmentation in unipolar depression: a guide to the guidelines. Int J Neuropsychopharmacol 23(9):587–625, 2020 32402075

Temple RO, Carvalho J, Tremont G: A national survey of physicians' use of and satisfaction with neuropsychological services. Arch Clin Neuropsychol 21(5):371–382, 2006 16844340

Ten Doesschate F, van Wingen GA, de Pont BJHB, et al: The longitudinal effects of electroconvulsive therapy on ictal interhemispheric coherence and its associations with treatment outcome: a naturalistic cohort study. Clin EEG Neurosci 50(1):44–50, 2019 29929395

Tenenbaum J: ECT regulation reconsidered. Medical Disability Law Reporter 7(2):148–159, 211, 1983

Teodorczuk A, Emmerson B, Robinson G: Revisiting the role of electroconvulsive therapy in schizophrenia: where are we now? Australas Psychiatry 27(5):477–479, 2019 31287328

Teraishi T, Nakatake M, Hirano J, et al: Electroconvulsive therapy and meningioma: a brief review. Nihon Shinkei Seishin Yakurigaku Zasshi 32(2):57–61, 2012 22708257

Tess AV, Smetana GW: Medical evaluation of patients undergoing electroconvulsive therapy. N Engl J Med 360(14):1437–1444, 2009 19339723

Tew JD Jr, Mulsant BH, Haskett RF, et al: Acute efficacy of ECT in the treatment of major depression in the old-old. Am J Psychiatry 156(12):1865–1870, 1999 10588398

Tew JD Jr, Mulsant BH, Haskett RF, et al: Relapse during continuation pharmacotherapy after acute response to ECT: a comparison of usual care versus protocolized treatment. Ann Clin Psychiatry 19(1):1–4, 2007 17453654

Tezuka N, Egawa H, Fukagawa D, et al: Assessment of QT interval and QT dispersion during electroconvulsive therapy using computerized measurements. J ECT 26(1):41–46, 2010 20190602

Tharyan P, Adams CE: Electroconvulsive therapy for schizophrenia. Cochrane Database Syst Rev (2):CD000076, 2005 15846598

Therrien Z, Hunsley J: Assessment of anxiety in older adults: a systematic review of commonly used measures. Aging Ment Health 16(1):1–16, 2012 21838650

Thienhaus OJ, Margletta S, Bennett JA: A study of the clinical efficacy of maintenance ECT. J Clin Psychiatry 51(4):141–144, 1990 2324077

Thiery M; Medical Research Council: Clinical trial of the treatment of depressive illness: report to the Medical Research Council by its Clinical Psychiatry Committee. BMJ 1(5439):881–886, 1965 14257398

Thirthalli J, Rakesh G, Gangadhar BN: Antiepileptic drugs–ECT combination: need for systematic studies. World J Biol Psychiatry 11(7):919–920, 2010 20726826

Thirthalli J, Harish T, Gangadhar BN: A prospective comparative study of interaction between lithium and modified electroconvulsive therapy. World J Biol Psychiatry 12(2):149–155, 2011 20645670

Thiruvenkatarajan V, Dharmalingam A, Armstrong-Brown A, et al: Uninterrupted anesthesia support and technique adaptations for patients presenting for electroconvulsive therapy during the COVID-19 era. J ECT 36(3):156–157, 2020 32511113

Thomas SJ, Shin M, McInnis MG, et al: Combination therapy with monoamine oxidase inhibitors and other antidepressants or stimulants: strategies for the management of treatment-resistant depression. Pharmacotherapy 35(4):433–449, 2015 25884531

Thompson D, Hylan TR, McMullen W, et al: Predictors of a medical-offset effect among patients receiving antidepressant therapy. Am J Psychiatry 155(6):824–827, 1998 9619157

Thornton JE, Mulsant BH, Dealy R, et al: A retrospective study of maintenance electroconvulsive therapy in a university-based psychiatric practice. Convuls Ther 6(2):121–129, 1990 11941053

Thukral-Mahajan P, Shah N, Kalra G, et al: Electroconvulsive therapy for medication-refractory depression in a patient with ruptured intracranial dermoid cyst, meningioma, and neurofibromatosis. Indian J Psychiatry 59(4):493–495, 2017 29497194

Tielkes CE, Comijs HC, Verwijk E, et al: The effects of ECT on cognitive functioning in the elderly: a review. Int J Geriatr Psychiatry 23(8):789–795, 2008 18311845

Tiller JW, Ingram N: Seizure threshold determination for electroconvulsive therapy: stimulus dose titration versus age-based estimations. Aust N Z J Psychiatry 40(2):188–192, 2006 16476138

Títoff V, Moury HN, Títoff IB, et al: Seizures, antiepileptic drugs, and CKD. Am J Kidney Dis 73(1):90–101, 2019 29784616

Tomimatsu T, Kakigano A, Mimura K, et al: Maternal carbon dioxide level during labor and its possible effect on fetal cerebral oxygenation: mini review. J Obstet Gynaecol Res 39(1):1–6, 2013 22765270

Toprak HI, Gedik E, Begeç Z, et al: Sevoflurane as an alternative anaesthetic for electroconvulsive therapy. J ECT 21(2):108–110, 2005 15905753

Tor PC, Bautovich A, Wang MJ, et al: A systematic review and meta-analysis of brief versus ultrabrief right unilateral electroconvulsive therapy for depression. J Clin Psychiatry 76(9):e1092–e1098, 2015 26213985

Tor PC, Tan XW, Martin D, et al: Comparative outcomes in electroconvulsive therapy (ECT): a naturalistic comparison between outcomes in psychosis, mania, depression, psychotic depression and catatonia. Eur Neuropsychopharmacol 51:43–54, 2021 34034099

Tornhamre E, Ekman CJ, Hammar Å, et al: The effect of pulse width on subjective memory impairment and remission rate 6 months after electroconvulsive therapy. J ECT 36(4):272–278, 2020 32453190

Torrico T, Kiong T, D'Assumpcao C, et al: Postinfectious COVID-19 catatonia: a report of two cases. Front Psychiatry 12:696347, 2021 34381391

Tørring N, Sanghani SN, Petrides G, et al: The mortality rate of electroconvulsive therapy: a systematic review and pooled analysis. Acta Psychiatr Scand 135(5):388–397, 2017 28332236

Trakada G, Velentza L, Konsta A, et al: Complications of anesthesia during electroconvulsive therapy due to undiagnosed obstructive sleep apnea: a casestudy. Respir Med Case Rep 20:145–149, 2017 28224078

Triplett P, Gerstenblith A, Reti IM, et al: Treatment of catatonic symptoms in a patient with autism spectrum disorder and Addison disease: a case report. J ECT 36(2):e10–e12, 2020 32108665

Tripodi B, Barbuti M, Novi M, et al: Clinical features and predictors of non-response in severe catatonic patients treated with electroconvulsive therapy. Int J Psychiatry Clin Pract 25(3):299–306, 2021 34382488

Trivedi C, Motiwala F, Mainali P, et al: Trends for electroconvulsive therapy utilization in children and adolescents in the United States from 2002 to 2017: a nationwide inpatient sample analysis. J ECT 37(2):100–106, 2021 33625175

Trivedi MH, Rush AJ, Wisniewski SR, et al: Evaluation of outcomes with citalopram for depression using measurement-based care in STAR*D: implications for clinical practice. Am J Psychiatry 163(1):28–40, 2006 16390886

Trollor JN, Sachdev PS: Electroconvulsive treatment of neuroleptic malignant syndrome: a review and report of cases. Aust N Z J Psychiatry 33(5):650–659, 1999 10544988

Trzepacz PT, Weniger FC, Greenhouse J: Etomidate anesthesia increases seizure duration during ECT: a retrospective study. Gen Hosp Psychiatry 15(2):115–120, 1993 8472938

Tsai J, Huang M, Rosenheck RA, et al: A randomized controlled trial of video psychoeducation for electroconvulsive therapy in the United States. Psychiatr Serv 71(6):562–569, 2020 32151214

Tsao C, Nusbaum A: Successful ECT course for catatonia after large pulmonary embolus and placement of inferior vena cava filter. Gen Hosp Psychiatry 29(4):374, 2007 17591515

Tsuang MT, Dempsey GM, Fleming JA: Can ECT prevent premature death and suicide in "schizoaffective" patients? J Affect Disord 1(3):167–171, 1979 162499

Tsujii T, Uchida T, Suzuki T, et al: Factors associated with delirium following electroconvulsive therapy: a systematic review. J ECT 35(4):279–287, 2019 31764452

Tubi N, Calev A, Higal D, et al: Subjective symptoms in depression and during the course of electroconvulsive therapy. Neuropsychiatry Neuropsychol Behav Neurol 6:187–192, 1993

Turner AD, Furey ML, Drevets WC, et al: Association between subcortical volumes and verbal memory in unmedicated depressed patients and healthy controls. Neuropsychologia 50(9):2348–2355, 2012 22714007

Tzabazis A, Schmitt HJ, Ihmsen H, et al: Postictal agitation after electroconvulsive therapy: incidence, severity, and propofol as a treatment option. J ECT 29(3):189–195, 2013 23792779

Uçok A, Uçok G: Maintenance ECT in a patient with catatonic schizophrenia and tardive dyskinesia. Convuls Ther 12(2):108–112, 1996 8744171

Ueda S, Koyama K, Okubo Y: Marked improvement of psychotic symptoms after electroconvulsive therapy in Parkinson disease. J ECT 26(2):111–115, 2010 20386461

Ujkaj M, Davidoff DA, Seiner SJ, et al: Safety and efficacy of electroconvulsive therapy for the treatment of agitation and aggression in patients with dementia. Am J Geriatr Psychiatry 20(1):61–72, 2012 22143072

Ukpong DI, Makanjuola RO, Morakinyo O: A controlled trial of modified electroconvulsive therapy in schizophrenia in a Nigerian teaching hospital. West Afr J Med 21(3):237–240, 2002 12744577

Ulett GA, Gleser GC, Caldwell BM, et al: The use of matched groups in the evaluation of convulsive and subconvulsive photoshock. Bull Menninger Clin 18(4):138–146, 1954 13160697

Ulett GA, Smith K, Gleser GC: Evaluation of convulsive and subconvulsive shock therapies utilizing a control group. Am J Psychiatry 112(10):795–802, 1956 13302483

Ulrich S, Ricken R, Adli M: Tranylcypromine in mind (part I): review of pharmacology. Eur Neuropsychopharmacol 27(8):697–713, 2017 28655495

Unal A, Bulbul F, Alpak G, et al: Effective treatment of catatonia by combination of benzodiazepine and electroconvulsive therapy. J ECT 29(3):206–209, 2013 23965606

Unal A, Altindag A, Demir B, et al: The use of lorazepam and electroconvulsive therapy in the treatment of catatonia: treatment characteristics and outcomes in 60 patients. J ECT 33(4):290–293, 2017 28640169

Unal G, Swami JK, Canela C, et al: Adaptive current-flow models of ECT: explaining individual static impedance, dynamic impedance, and brain current density. Brain Stimul 14(5):1154–1168, 2021 34332156

Ungvari GS, Caroff SN, Gerevich J: The catatonia conundrum: evidence of psychomotor phenomena as a symptom dimension in psychotic disorders. Schizophr Bull 36(2):231–238, 2010 19776208

U.S. Centers for Medicare and Medicaid Services: CMS Interoperability and Patient Access Final Rule. Available at: www.cms.gov/Regulations-and-Guidance/Guidance/Interoperability/index. Accessed October 11, 2020.

U.S. Centers for Medicare and Medicaid Services: Vagus Nerve Stimulation (VNS) for Treatment Resistant Depression (TRD). Available at: www.cms.gov/Medicare/Coverage/Coverage-with-Evidence-Development/VNS. Accessed June 25, 2022.

U.S. Department of Health and Human Services: Food and Drug Administration Reviewer Guidance Evaluating the Risks of Drug Exposure in Human Pregnancies. April 2005. Available at: www.fda.gov/media/71368/download. Accessed May 15, 2022.

U.S. Department of Health and Human Services: Summary of the HIPAA Security Rule. Office for Civil Rights, 2013. Available at: www.hhs.gov/hipaa/for-professionals/security/laws-regulations/index.html. Accessed October 11, 2020.

U.S. Food and Drug Administration: Neurological Devices; Reclassification of Electroconvulsive Therapy Devices Intended for Use in Treating Severe Major Depressive Episode in Patients 18 Years of Age and Older Who Are Treatment Resistant or Require a Rapid Response; Effective Date of Requirement for Premarket Approval for Electroconvulsive Therapy for Certain Specified Intended Uses. Federal Register 80 FR 81223, 2015. Available at: www.federalregister.gov/documents/2015/12/29/2015-32592/neurological-devices-reclassification-of-electroconvulsive-therapy-devices-intended-for-use-in. Accessed January 14, 2022.

U.S. Food and Drug Administration: FDA Drug Safety Communication: FDA Review Results in New Warnings About Using General Anesthetics and Sedation Drugs in Young Children and Pregnant Women. January 14, 2016. Available at: www.fda.gov/drugs/drug-safety-and-availability/fda-drug-safety-communication-fda-review-results-new-warnings-about-using-general-anesthetics-and. Accessed January 17, 2021.

U.S. Food and Drug Administration: FDA Drug Safety Communication: FDA Approves Label Changes for Use of General Anesthetic and Sedation Drugs in Young Children. April 17, 2017. Available at: www.fda.gov/drugs/drug-safety-and-availability/fda-drug-safety-communication-fda-approves-label-changes-use-general-anesthetic-and-sedation-drugs. Accessed January 17, 2021.

U.S. Food and Drug Administration: De Novo Classification Request for Monarch eTNS System. 2018a. Available at: www.accessdata.fda.gov/cdrh_docs/reviews/DEN180041.pdf. Accessed June 26, 2022.

U.S. Food and Drug Administration: Neurological devices; reclassification of electroconvulsive therapy devices; effective date of requirement for premarket approval for electroconvulsive therapy devices for certain specified intended uses. Fed Regist 83(246):66103–66124, 2018b 30596410

U.S. Food and Drug Administration: Benefits and Risks of Cochlear Implants. February 9, 2021. Available at: www.fda.gov/medical-devices/cochlear-implants/benefits-and-risks-cochlear-implants. Accessed May 12, 2022.

U.S. Food and Drug Administration: 510(k) Premarket Notification. K211856. June 6, 2022. Available at: www.accessdata.fda.gov/scripts/cdrh/cfdocs/cfpmn/pmn.cfm?ID=K211856. Accessed June 26, 2022.

U.S. Food and Drug Administration: Letter to Magnus Neuromodulation System (MNS) With SAINT Technology. 2023. Available at: www.accessdata.fda.gov/cdrh_docs/pdf22/K220177.pdf. Accessed July 16, 2023.

Usta Saglam NG, Aksoy Poyraz C, Yalcin M, et al: ECT augmentation of antipsychotics in severely ill schizophrenia: a naturalistic, observational study. Int J Psychiatry Clin Pract 24(4):392–397, 2020 32538214

Usui C, Hatta K, Doi N, et al: Improvements in both psychosis and motor signs in Parkinson's disease, and changes in regional cerebral blood flow after electroconvulsive therapy. Prog Neuropsychopharmacol Biol Psychiatry 35(7):1704–1708, 2011 21605615

Vaidya PV, Anderson EL, Bobb A, et al: A within-subject comparison of propofol and methohexital anesthesia for electroconvulsive therapy. J ECT 28(1):14–19, 2012 22330701

Valentí M, Benabarre A, García-Amador M, et al: Electroconvulsive therapy in the treatment of mixed states in bipolar disorder. Eur Psychiatry 23(1):53–56, 2008 18191551

Valentine M, Keddie KM, Dunne D: A comparison of techniques in electroconvulsive therapy. Br J Psychiatry 114(513):989–996, 1968 4879295

Valentine SJ, Marjot R, Monk CR: Preoxygenation in the elderly: a comparison of the four-maximal-breath and three-minute techniques. Anesth Analg 71(5):516–519, 1990 2221412

van Bronswijk S, Moopen N, Beijers L, et al: Effectiveness of psychotherapy for treatment-resistant depression: a meta-analysis and meta-regression. Psychol Med 49(3):366–379, 2019 30139408

Van Den Berg AA, Honjol NM: Electroconvulsive therapy and intraocular pressure. Middle East J Anaesthesiol 14(4):249–258, 1998 9557912

van den Broek WW, Groenland TH, Kusuma A, et al: Double-blind placebo controlled study of the effects of etomidate-alfentanil anesthesia in electroconvulsive therapy. J ECT 20(2):107–111, 2004 15167427

van den Broek WW, Birkenhäger TK, Mulder PG, et al: Imipramine is effective in preventing relapse in electroconvulsive therapy-responsive depressed inpatients with prior pharmacotherapy treatment failure: a randomized, placebo-controlled trial. J Clin Psychiatry 67(2):263–268, 2006 16566622

Van den Eynde V, Gillman PK, Blackwell BB: The prescriber's guide to the MAOI diet—thinking through tyramine troubles. Psychopharmacol Bull 52(2):73–116, 2022 35721816

Van de Velde N, Geerts PJ, Tandt H, et al: Discontinuation of continuation or maintenance electroconvulsive therapy caused by the COVID-19 pandemic: a naturalistic study investigating relapse in patients with major depressive disorder. J ECT 37(4):230–237, 2021 34145171

Vande Voort JL, Morgan RJ, Kung S, et al: Continuation phase intravenous ketamine in adults with treatment-resistant depression. J Affect Disord 206:300–304, 2016 27656788

van Diermen L, van den Ameele S, Kamperman AM, et al: Prediction of electroconvulsive therapy response and remission in major depression: meta-analysis. Br J Psychiatry 212(2):71–80, 2018 29436330

van Diermen L, Poljac E, Van der Mast R, et al: Toward targeted ECT: the interdependence of predictors of treatment response in depression further explained. J Clin Psychiatry 82(1):20m13287, 2020 33326710

Vanelle JM, Loo H, Galinowski A, et al: Maintenance ECT in intractable manic-depressive disorders. Convuls Ther 10(3):195–205, 1994 7834256

van Haelst IM, van Klei WA, Doodeman HJ, et al: Antidepressive treatment with monoamine oxidase inhibitors and the occurrence of intraoperative hemodynamic events: a retrospective observational cohort study. J Clin Psychiatry 73(8):1103–1109, 2012 22938842

van Herck E, Sienaert P, Hagon A: Electroconvulsive therapy for patients with intracranial aneurysms: a case study and literature review [in Dutch]. Tijdschr Psychiatr 51(1):43–51, 2009 19194845

Vann Jones S, McCollum R: Subjective memory complaints after electroconvulsive therapy: systematic review. BJPsych Bull 43(2):73–80, 2019 30860456

van Rooijen G, Denys D, Fliers E, et al: Effective electroconvulsive therapy in a patient with psychotic depression with active Cushing Disease. J ECT 32(3):e20–e21, 2016 27379791

van Waarde JA, Stolker JJ, van der Mast RC: ECT in mental retardation: a review. J ECT 17(4):236–243, 2001 11731724

van Waarde JA, Tuerlings JH, Verwey B, et al: Electroconvulsive therapy for catatonia: treatment characteristics and outcomes in 27 patients. J ECT 26(4):248–252, 2010 19935090

van Waarde JA, Scholte HS, van Oudheusden LJ, et al: A functional MRI marker may predict the outcome of electroconvulsive therapy in severe and treatment-resistant depression. Mol Psychiatry 20(5):609–614, 2015 25092248

Vasavada MM, Leaver AM, Njau S, et al: Short- and long-term cognitive outcomes in patients with major depression treated with electroconvulsive therapy. J ECT 33(4):278–285, 2017 28617690

Veltman EM, de Boer A, Dols A, et al: Melancholia as predictor of electroconvulsive therapy outcome in later life. J ECT 35(4):231–237, 2019 31764445

Verdijk JPAJ, van Kessel MA, Oud M, et al: Pharmacological interventions to diminish cognitive side effects of electroconvulsive therapy: a systematic review and meta-analysis. Acta Psychiatr Scand 145(4):343–356, 2022 35075641

Verrier RL, Nearing BD, D'Avila A: Spectrum of clinical applications of inter-lead ECG heterogeneity assessment: from myocardial ischemia detection to sudden cardiac death risk stratification. Ann Noninvasive Electrocardiol 26(6):e12894, 2021 34592018

Versiani M, Cheniaux E, Landeira-Fernandez J: Efficacy and safety of electroconvulsive therapy in the treatment of bipolar disorder: a systematic review. J ECT 27(2):153–164, 2011 20562714

Verwijk E, Comijs HC, Kok RM, et al: Neurocognitive effects after brief pulse and ultrabrief pulse unilateral electroconvulsive therapy for major depression: a review. J Affect Disord 140(3):233–243, 2012 22595374

Verwijk E, Comijs HC, Kok RM, et al: Short- and long-term neurocognitive functioning after electroconvulsive therapy in depressed elderly: a prospective naturalistic study. Int Psychogeriatr 26(2):315–324, 2014 24280446

Vicheva P, Butler M, Shotbolt P: Deep brain stimulation for obsessive-compulsive disorder: a systematic review of randomised controlled trials. Neurosci Biobehav Rev 109:129–138, 2020 31923474

Vieta E: The treatment of mixed states and the risk of switching to depression. Eur Psychiatry 20(2):96–100, 2005 15797692

Viguera A, Rordorf G, Schouten R, et al: Intracranial haemodynamics during attenuated responses to electroconvulsive therapy in the presence of an intracerebral aneurysm. J Neurol Neurosurg Psychiatry 64(6):802–805, 1998 9647316

Viguera AC, Nonacs R, Cohen LS, et al: Risk of recurrence of bipolar disorder in pregnant and nonpregnant women after discontinuing lithium maintenance. Am J Psychiatry 157(2):179–184, 2000 10671384

Vila-Rodriguez F, McGirr A, Tham J, et al: Electroconvulsive therapy in patients with deep brain stimulators. J ECT 30(3):e16–e18, 2014 24625701

Virupaksha HS, Shashidhara B, Thirthalli J, et al: Comparison of electroconvulsive therapy (ECT) with or without anti-epileptic drugs in bipolar disorder. J Affect Disord 127(1–3):66–70, 2010 20557948

Vishne T, Amiaz R, Grunhaus L: Promethazine for the treatment of agitation after electroconvulsive therapy: a case series. J ECT 21(2):118–121, 2005a 15905755

Vishne T, Aronov S, Amiaz R, et al: Remifentanil supplementation of propofol during electroconvulsive therapy: effect on seizure duration and cardiovascular stability. J ECT 21(4):235–238, 2005b 16301884

Voineskos D, Daskalakis ZJ, Blumberger DM: Management of treatment-resistant depression: challenges and strategies. Neuropsychiatr Dis Treat 16:221–234, 2020 32021216

Volkaerts L, Roels R, Bouckaert F: Motor function improvement after electroconvulsive therapy in a Parkinson's disease patient with deep brain stimulator. J ECT 36(1):66–68, 2020 31652177

Volpe FM, Tavares A, Correa H: Naturalistic evaluation of inpatient treatment of mania in a private Brazilian psychiatric hospital. Braz J Psychiatry 25(2):72–77, 2003 12975702

Vuksan Ćusa B, Klepac N, Jakšić N, et al: The effects of electroconvulsive therapy augmentation of antipsychotic treatment on cognitive functions in patients with treatment-resistant schizophrenia. J ECT 34(1):31–34, 2018 29053485

Wachtel LE: Treatment of catatonia in autism spectrum disorders. Acta Psychiatr Scand 139(1):46–55, 2019 30506668

Wachtel LE, Reti IM, Ying H: Stability of intraocular pressure after retinal reattachment surgery during electroconvulsive therapy for intractable self-injury in a 12-year-old autistic boy. J ECT 30(1):73–76, 2014 23812023

Wade BSC, Hellemann G, Espinoza RT, et al: Depressive symptom dimensions in treatment-resistant major depression and their modulation with electroconvulsive therapy. J ECT 36(2):123–129, 2020 31464814

Wagner E, Kane JM, Correll CU, et al: Clozapine combination and augmentation strategies in patients with schizophrenia: recommendations from an international expert survey among the Treatment Response and Resistance In Psychosis (TRRIP) working group. Schizophr Bull 46(6):1459–1470, 2020 32421188

Wagner GS, McClintock SM, Rosenquist PB, et al: Major depressive disorder with psychotic features may lead to misdiagnosis of dementia: a case report and review of the literature. J Psychiatr Pract 17(6):432–438, 2011 22108402

Wainwright AP, Brodrick PM: Suxamethonium in myasthenia gravis. Anaesthesia 42(9):950–957, 1987 3674355

Wajima Z, Shiga T, Yoshikawa T, et al: Propofol alone, sevoflurane alone, and combined propofol-sevoflurane anaesthesia in electroconvulsive therapy. Anaesth Intensive Care 31(4):396–400, 2003 12973963

Walter G, Rey JM: An epidemiological study of the use of ECT in adolescents. J Am Acad Child Adolesc Psychiatry 36(6):809–815, 1997 9183136

Walter G, Rey JM, Starling J: Experience, knowledge and attitudes of child psychiatrists regarding electroconvulsive therapy in the young. Aust N Z J Psychiatry 31(5):676–681, 1997 9400873

Walter-Ryan WG: ECT regulation and the two-tiered care system. Am J Psychiatry 142(5):661–662, 1985 3985213

Wang G, Zheng W, Li XB, et al: ECT augmentation of clozapine for clozapine-resistant schizophrenia: a meta-analysis of randomized controlled trials. J Psychiatr Res 105:23–32, 2018 30144667

Wang HN, Wang XX, Zhang RG, et al: Clustered repetitive transcranial magnetic stimulation for the prevention of depressive relapse/recurrence: a randomized controlled trial. Transl Psychiatry 7(12):1292, 2017 29249805

Wang N, Wang XH, Lu J, et al: The effect of repeated etomidate anesthesia on adrenocortical function during a course of electroconvulsive therapy. J ECT 27(4):281–285, 2011 22080238

Wang WL, Wang SY, Hung HY, et al: Safety of transcranial magnetic stimulation in unipolar depression: A systematic review and meta-analysis of randomized-controlled trials. J Affect Disord 301:400–425, 2022 35032510

Wang X, Chen Y, Zhou X, et al: Effects of propofol and ketamine as combined anesthesia for electroconvulsive therapy in patients with depressive disorder. J ECT 28(2):128–132, 2012 22622291

Wang Z, Cai X, Qiu R, et al: Case report: Lateral habenula deep brain stimulation for treatment-resistant depression. Front Psychiatry 11:616501, 2021 33519557

Ward HB, Fromson JA, Cooper JJ, et al: Recommendations for the use of ECT in pregnancy: literature review and proposed clinical protocol. Arch Womens Ment Health 21(6):715–722, 2018 29796968

Ware JE, Gandek B: The SF-36 Health Survey: development and use in mental health research and the IQOLA Project. Int J Ment Health 23:49–73, 1994

Ware JE Jr, Sherbourne CD: The MOS 36-item short-form health survey (SF-36). I. Conceptual framework and item selection. Med Care 30(6):473–483, 1992 1593914

Warmflash VL, Stricks L, Sackeim HA, et al: Reliability and validity of measures of seizure duration. Convuls Ther 3(1):18–25, 1987 11940885

Warnell RL, Elahi N: Introduction of vagus nerve stimulation into a maintenance electroconvulsive therapy regimen: a case study and cost analysis. J ECT 23(2):114–119, 2007 17548984

Warnell RL, Duk AD, Christison GW, et al: Teaching electroconvulsive therapy to medical students: effects of instructional method on knowledge and attitudes. Acad Psychiatry 29(5):433–436, 2005 16387965

Warren MB, Elder S, Litchfield NP: Electroconvulsive therapy for depression comorbid with myasthenia gravis: a case report and review of the literature. J ECT 34(1):50–54, 2018 28796013

Warren N, Grote V, O'Gorman C, et al: Electroconvulsive therapy for anti-N-methyl-D-aspartate (NMDA) receptor encephalitis: a systematic review of cases. Brain Stimul 12(2):329–334, 2019 30528383

Warren N, Eyre-Watt B, Pearson E, et al: Tardive seizures after electroconvulsive therapy. J ECT 38(2):95–102, 2022 35093969

Watanabe S, Yasuda K, Tada T, et al: Electroconvulsive therapy in a patient with depression on hemodialysis: a review of the literature. J ECT 39(2):71–73, 2023 35536991

Wattjes MP, Ciccarelli O, Reich DS, et al: 2021 MAGNIMS-CMSC-NAIMS consensus recommendations on the use of MRI in patients with multiple sclerosis. Lancet Neurol 20(8):653–670, 2021 34139157

Watts BV: A time-out before every ECT treatment. J ECT 32(4):224, 2016 27564425

Watts BV, Groft A, Bagian JP, et al: An examination of mortality and other adverse events related to electroconvulsive therapy using a national adverse event report system. J ECT 27(2):105–108, 2011 20966769

Watts BV, Peltzman T, Shiner B: Mortality after electroconvulsive therapy. Br J Psychiatry 219(5):588–593, 2021 35048831

Watts BV, Peltzman T, Shiner B: Electroconvulsive therapy and death by suicide. J Clin Psychiatry 83(3):21m13886, 2022 35421285

Webb MC, Coffey CE, Saunders WR, et al: Cardiovascular response to unilateral electroconvulsive therapy. Biol Psychiatry 28(9):758–766, 1990 2257285

Wechsler B, Desai MS, Khurshid KA: Electroconvulsive therapy in a patient with psychotic depression and recent subarachnoid hemorrhage. J ECT 37(4):e39–e40, 2021 34699389

Wechsler D: Wechsler Memory Scale, 4th Edition (WMS-IV). San Antonio, TX, Pearson Clinical Assessment, 2009

Weiner R, Lisanby SH, Husain MM, et al: Electroconvulsive therapy device classification: response to FDA advisory panel hearing and recommendations. J Clin Psychiatry 74(1):38–42, 2013 23419224

Weiner RD: The psychiatric use of electrically induced seizures. Am J Psychiatry 136(12):1507–1517, 1979 389068

Weiner RD: ECT and seizure threshold: effects of stimulus wave form and electrode placement. Biol Psychiatry 15(2):225–241, 1980 7417613

Weiner RD: Does ECT cause brain damage? Behav Brain Sci 7:1–53, 1984

Weiner RD, Sibert TE: Use of ECT in treatment of depression in patients with diabetes mellitus. J Clin Psychiatry 57(3):138, 1996 8617703

Weiner RD, Volow MR, Gianturco DT, et al: Seizures terminable and interminable with ECT. Am J Psychiatry 137(11):1416–1418, 1980a 6776828

Weiner RD, Whanger AD, Erwin CW, et al: Prolonged confusional state and EEG seizure activity following concurrent ECT and lithium use. Am J Psychiatry 137(11):1452–1453, 1980b 7435687

Weiner RD, Rogers HJ, Davidson JR, et al: Effects of electroconvulsive therapy upon brain electrical activity. Ann N Y Acad Sci 462:270–281, 1986a 3458408

Weiner RD, Rogers HJ, Davidson JR, et al: Effects of stimulus parameters on cognitive side effects. Ann N Y Acad Sci 462:315–325, 1986b 3458412

Weiner RD, Coffey CE, Krystal AD: The monitoring and management of electrically induced seizures. Psychiatr Clin North Am 14(4):845–869, 1991 1771151

Weiner RD, Coffey CE, Krystal AD: Electroconvulsive therapy in the medical and neurologic patient, in Psychiatric Care of the Medical Patient, 2nd Edition. Edited by Stoudemire A, Fogel BS, Grenberg D. New York, Oxford University Press, 2000, pp 419–428

Weiner RD, Husain MM, Young JR, et al: Electroconvulsive therapy and other forms of brain stimulation, in The American Psychiatric Association Publishing Textbook of Geriatric Psychiatry, 6th Edition. Edited by Steffens DC, Zdanys K. Washington, DC, American Psychiatric Publishing, 2023, pp 601–642

Weiner SJ, Ward TN, Ravaris CL: Headache and electroconvulsive therapy. Headache 34(3):155–159, 1994 8200790

Weinstein RM: Migraine occurring as sequela of electroconvulsive therapy. Headache 33(1):45, 1993 8436500

Weintraub D, Lippmann SB: Electroconvulsive therapy in the acute poststroke period. J ECT 16(4):415–418, 2000 11314880

Weisberg LA, Elliott D, Mielke D: Intracerebral hemorrhage following electroconvulsive therapy. Neurology 41(11):1849, 1991 1944925

Weiss A: The Electroconvulsive Therapy Workbook: Clinical Applications. New York, Routledge, 2018

Weiss A, Hussain S, Ng B, et al: Royal Australian and New Zealand College of Psychiatrists professional practice guidelines for the administration of electroconvulsive therapy. Aust N Z J Psychiatry 53(7):609–623, 2019 30966782

Welch CA, Drop LJ: Cardiovascular effects of ECT. Convuls Ther 5(1):35–43, 1989 11940992

Weller M, Kornhuber J: Electroconvulsive therapy in a geriatric patient with multiple bone fractures and generalized plasmocytoma. Pharmacopsychiatry 25(6):278–280, 1992 1494595

Wells DA: Electroconvulsive treatment for schizophrenia: a ten-year survey in a university hospital psychiatric department. Compr Psychiatry 14(4):291–298, 1973 4724657

Wells DG, Bjorksten AR: Monoamine oxidase inhibitors revisited. Can J Anaesth 36(1):64–74, 1989 2563341

Wengel SP, Burke WJ, Pfeiffer RF, et al: Maintenance electroconvulsive therapy for intractable Parkinson's disease. Am J Geriatr Psychiatry 6(3):263–269, 1998 9659959

Wesner RB, Winokur G: The influence of age on the natural history of unipolar depression when treated with electroconvulsive therapy. Eur Arch Psychiatry Neurol Sci 238(3):149–154, 1989 2721532

Wessels WH: A comparative study of the efficacy of bilateral and unilateral electroconvulsive therapy with thioridazine in acute schizophrenia. S Afr Med J 46(26):890–892, 1972 5057333

West ED: Electric convulsion therapy in depression: a double-blind controlled trial. Br Med J (Clin Res Ed) 282(6261):355–357, 1981 6780021

Westreich L, Levine S, Ginsburg P, et al: Patient knowledge about electroconvulsive therapy: effect of an informational video. Convuls Ther 11(1):32–37, 1995 7796066

Wettstein RM, Roth LH: The psychiatrist as legal guardian. Am J Psychiatry 145(5):600–604, 1988 3358464

White PF, Purdue L, Downing M, et al: Intranasal sumatriptan for prevention of post-ECT headaches. Headache 46(4):692, 2006 16643571

Wiest DB, Haney JS: Clinical pharmacokinetics and therapeutic efficacy of esmolol. Clin Pharmacokinet 51(6):347–356, 2012 22515557

Wijeratne C, Shome S: Electroconvulsive therapy and subdural hemorrhage. J ECT 15(4):275–279, 1999 10614035

Wilkening J, Witteler F, Goya-Maldonado R: Suicidality and relief of depressive symptoms with intermittent theta burst stimulation in a sham-controlled randomized clinical trial. Acta Psychiatr Scand 146(6):540–556, 2022 36163686

Wilkins KM, Ostroff R, Tampi RR: Efficacy of electroconvulsive therapy in the treatment of nondepressed psychiatric illness in elderly patients: a review of the literature. J Geriatr Psychiatry Neurol 21(1):3–11, 2008 18287164

Wilkinson ST, Ostroff RB, Sanacora G: Computer-assisted cognitive behavior therapy to prevent relapse following electroconvulsive therapy. J ECT 33(1):52–57, 2017 27564424

Wille PD: Electroconvulsive therapy in a patient on chronic hemodialysis. Nephrol Nurs J 34(4):441–443, 2007 17891913

Williams JB, Arvidson MM: Resource document for electroconvulsive therapy in adult correctional settings. J ECT 37(1):18–23, 2021 32558763

Williams K, Smith J, Glue P, et al: The effects of electroconvulsive therapy on plasma insulin and glucose in depression. Br J Psychiatry 161:94–98, 1992 1638337

Williams NR, Bentzley BS, Sahlem GL, et al: Unilateral ultra-brief pulse electroconvulsive therapy for depression in Parkinson's disease. Acta Neurol Scand 135(4):407–411, 2017 27241213

Williams NR, Sudheimer KD, Bentzley BS, et al: High-dose spaced theta-burst TMS as a rapid-acting antidepressant in highly refractory depression. Brain 141(3):e18, 2018 29415152

Williams S, Ostroff R: Chronic renal failure, hemodialysis, and electroconvulsive therapy: a case report. J ECT 21(1):41–42, 2005 15791177

Wilson IC, Vernon JT, Sandifer MG Jr, et al: A controlled study of treatments of depression. J Neuropsychiatry 4:331–337, 1963 14054810

Wilson S, Croarkin PE, Aaronson ST, et al: Systematic review of preservation TMS that includes continuation, maintenance, relapse-prevention, and rescue TMS. J Affect Disord 296:79–88, 2022 34592659

Wilson-Baig N, Badminton M, Schulenburg-Brand D: Acute hepatic porphyria and anaesthesia: a practical approach to the prevention and management of acute neurovisceral attacks. BJA Educ 21(2):66–74, 2021 33889432

Wingate BJ, Hansen-Flaschen J: Anxiety and depression in advanced lung disease. Clin Chest Med 18(3):495–505, 1997 9329872

Winslade WJ: Electroconvulsive therapy: legal regulations, ethical concerns, in Review of Psychiatry, Vol 7. Edited by Frances AJ, Hales RE. Washington, DC, American Psychiatric Press, 1988, pp 513–525

Winslade WJ, Liston EH, Ross JW, et al: Medical, judicial, and statutory regulation of ECT in the United States. Am J Psychiatry 141(11):1349–1355, 1984 6496778

Wolff GE: Electric shock treatment: a "must" for chronic patients in mental hospitals. Am J Psychiatry 111(10):748–750, 1955 14361758

Wolff GE: Results of four year active therapy for chronic mental patients and the value of an individual maintenance dose of ECT. Am J Psychiatry 114(5):453–456, 1957 13470118

Woodward MR, Doddi S, Marano C, et al: Evaluating salvage electroconvulsive therapy for the treatment of prolonged super refractory status epilepticus: a case series. Epilepsy Behav 144:109286, 2023 37276802

World Health Organization: Development of the World Health Organization WHOQOL-BREF quality of life assessment. Psychol Med 28(3):551–558, 1998a 9626712

World Health Organization: World Health Organization Quality of Life Assessment (WHOQOL): development and general psychometric properties. Soc Sci Med 46(12):1569–1585, 1998b 9672396

World Health Organization: Measuring Health and Disability: Manual for WHO Disability Assessment Schedule (WHODAS 2.0). Edited by Üstün TB, Kostanjsek N, Chatterji S, et al. Geneva, WHO Press, 2010. Available at: www.who.int/publications/i/item/measuring-health-and-disability-manual-for-who-disability-assessment-schedule-(-whodas-2.0). Accessed July 23, 2022.

Wyatt RJ: Neuroleptics and the natural course of schizophrenia. Schizophr Bull 17(2):325–351, 1991 1679255

Wyatt RJ: Early intervention for schizophrenia: can the course of the illness be altered? Biol Psychiatry 38(1):1–3, 1995 7548467

Yahya AS, Khawaja S: Electroconvulsive therapy in multiple sclerosis: a review of current evidence. Prim Care Companion CNS Disord 23(2):20r02717, 2021 34000115

Yamaguchi S, Nagao M, Ikeda T, et al: QT dispersion and rate-corrected QT dispersion during electroconvulsive therapy in elderly patients. J ECT 27(3):183–188, 2011 21865956

Ye L, Karlapati SK, Lippmann S: Topiramate for post-electroconvulsive therapy headaches. J ECT 29(3):e49, 2013 23965610

Ye L, Xiao X, Zhu L: The comparison of etomidate and propofol anesthesia in patients undergoing gastrointestinal endoscopy: a systematic review and meta-analysis. Surg Laparosc Endosc Percutan Tech 27(1):1–7, 2017 28079763

Yeoh SY, Roberts E, Scott F, et al: Catatonic episodes related to substance use: a cross-sectional study using electronic healthcare records. J Dual Diagn 18(1):52–58, 2022 35001837

Ying YB, Jia LN, Wang ZY, et al: Electroconvulsive therapy is associated with lower readmission rates in patients with schizophrenia. Brain Stimul 14(4):913–921, 2021 34044182

Yoldi-Negrete M, Gill LN, Olivares S, et al: The effect of continuation and maintenance electroconvulsive therapy on cognition: a systematic review of the literature and meta-analysis. J Affect Disord 316:148–160, 2022 35952935

Yonkers KA, Wisner KL, Stowe Z, et al: Management of bipolar disorder during pregnancy and the postpartum period. Am J Psychiatry 161(4):608–620, 2004 15056503

Yonkers KA, Wisner KL, Stewart DE, et al: The management of depression during pregnancy: a report from the American Psychiatric Association and the American College of Obstetricians and Gynecologists. Obstet Gynecol 114(3):703–713, 2009 19701065

Yoosefi A, Sepehri AS, Kargar M, et al: Comparing effects of ketamine and thiopental administration during electroconvulsive therapy in patients with major depressive disorder: a randomized, double-blind study. J ECT 30(1):15–21, 2014 24091902

Youn T, Jeong SH, Kim YS, et al: Long-term clinical efficacy of maintenance electroconvulsive therapy in patients with treatment-resistant schizophrenia on clozapine. Psychiatry Res 273:759–766, 2019 31207863

Young RC, Biggs JT, Ziegler VE, et al: A rating scale for mania: reliability, validity and sensitivity. Br J Psychiatry 133:429–435, 1978 728692

Youssef NA, Casola B, Rosenquist PB, et al: Safe administration of ECT in a suicidal patient with a space-occupying astrocytoma. J ECT 37(3):207–208, 2021a 33625177

Youssef NA, George MS, McCall WV, et al: The effects of focal electrically administered seizure therapy compared with ultrabrief pulse right unilateral electroconvulsive therapy on suicidal ideation: a 2-site clinical trial. J ECT 37(4):256–262, 2021b 34015791

Yuan S, Tirrell E, Gobin AP, et al: Effect of previous electroconvulsive therapy on subsequent response to transcranial magnetic stimulation for major depressive disorder. Neuromodulation 23(3):393–398, 2020 31588659

Yuzda E, Parker K, Parker V, et al: Electroconvulsive therapy training in Canada: a call for greater regulation. Can J Psychiatry 47(10):938–944, 2002 12553129

Zahavi GS, Dannon P: Comparison of anesthetics in electroconvulsive therapy: an effective treatment with the use of propofol, etomidate, and thiopental. Neuropsychiatr Dis Treat 10:383–389, 2014 24591833

Zaizar ED, Papini S, Gonzalez-Lima F, et al: Singular and combined effects of transcranial infrared laser stimulation and exposure therapy on pathological fear: a randomized clinical trial. Psychol Med 53(3):908–917, 2023 34284836

Zakzanis KK, Leach L, Kaplan E: On the nature and pattern of neurocognitive function in major depressive disorder. Neuropsychiatry Neuropsychol Behav Neurol 11(3):111–119, 1998 9742509

Zandi PP, Morreale M, Reti IM, et al: National Network of Depression Centers' recommendations on harmonizing clinical documentation of electroconvulsive therapy. J ECT 38(3):159–164, 2022 35704844

Zarate CA Jr, Singh JB, Carlson PJ, et al: A randomized trial of an N-methyl-D-aspartate antagonist in treatment-resistant major depression. Arch Gen Psychiatry 63(8):856–864, 2006 16894061

Zeifert M: Results obtained from the administration of 12,000 doses of metrazol to mental patients. Psychiatr Q 15:772–778, 1941

Zeiler FA, Matuszczak M, Teitelbaum J, et al: Electroconvulsive therapy for refractory status epilepticus: a systematic review. Seizure 35:23–32, 2016 26789495

Zervas IM, Fink M: ECT for refractory Parkinson's disease (letter). Convuls Ther 7(3):222–223, 1991 11941126

Zervas IM, Fink M: ECT and delirium in Parkinson's disease. Am J Psychiatry 149(12):1758, author reply 1759–1760, 1992 1443265

Zervas IM, Jandorf L: The Randt Memory Test in electroconvulsive therapy: relation to illness and treatment parameters. Convuls Ther 9(1):28–38, 1993 11941189

Zervas IM, Theleritis C, Soldatos CR: Using ECT in schizophrenia: a review from a clinical perspective. World J Biol Psychiatry 13(2):96–105, 2012 21486108

Zhang J, Wang G, Yang X, et al: Efficacy and safety of electroconvulsive therapy plus medication versus medication alone in acute mania: a meta-analysis of randomized controlled trials. Psychiatry Res 302:114019, 2021 34058715

Zhang Y, White PF, Thornton L, et al: The use of nicardipine for electroconvulsive therapy: a dose-ranging study. Anesth Analg 100(2):378–381, 2005 15673861

Zhang ZJ, Chen YC, Wang HN, et al: Electroconvulsive therapy improves antipsychotic and somnographic responses in adolescents with first-episode psychosis—a case-control study. Schizophr Res 137(1-3):97–103, 2012 22341901

Zheng W, Cao XL, Ungvari GS, et al: Electroconvulsive therapy added to nonclozapine antipsychotic medication for treatment resistant schizophrenia: meta-analysis of randomized controlled trials. PLoS One 11(6):e0156510, 2016 27285996

Zielinski RJ, Roose SP, Devanand DP, et al: Cardiovascular complications of ECT in depressed patients with cardiac disease. Am J Psychiatry 150(6):904–909, 1993 8494067

Zimmerman M, McGlinchey JB: Depressed patients' acceptability of the use of self-administered scales to measure outcome in clinical practice. Ann Clin Psychiatry 20(3):125–129, 2008 18633738

Zimmerman M, Coryell W, Pfohl B: The treatment validity of DSM-III melancholic subtyping. Psychiatry Res 16(1):37–43, 1985 3864174

Zimmerman M, Coryell W, Stangl D, et al: An American validation study of the Newcastle scale. III. Course during index hospitalization and six-month prospective follow-up. Acta Psychiatr Scand 73(4):412–415, 1986 3728067

Zimmerman M, Posternak MA, Chelminski I: Is it time to replace the Hamilton Depression Rating Scale as the primary outcome measure in treatment studies of depression? J Clin Psychopharmacol 25(2):105–110, 2005 15738740

Zimmerman M, Clark HL, Multach MD, et al: Have treatment studies of depression become even less generalizable? A review of the inclusion and exclusion criteria in placebo controlled antidepressant efficacy trials published during the past 20 years. Mayo Clin Proc 90(9):1180–1186, 2015 26276679

Zimmerman M, Walsh E, Friedman M, et al: Are self-report scales as effective as clinician rating scales in measuring treatment response in routine clinical practice? J Affect Disord 225:449–452, 2018 28858659

Zimmermann R, Schmitt H, Rotter A, et al: Transient increase of plasma concentrations of amyloid β peptides after electroconvulsive therapy. Brain Stimul 5(1):25–29, 2012 22037136

Zink M, Sartorius A, Lederbogen F, et al: Electroconvulsive therapy in a patient receiving rivastigmine. J ECT 18(3):162–164, 2002 12394536

Zis AP: Acute administration of fluoxetine and the duration of electrically induced seizures. Convuls Ther 8(1):38–39, 1992 11941148

Zis AP, McGarvey KA, Clark CM, et al: Effect of stimulus energy on electroconvulsive therapy-induced prolactin release. Convuls Ther 9(1):23–27, 1993 11941188

Zisselman MH, Jaffe RL: ECT in the treatment of a patient with catatonia: consent and complications. Am J Psychiatry 167(2):127–132, 2010 20123920

Zlatar ZZ, Muniz M, Galasko D, et al: Subjective cognitive decline correlates with depression symptoms and not with concurrent objective cognition in a clinic-based sample of older adults. J Gerontol B Psychol Sci Soc Sci 73(7):1198–1202, 2018 28329816

Zorumski CF, Rutherford JL, Burke WJ, et al: ECT in primary and secondary depression. J Clin Psychiatry 47(6):298–300, 1986 3711027

Zwil AS, Pelchat RJ: ECT in the treatment of patients with neurological and somatic disease. Int J Psychiatry Med 24(1):1–29, 1994 8077081

Zwil AS, Bowring MA, Price TRP, et al: Prospective electroconvulsive therapy in the presence of intracranial tumor. Convuls Ther 6(4):299–307, 1990 11941083

Index

*Page numbers printed in **boldface** type refer to tables or figures.*

Diuretics, 164
Documentation, 43–49
  of adverse effects, 46, 48–49
  after completion of ECT course,
    46, 49
  of consent discussion, 129, 133
  during ECT course, 45–48
  between ECT treatment sessions,
    45, 47–48
  facility responsibilities, 43, 46
  of ictal motor response, 202–203
  pre-ECT evaluation, 44, 70
  prior to ECT course, 44, 47
  privileging actions, 66
  recommendations, 46–49
  at time of each ECT treatment, 45–
    46, 48
Dolasetron, 246, 251
Dopamine-blocking agents, 22, 174,
    246, 251
Dopaminergic medications, 165
Double stimulation, 276
Doxylamine-pyridoxine, 105–106
Dynamic impedance, 277
Dysthymia, 13

ECT devices, 34–35
  electrical safety, 35, 38–39
  FDA classification, 5, 16, 34
  impedance testing, 190–191, 198–
    199
  maximum output, 181, 187
  physiological monitoring of
    motor response, 202
  recommendations, 38–39
  retesting, 34–35, 38–39
  stimulus controls, 181–182, 196
  warnings, 257
ECT psychiatrist
  maintenance ECT evaluation, 291,
    295
  patient preparation
    responsibilities, 140–143
  responsibilities of, 26, 30
ECT treatment nurse
  recovery nurse, 28–29, 31–32

responsibilities, 27–28, 31
ECT treatment team
  anesthesia providers, 26–27, 30
  ECT psychiatrist, 26, 30
  ECT treatment nurse, 27–28
  members, 25, 29–30
  recommendations, 29–32
  responsibilities, 26–29, 30–32
ECT-Related Anxiety Questionnaire
    (ERAQ), 218, 221, **222**
Education and training, 51–63
  anesthesiology residency
    programs, 55–56, 61–62
  board examinations, 57, 62–63
  continuing education programs,
    57–58, 63
  general considerations, 51
  geriatric psychiatry training
    programs, 55, 61
  medical school training, 52, 58–59
  nursing schools, 57, 62
  privileging, 65–66
  psychiatry residency programs,
    52–55
  recommendations, 58–63
EEG. See Electroencephalography
Efficacy of ECT, 7–10
Electrical stimulus
  parameters, 181–184, 196
  waveform characteristics, 179–181,
    180, 196
Electroconvulsive Therapy Cognitive
    Assessment (ECCA), 259
Electrode placement, 184–189, **185,**
    196–197, 313, 318–319
  changing, 235, 237
  choice of, 184–187, **185,** 196–197
  modifying, 277, 279
  shift for missed seizures, 274, 279
Electrode positioning, 188–189, 197
Electrode site placement, 190, 198
Electrode types, 189–190, 197
Electroencephalography (EEG)
  amplification setting, 205
  determination of EEG seizure
    endpoint, 205